Recent Results in Cancer Research

Fortschritte der Krebsforschung

Progrès dans les recherches sur le cancer

40

Edited by

V. G. Allfrey, New York · M. Allgöwer, Basel · K. H. Bauer, Heidelberg
I. Berenblum, Rehovoth · F. Bergel, Jersey · J. Bernard, Paris
W. Bernhard, Villejuif · N. N. Blokhin, Moskva · H. E. Bock, Tübingen
P. Bucalossi, Milano · A. V. Chaklin, Moskva
M. Chorazy, Gliwice · G. J. Cunningham, Richmond · M. Dargent, Lyon
G. Della Porta, Milano · P. Denoix, Villejuif · R. Dulbecco, La Jolla
H. Eagle, New York · E. Eker, Oslo · R. A. Good, New York
P. Grabar, Paris · H. Hamperl, Bonn · R. J. C. Harris, Salisbury
E. Hecker, Heidelberg · R. Herbeuval, Nancy · J. Higginson, Lyon
W. C. Hueper, Fort Myers · H. Isliker, Lausanne
J. Kieler, København · G. Klein, Stockholm · H. Koprowski, Philadelphia
L. G. Koss, New York · G. Martz, Zürich · G. Mathé, Villejuif
O. Mühlbock, Amsterdam · W. Nakahara, Tokyo · L. J. Old, New York
V. R. Potter, Madison · A. B. Sabin, Rehovoth · L. Sachs, Rehovoth
E. A. Saxén, Helsinki · C. G. Schmidt, Essen · S. Spiegelman, New York
W. Szybalski, Madison · H. Tagnon, Bruxelles · R. M. Taylor, Toronto
A. Tissières, Genève · E. Uehlinger, Zürich · R. W. Wissler, Chicago
T. Yoshida, Tokyo

Editor in chief
P. Rentchnick, Genève

Recent Results in Cancer Research

F. A. Langley · A. C. Crompton

Epithelial Abnormalities of the Cervix Uteri

With 81 Figures

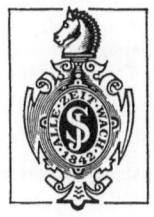

Springer-Verlag Berlin Heidelberg GmbH 1973

F. A. Langley, M.Sc., M.D., F.R.C.Path., F.R.C.O.G.,

Professor of Obstetrical and Gynaecological Pathology, University of Manchester.
Consultant Pathologist, St. Mary's Hospital for Women and Children, Manchester

A. C. Crompton, M.D., F.R.C.S.Ed., M.R.C.O.G.,

Consultant Obstetrician and Gynaecologist, Leeds (St. James's) University Hospital.
Sometime Lecturer in Obstetrics and Gynaecology, University of Manchester

Sponsored by the Swiss League against Cancer

ISBN 978-3-662-07070-3   ISBN 978-3-662-07068-0 (eBook)
DOI 10.1007/978-3-662-07068-0

Contents

Introduction

The introduction of colposcopy and exfoliative cytology as a means of examining the cervix uteri has opened up the possibility of studying the preceding and early stages of invasive carcinoma of the cervix and has also brought to light a number of conditions which are possibly only indirectly related, if related at all, to cervical neoplasia. Using these methods combined with histological evaluation it is possible to gain some insight into the natural history of cervical carcinoma. The importance of this is not confined to the cervix for, in this respect, the cervical lesions may prove a paradigm for those of the bladder, stomach and elsewhere.

At present the broad outline of the natural history of these cervical lesions is emerging but the temporal and spatial relationships of the various phases is unclear, largely because of the number of possibilities envisaged which involves more variables than can be controlled in any one investigation. In this monograph we have endeavoured to indicate the limitations of the various approaches and to stress the need for controlling the accuracy of assessment whether it be histological, cytological or colposcopic.

It is well sometimes to sit back and view a disease as a biological experiment in order to improve our understanding of its evolution and thereby gain some insight into its possible control. This has been our aim in this monograph rather than to present a comprehensive account of the present state of our knowledge of cervical abnormalities which would be both tedious and disjointed.

We have only lightly touched on treatment and we have avoided discussing the value of mass screening, rather presenting the abnormalities in broad biological terms. For it seems to us that these lesions are probably multifactorial in origin and that a variety of factors outside the immediate control of the gynaecologist may affect the patterns of these lesions in the future, especially changing customs of marriage and sexual mores.

We would like to thank Professor W. I. C. Morris for the facilities of the Department of Obstetrics and Gynaecology, Manchester University, which have made this study possible. We are grateful to Mr. B. Figg for preparing the photomicrographs and Dr. Ollerenshaw, together with his staff in the Department of Medical Illustration, United Manchester Hospitals, for drawing the diagrams. The editor of the Journal of Clinical Pathology has kindly given us permission to reproduce Figs. 2.1., 3.13., 3.14. and 3.15., and the editor of the Journal of Obstetrics and Gynaecology of the British Commonwealth has courteously allowed us to include Figs. 3.9., 3.10. and 3.11. Those of our colleagues who from time to time have read portions of the text whilst it was in preparation have rendered us a valuable service in their critical and constructive comments. Finally we would thank Mrs. D. Shaw and Miss S. Hamilton and Miss A. Godsell for typing drafts of various chapters and Mrs. J. Edwards for the typing of the completed manuscript.

F. A. Langley, A. C. Crompton, 1973.

Chapter 1

The Normal Cervix

The cervix uteri is covered by two types of epithelium, the portio vaginalis by stratified squamous epithelium and the endocervix by columnar epithelium. The purpose of this chapter is to examine the normal structure and function of these two epithelia in broad biological terms as a background to a consideration of their pathology.

1. The Development of the Cervix Uteri

The development of the cervix has been extensively reviewed by HORSTMANN and STEGNER (1966) and modern views are discussed by DAVIES and KUSAMA (1962). In the classical view, the cervix and the upper part of the vagina are Müllerian in

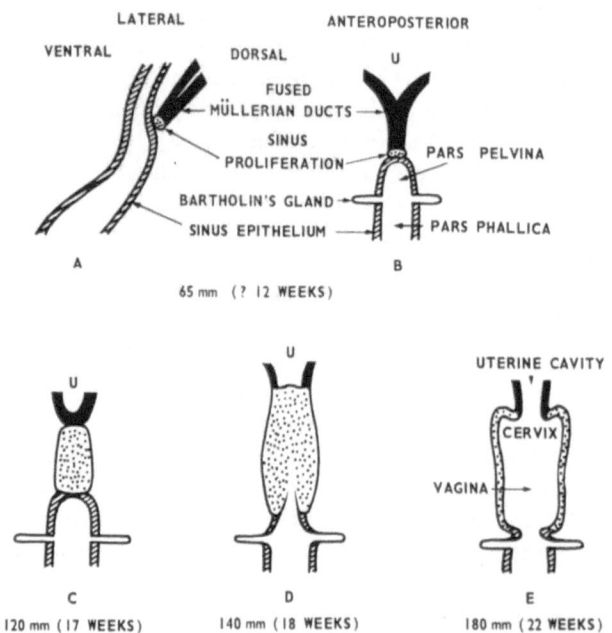

Fig. 1.1. A schematic representation of the development of the human vagina and cervix, after BULMER (1957) and DAVIES and KUSAMA (1962). The area shaded black represents the fused Müllerian ducts; the stippled area is the sinus proliferation and the cross hatched area is the epithelium of the urogenital sinus

origin whilst the lower end of the vagina is developed from the urogenital sinus (KOFF 1933). BULMER (1957) has brought forward evidence that the human vagina is developed entirely from the urogenital sinus, the uterus and an indeterminate part of the cervix being of Müllerian origin. He has shown that the vagina arises as a proliferation of the epithelium in the posterior wall of the pars pelvina of the urogenital sinus and is therefore endodermal. The pars pelvina of the sinus is the narrowed and elongated part, distal to the bladder, which is succeeded at the level of

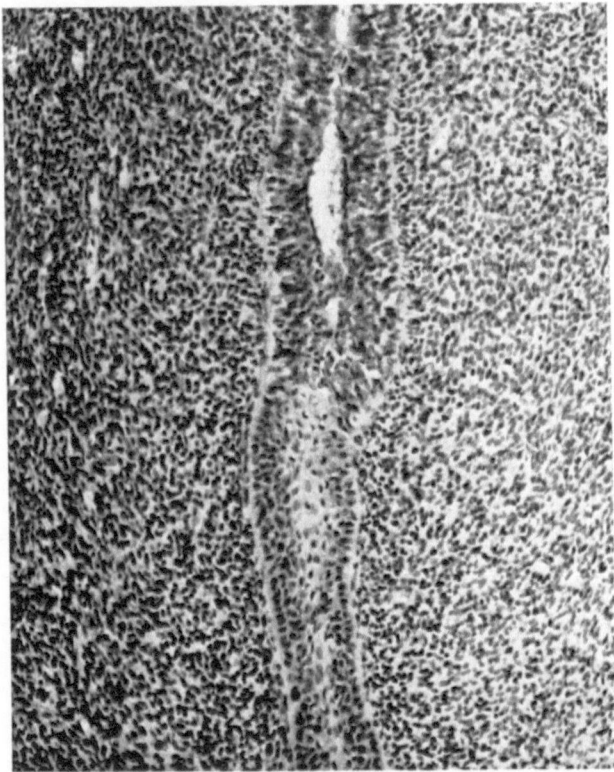

Fig. 1.2. In the upper part of the field the fused Müllerian ducts are developing a cavity, later to form the lumen of the uterus. In the lower part of the field is the solid core of epithelial cells formed from the sinus proliferation. From a fifteen-week foetus. (H. & E. ×120)

Bartholin's gland by the pars phallica of the sinus. The proliferation forms a solid cord of cells which displaces the Müllerian ducts cranially and dorsally. The vagina is formed by canalization of this cord between the eighteenth and twenty-second week of gestation. The junction between the epithelium of the sinus proliferation and the fused Müllerian ducts probably lies in the region of the cervix. The demarcation of the cervix from the vagina is established during the fifth month by massing of mesoderm round the lower end of the fused Müllerian ducts and the formation of the vaginal fornices as proliferations of the stratified squamous epithelium. The sequence of changes is shown in Figs. 1.1., 1.2. and 1.3.

DAVIES and KUSAMA (1962) have shown that at thirty weeks the junction between
the vaginal and cervical epithelium is well defined (Fig. 1.4.) but variable in site. In
some areas the squamous epithelium extends up to the level of the external os but
in other areas of the same cervix the junction between squamous and columnar epithelium lies far out laterally in the vaginal fornix. At the junction the basal layer of
the vaginal epithelium may disappear abruptly and the intermediate layer become
continuous with the cervical epithelium. The cervical epithelium at this junctional

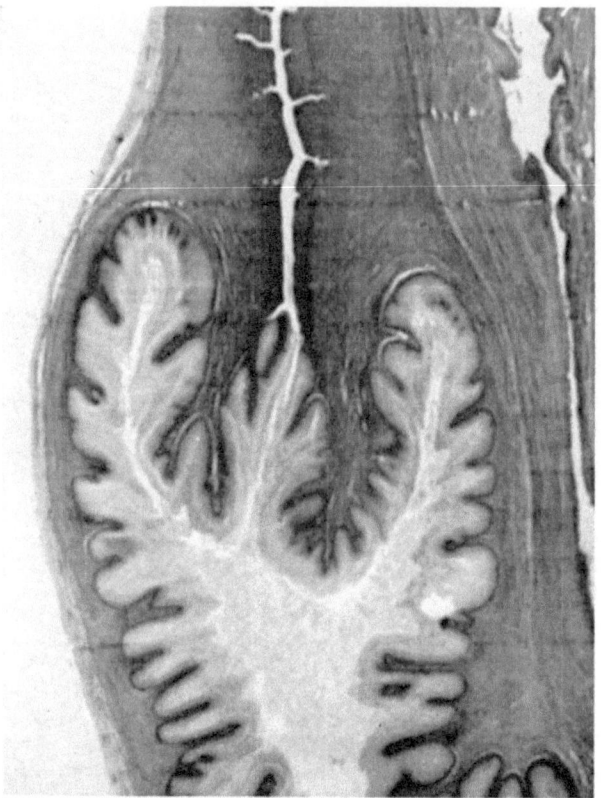

Fig. 1.3. A section from a twenty-seven week foetus. The vagina and fornices are now well formed.
(H. & E. ×8)

zone is of stratified, or pseudostratified, columnar type. They consider it to differ
from squamous metaplastic epithelium in that the nuclei of the basal layers are arranged
at right angles to the basement membrane. GRUENAGEL (1957), MATĚJKA (1963) and
HORSTMANN and STEGNER (1966) regard these subcylindrical cells as "reserve cells",
corresponding to the reserve cells described by HOWARD et al. (1949, 1951) in older
women. According to GRUENAGEL there are no intercellular bridges between these
reserve cells, the cytoplasm stains lightly, the nuclei are round and vesicular. The
cytoplasm of many of the cells gives an alcian blue positive reaction which may indicate a relationship to the columnar cells.

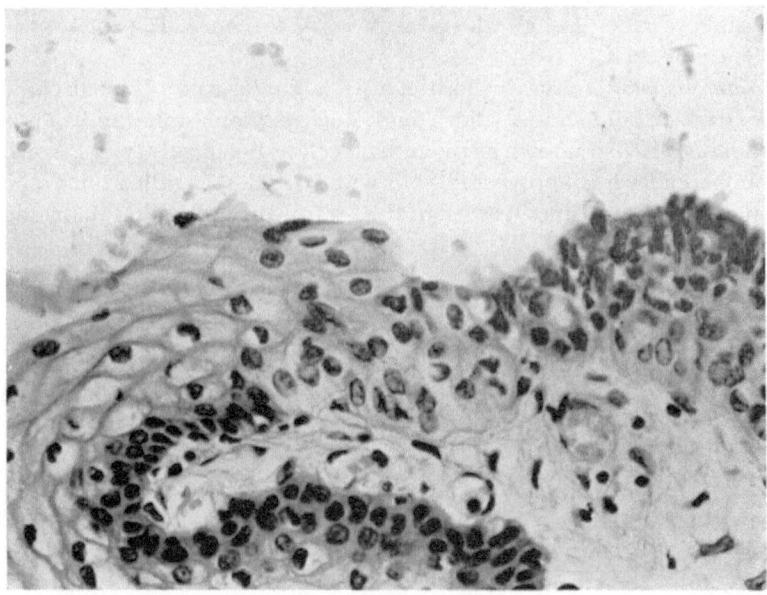

Fig. 1.4. A section from the squamo-columnar junction of a thirty-week foetus. The cells of the basal and parabasal layer stop abruptly but those of the intermediate layer are continued beneath the columnar layer of the endocervix. (H. & E. ×300)

In late foetal and early neonatal life the squamous epithelium of the vagina and cervix is very thick but it is rapidly shed in the first few weeks after birth. This change is probably caused by the fall in circulating hormones derived from the mother, and in particular by the fall in oestrogen level. The complex pattern of the endocervical epithelium in late foetal and early neonatal life in many ways resembles that seen in cervical polypi resulting from the use of oral contraceptives and is a reminder that the effects of both oestrogen and progesterone must be considered.

2. The Squamous Epithelium of the Cervix

a) The Histological Pattern

The preceding discussion emphasises that a close relationship exists between the squamous epithelium of the vagina and the cervix while the differences, as in the response to hormonal stimuli, are usually only ones of degree. Although this squamous epithelium is endodermal in origin it will also be profitable in our subsequent discussions to compare it with that of the epidermis.

The squamous epithelium of the vagina and cervix is not usually keratinized. Indeed the keratinization of vulvar epithelium sharply distinguishes it from vaginal epithelium at the vulvo-vaginal junction. Nevertheless in uterine prolapse and certain pathological states the cervico-vaginal epithelium may keratinize. DIERKS (1927) originally described five zones or layers of cells in this epithelium. This system is usually followed for descriptive purposes, although with some variation in terminology according to the author. As KRANTZ and PHILLIPS (1962) point out it is not usually possible to recognize all the layers in every specimen. Table 1.1. summarizes some of the terms used.

The *stratum basale* (stratum cylindricum) is a single row of small cubical cells with large, dark-staining nuclei and a high nucleo-cytoplasmic ratio. The *stratum spinosum profundum* is also known as the prickle-cell or parabasal layer. It consists of a varying number of layers of polyhedral cells with large dark-staining nuclei. Normally mitotic figures may sometimes be seen in this stratum as in the stratum basale. In the

Table 1.1. The layers of the squamous epithelium of the cervix uteri

Terms used in the text	Synonyms	
Stratum basale	Stratum cylindricum	Stratum germinativum (HACKEMANN *et al.*)
Stratum spinosum profundum parabasal layer	Dark Zone (TRAUT *et al.*)	Stratum spinosum (HACKEMANN *et. al.*)
Stratum spinosum superficiale, intermediate layer	Light Zone (TRAUT *et al.*)	
Intraepithelial zone stratum granulosum	Verdichtungszone (STEMSHORN) Verhornungszone (DIERKS)	Stratum functionalis (HACKEMANN *et. al.*)
Stratum superficiale	Stratum corneum (PAPANICOLAOU) Stratum functionalis (DIERKS)	

stratum spinosum superficiale the cells tend to be flattened. The cytoplasm of the cells contains glycogen and may be vacuolated and the nuclei stain less darkly than in the deeper layers and are vesicular. Mitoses are rarely, if ever, seen. This zone is sometimes known as the intermediate, navicular or clear-cell layer (KRANTZ and PHILLIPS 1962). HORSTMANN and STEGNER (1966) term the whole stratum spinosum the *Intermediarzone*, whilst DIERKS (1927) terms all the first three zones the *stratum basalis*. Between these three layers and the superficial layer lies a narrow, inconstant zone, the intraepithelial or condensation zone. It consists of closely packed, flattened cells in which both the nuclei and cytoplasm tend to stain darkly and if the superficial zone is keratinized keratohyaline granules are seen, the layer is then termed the *stratum granulosum*. The fifth and outermost layer is the *stratum superficiale*. This consists of several layers of flat, elongated cells, with pyknotic nuclei but if keratinization occurs nuclei will be absent. PAPANICOLAOU *et al.* (1948) distinguish two types of superficial layer — cornified and keratinized. The use of these two terms has caused some confusion, which has been discussed at length in Acta Cytologica 4, (1960). The terms are not strictly synonymous since they describe differing appearances of this outer layer (see Fig. 1.5.).

From this brief description of the layers of the squamous epithelium of the portio vaginalis it will be seen that the terminology used varies with the author and is not conducive to the maximum degree of clarity. Moreover, the boundary between the layers is often not sharply defined, particularly between the stratum spinosum profundum and the stratum spinosum superficiale. HACKEMANN *et al.* (1968) found that the electron microscope failed to reveal five clear-cut succesive layers and proposed to speak of a basal layer or stratum germinativum, a wide stratum spinosum and a superficial multilayered stratum functionalis.

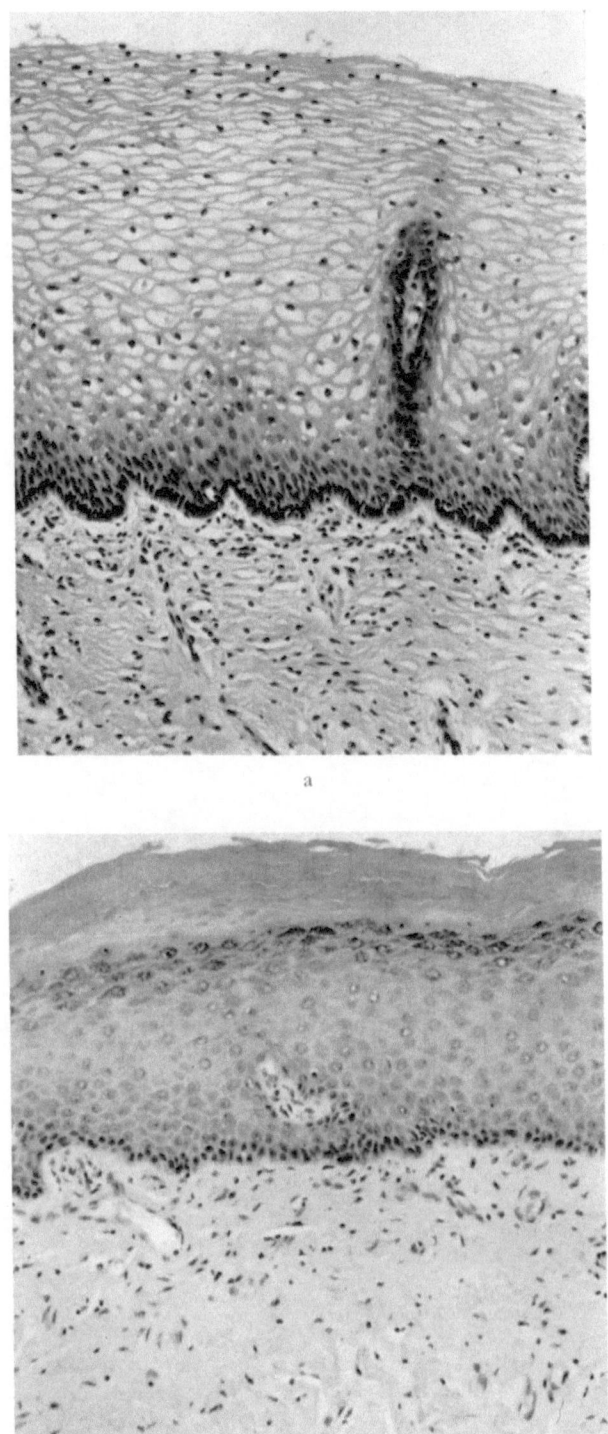

a

b

Fig. 1.5.a Typical cornified squamous epithelium of the ectocervix. The basal (germinative) layer is well defined, the other layers gradually merge into each other, b Keratinized epithelium of the ectocervix. The granular, or intraepithelial, zone is well defined. (H. & E. ×120)

The pattern of cervical squamous epithelium varies from epoch to epoch of a woman's life and at any period it may vary from place to place in the same cervix. At birth the squamous epithelium of the cervix is very thick and has a basket-weave

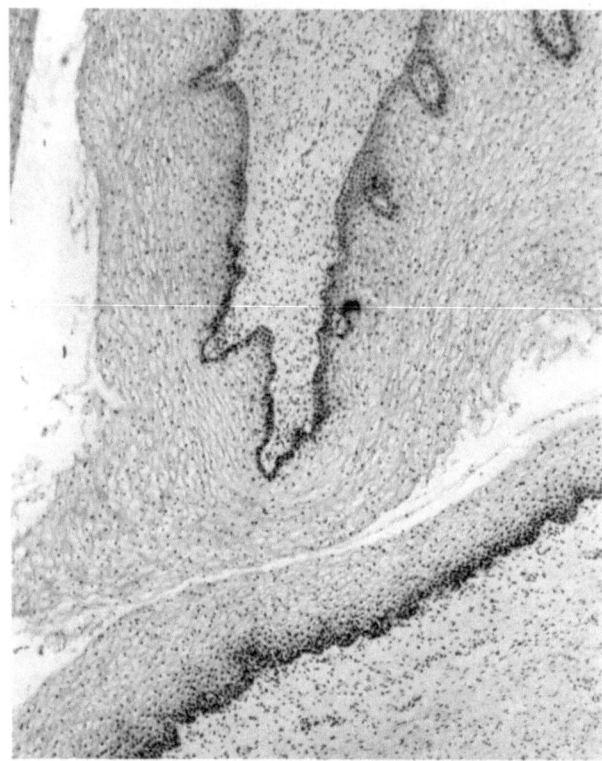

Fig. 1.6. The squamous epithelium of the ectocervix and vagina of a newborn infant. The epithelium is thick and the superficial layers are exfoliating. (H. & E. ×50)

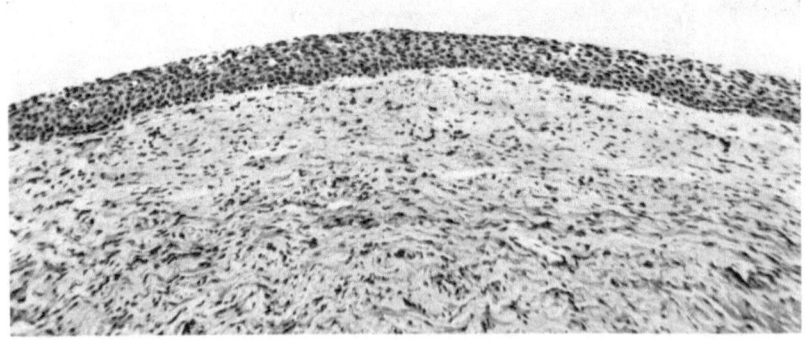

Fig. 1.7. Atrophic squamous epithelium from the ectocervix. Note the loss of stratification but the relative cellularity. From a woman of sixty-one years whose menopause was eleven years previously. (H. & E. × 125)

structure (Fig. 1.6.) presumably as a result of oestrogenic stimulation. The greater part of this epithelium exfoliates as the oestrogenic effect is lost and it is remodelled as a thin menbrane. After the menopause the squamous epithelium becomes atrophic (Fig. 1.7.); it is thin, stratification is reduced or almost lost, the nuclei are dark and the cytoplasm of the cells is scanty and hence they are more closely packed together. The rate of atrophy varies considerably from woman to woman. In some, atrophy occurs soon after the cessation of menstruation but in others there may be very little atrophy even ten years after the menopause. The cause of these differences is uncertain, it may depend on differences in steroid hormone production by extragenital sources or on differences in sexual activity.

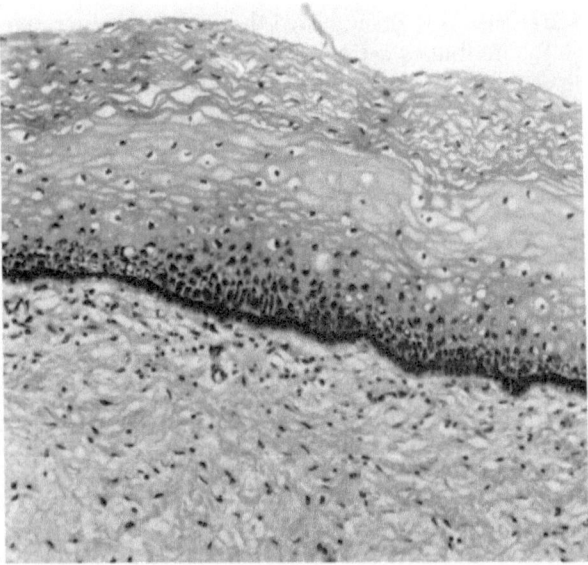

Fig. 1.8. Squamous epithelium showing a "basket-weave" arrangement of the cells of the superficial layer. (H. & E. × 120)

During the childbearing period the squamous epithelium of the portio vaginalis of the cervix is not static but varies with the phase of the menstrual cycle, in pregnancy and during the puerperium. Normally during this epoch the squamous epithelium is well glycogenated in the upper layers but patches of glycogenated epithelium may sometimes be seen sitting next to non-glycogenated epithelium. Often the cells in the more superficial layers are loosely attached to the underlying cells giving a basket-weave pattern (Fig. 1.8.) and patches of such epithelium may be interspersed with more compact epithelium. The contour of the epithelial-connective tissue junction varies; sometimes it is straight and flat but often wavy. This waviness is determined by the underlying vascular pattern and is usually associated with squamous metaplasia but sometimes it persists far out on the portio vaginalis reaching almost to the fornix and in such a site it is unlikely always to be the result of prior squamous metaplasia.

b) Special Cells in the Squamous Epithelium of the Portio Vaginalis Uteri

ZWILLENBERG (1958, 1959) described mast cells in the stratified squamous epithelium of the vagina and cervix. They may have migrated into the epithelium from the cervical stroma. IVERSEN (1960) described mast cells in the stroma of the human cervix and found them most plentiful during the secretory phase of the menstrual cycle. NOZAKA and SIMPSON (1962) also found mast cells beneath the squamous epithelium and VANTSA et al. (1963) found them predominantly round the blood vessels of the cervix.

The function of the mast cells at this site is unknown. They may regulate local blood clotting through heparin production or vasoconstriction and capillary permeability mediated by the secretion of histamine (SELYE 1965). ASBOE-HANSEN (1954) suggested that under various hormonal stimuli mast cells may secrete hyaluronic acid. HORSTMANN and STEGNER (1966) suggested that an antiproliferative action might be mediated through the inhibitory action of heparin on phosphatases.

Dendritic cells were first described in the epidermis by LANGERHANS (1868). The nature and function of these cells is uncertain; BREATHNACH (1965) has critically reviewed the literature. Conventional staining methods including gold impregnation are capricious but JARRETT and RILEY (1963) have shown that LANGERHANS cells can be visualized by virtue of their ATP-ase activity and CAMPO-AASEN and PEARSE (1966) have called the LANGERHANS cell "the epidermal macrophage" because of its pattern of hydrolytic enzymes.

By means of supravital staining and gold impregnation dentritic-like cells have been seen in the upper strata of the squamous epithelium of the vagina and portio vaginalis of the cervix (ZWILLENBERG 1959). SALERNO (1944) and POLAK (1949) found dopa-positive dendritic cells in the basal part of the portio vaginalis. These were presumably melanocytes. HACKEMANN et al. (1968), using electronmicroscopy, have described clear cells without desmosomal attachments in the basal and suprabasal layers. The morphological features of some of these cells correspond to those of LANGERHANS cells.

c) The Fine Structure of the Squamous Epithelium of the Cervix Uteri

α) Tonofibrils and the Structural Changes in Keratinization

In 1924 SCHMIDT demonstrated by polarizing microscopy the existence of a birefringent fibre system in keratinizing squamous epithelium indicating an orderly submicroscopic structural array. A similar system can be seen in keratinized squamous epithelium of the cervix and occasionally in the superficial layers of non-keratinized epithelium (Fig. 1.9.). Using the ferrocyanide reaction, GIROUD and BULLIARD (1932) found thiol groups in the germinative layer and disulphide groups in the cornified layer of skin. DERKSON et al. (1937) correlated the birefringence of the fibre system, the X-ray diffraction pattern and cytochemistry of keratinizing epithelium and their work has formed the basis of subsequent concepts.

Although the intracellular fibre system, or tonofibrils, can be studied to a limited extent by light microscopy, electron microscopy is more informative. MORICARD et al. (1958), MORICARD and CARTIER (1964) and HACKEMANN et al. (1960), among others, have described the fibre system in the cervix as did ODLAND (1964) in the skin. The

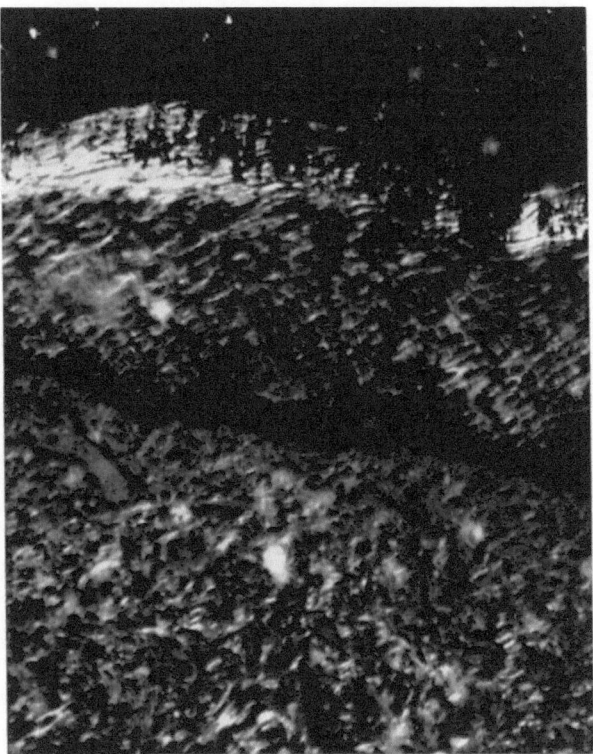

Fig. 1.9. Squamous epithelium of the ectocervix viewed in polarised light. The keratinized cells are strongly anisotropic. (H. & E. × 120)

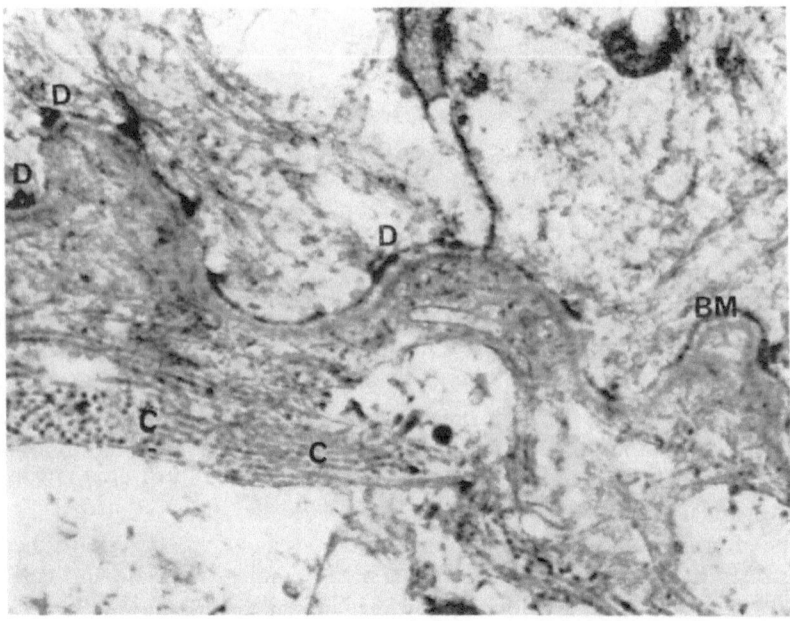

Fig. 1.10. An electron photomicrograph showing the basal cells and the underlying stroma. Note the undulating basement membrane (BM) and the half desmosomes (D). C indicates the collagen fibres of the stroma. (× 25,000)

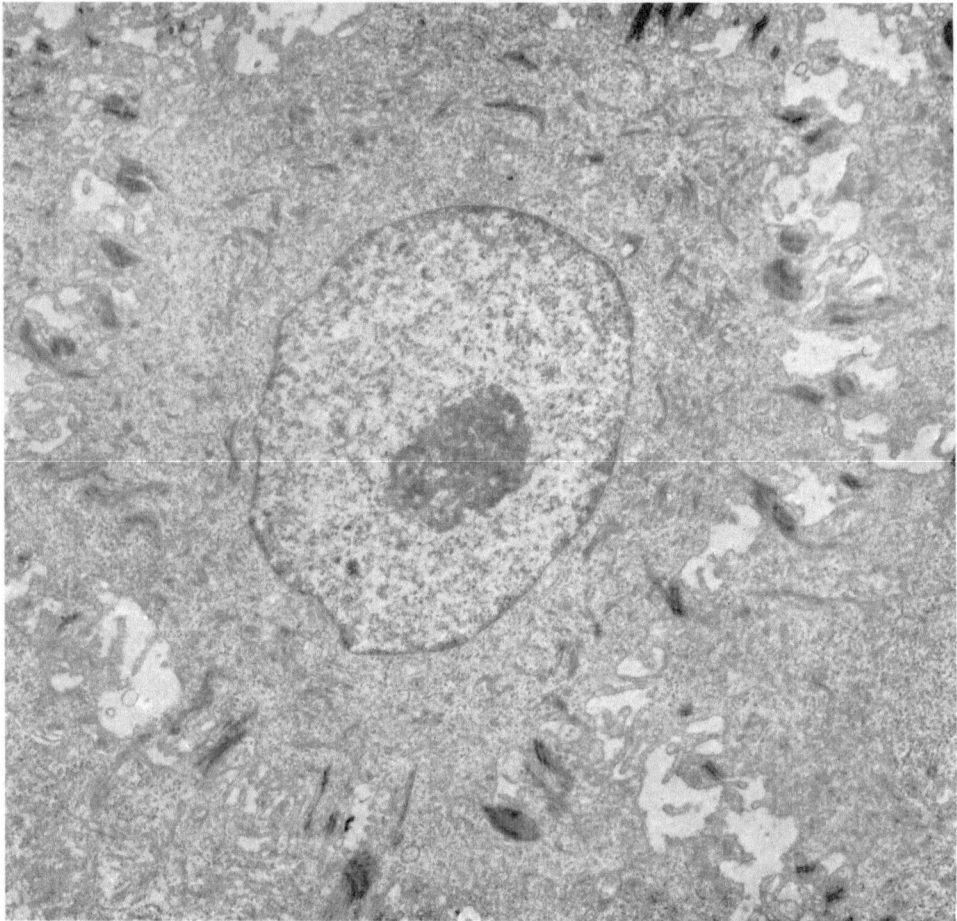

Fig. 1.11. An electron photomicrograph of a parabasal cell. Mitochondria are randomly dispersed in the cytoplasm. Clusters of microfibrils are readily seen. The desmosomal junctions between this and adjacent cells are conspicuous. ($\times$ 8,000)

cytoplasm of the basal cells contains tonofilaments some of which converge on the half-desmosomes at the base of the cells. Tonofilaments are organized into moderately dense fibrils for a short distance from the junctional desmosomes. However, tonofilaments are less conspicuous in the basal cells of the cervix than in those of the epidermis. In the stratum spinosum profundum the tonofilaments are more densely packed and conspicuous. In the stratum corneum, or functionalis, the tonofilaments are concentrated near and parallel to the cell borders (HACKEMANN *et al.* 1968) (Figs. 1.10., 1.11. and 1.12.).

In the stratum spinosum profundum GRUBB *et al.* (1968) have described small granules scattered through the cytoplasm. These granules are ovoid and vary in size from 900 to 2,400 Å. They are bounded by a trilaminar membrane and internally consist of both electron-dense and translucent areas. In the stratum spinosum superficiale they at first increase progressively in number, becoming aligned to the distal

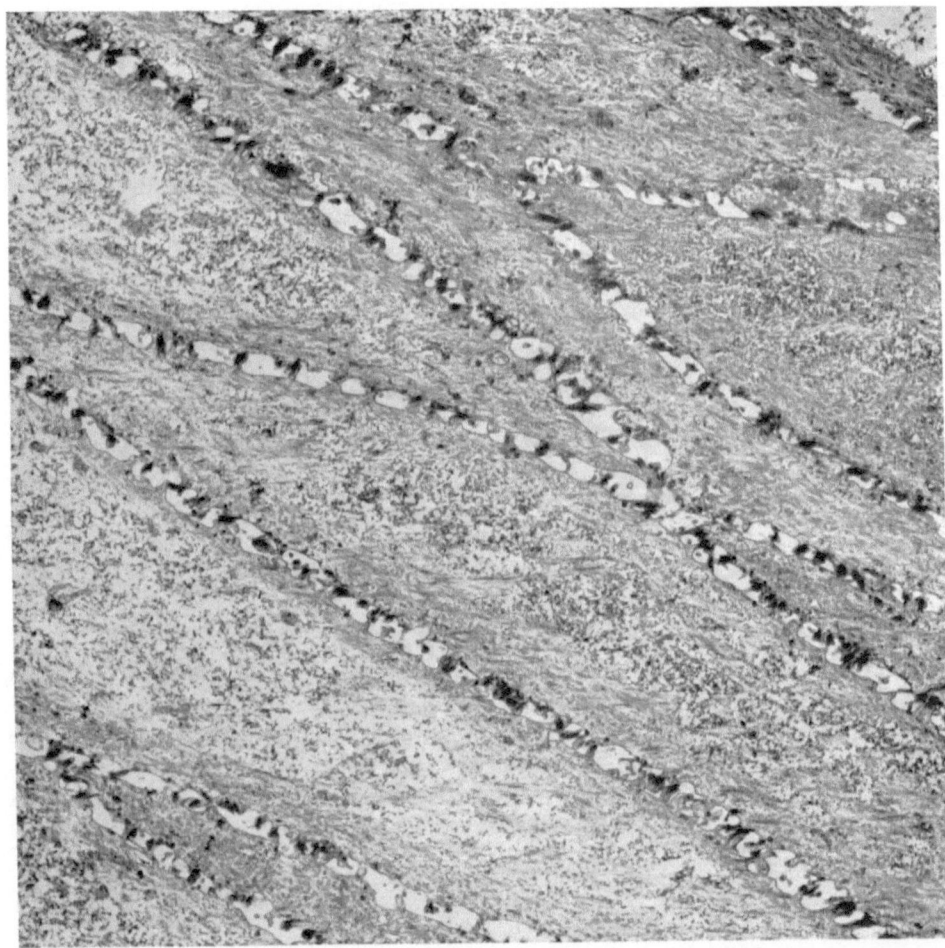

Fig. 1.12. An electron photomicrograph of the superficial layer. Note the numerous granules of glycogen and the intracellular fibre system. ($\times$ 6,000)

border of the cells, and then they gradually diminish in number until they are absent from the outermost cells of the zone. As these granules diminish in number, small osmiophilic bodies appear which are compatible with keratohyaline granules. In the cervix, cells of the stratum functionalis contain keratohyaline granules which in the epidermis are characteristically present in the granular layer. GRUBB et al. (1968) suggest that their small ovoid granules contribute to the development of keratohyaline granules.

It is pertinent to remark that the material used by HACKEMANN et al. (1968) consisted of seven biopsy specimens, one from a post-menopausal woman and six from women of childbearing age. None of these presumably showed keratinization It would be interesting and valuable to study material from cervices showing keratinization and to compare this with epidermis, despite JARRETT et al. (1966) suggesting that the mode of epidermal keratinization is still controversial. It is, therefore, only possible to understand keratinization of the cervix in the broadest terms. In the skin, ODLAND (1964) has described the development of keratohyaline granules near organelles associated with cellular synthesis and in the interstices of the mesh of pre-existing filaments. From the time of its appearance keratohyaline possesses an internal structure suggestive of ordered keratin. Thus it may be supposed that tonofilaments and keratohyaline are epidermal precursors of the two-component system of epidermal keratin. Similar views have also been developed by BRODY (1964a) but JARRETT *et al.* (1966) described epidermal keratinization in different terms. At the stage of transition from granular to horny layer there is a sudden appearance of hydrolytic enzymes. This sudden release of hydrolases causes rapid destruction of the non-keratinized cytoplasm leaving a hollow shell with a keratinized periphery. Care must be taken not to draw too close a parallel between cervical epithelium and epidermis.

β) The Organelles and Other Cell Inclusions of Cervical Squamous Epithelium

The following description is based on the accounts of MORICARD and CARTIER (1964) and HACKEMANN *et al.* (1968).

Pinocytic vesicles occur in the basal cells and are especially concentrated between the desmosomes. In these cells there are large numbers of mitochondria especially beneath the proximal pole of the nucleus. Lysosome-like structures are numerous, multivesicular bodies occasionally occur and ribosomes and small amounts of endoplasmic reticulum can be seen. The Golgi complex is well developed. In the stratum spinosum profundum the organelles seen in the basal cells are present but the mitochondria have no special distribution. MORICARD and CARTIER frequently found the Golgi complex at both ends of the nucleus in this zone, whilst in the stratum spinosum superficiale it was usually basally situated. In the more superficial layers the Golgi complex and endoplasmic reticulum are not seen, and degenerate mitochondria and lysosome-like bodies are seen only in small numbers.

γ) Cell Cohesion

One of the properties of malignant tumours is that the tissues fray because of lack of cohesion between the cells (COMAN 1944, 1953). In carcinoma *in situ cervicis* the cells often still cohere but a strip of epithelium may lose its adhesion to the underlying connective tissue. It is thus important to examine the normal mechanism of cohesion and adhesion.

The cells of squamous epithelium, whether epidermal, oesophageal or cervical, are not completely attached to their neighbours. Contact with other cells is made over small areas which give rise to the characteristic cytoplasmic bridges. These bridges are most clearly seen in the stratum spinosum and hence the synonym "the prickle-cell layer". At the middle of each of these bridges is a swelling called the node of Bizzozero, or desmosome. Electron microscopy shows that the desmosomes are small areas of contact at which the plasma membrane of each cell is thickened. Between the thickened plasma membrane lies a layer of interdesmosomal cement. The structure of the desmosomes of normal vaginal and cervical squamous epithelium has been described by a number of workers including KARRER (1960), PETRY *et al.* (1961), CARSTEN *et al.* (1962), MORICARD and CARTIER (1964) and more recently by HACKEMANN *et al.* (1968).

HACKEMANN *et al.* (1968) found a moderate number of desmosomes on the upper borders of the basal cells connecting them to the parabasal cells but on the lateral borders the desmosomes were scanty. In some specimens the intercellular space was wide and in others narrow. Large numbers of desmosomes anchored the cells together in the stratum spinosum: in the deeper part of this zone the intercellular spaces were wide but these were reduced in the more superficial part. In the micrographs of HACKEMANN *et al.* desmosomes can still be seen in the stratum functionalis; MORICARD and CARTIER described a dissociation of desmosomal structures in this region.

The integrity or cohesion of squamous epithelium appears to depend on the numerous desmosome-tonofilament complexes and on the intercellular cement. The complex organization of the desmosomes gives the impression of great stability. Evidence is accumulating that in the squamous epithelium of the skin the desmosome-tonofilament complex can readily be broken and reformed. Thus, EPSTEIN *et al.* (1966) have shown that in the skin during the process of epidermal regeneration keratinocytes can move towards the surface at different speeds and that cells must therefore lose contact in order to move past their neighbours. Likewise MISHMA and PINKUS (1968) have shown a loss of intercellular connections following stripping of the keratin layer of the skin by tape, whilst recovery is followed by a new formation of desmosomes rather than repair of old ones.

In skin a PAS-positive, diastase-resistant substance has been demonstrated on or between the cell membranes and in the intercellular bridges (BRAUN-FALCO 1954). These same sites also react positively with Hale's stain and alcian blue (BRAUN-FALCO 1958). These reactions suggest the presence of neutral and acid mucopolysaccharides at sites where the theoretical cement substance should be concentrated. No studies of this cement substance are recorded in the cervix but it is likely that a similar substance will be found. Further evidence in support of the role intercellular cement plays in cell cohesiveness is indicated in the experiments of KEMP (1968) which have shown that removal of sialic acid from cell surfaces *in vitro* (albeit chicken embryo muscle cells) by N-acetylneuraminate glycohydrolase reduces cell aggregation.

FLESCH and ESODA (1964) have produced evidence that abnormal mucopolysaccharide metabolism in the skin may be associated with the formation of pathological horny layers, as for example in psoriasis. A similar mechanism may play some part in pathological states of the cervix associated with hyperkeratinization.

In the cervix HACKEMANN *et al.* (1968) have seen non-desmosomal cell junctions and connections similar to those described by FARQUHAR and PALADE (1965) but the significance of these is not yet apparent.

δ) *Cell Adhesion*

There has been some dispute as to whether or not a basement membrane is present under the squamous epithelium of the cervix. The term basement membrane had a well defined connotation before the introduction of the electron microscope. With the advent of this instrument and fine analysis of the tissue immediately subjacent to the epithelium the term basement membrane has become imprecise. Starting from the connective tissue and moving towards the epithelium there are, according to MORICARD and CARTIER (1964), three successive layers: (a) the reticular basal membrane, approximately 2 μ in thickness, corresponding to the basement membrane of classical histology, (b) the basal lamella about 600 Å thick and (c) the plasma membrane of basal cells. The basal lamella has been called the "basement membrane" by ODLAND (1958) in his description of the epidermis and by DOUGHERTY and LOW (1958) in their description of the cervix. According to ASHWORTH *et al.* (1961) this basal lamella in the cervix is a homogeneous electron-dense membrane 300 Å thick, but on the stromal surface fine granules and fibrils are noted, suggesting a relationship to collagen fibrils and a space, 200 Å in width, is present between it and the plasma membrane of the basal cells. In normal epithelium the electron-dense membrane is folded and convoluted because of numerous footlike projections from the basal cells. BERGER (1961 a) and YOUNES *et al.* (1965) have described fibrils anchoring the electron-

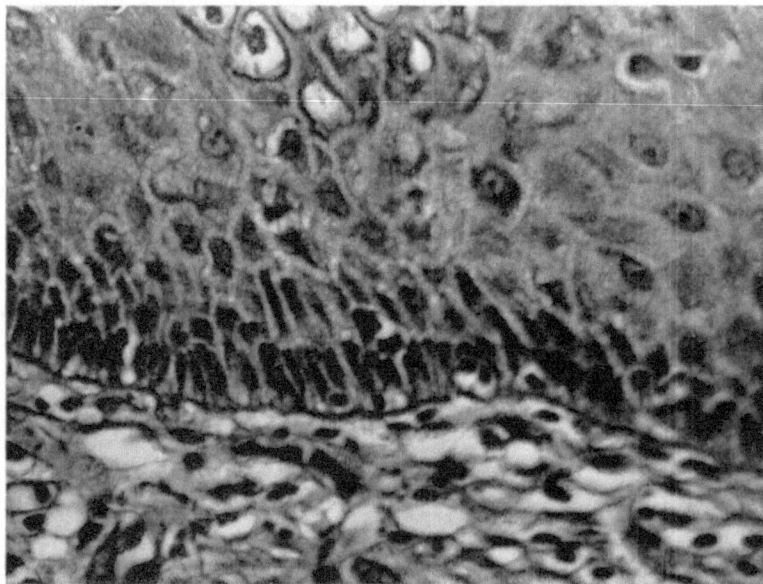

Fig. 1.13. This shows a well defined basement membrane between the squamous epithelium and the cervical stroma. Stained by the periodic acid Schiff method and Hale's colloidal iron. ($\times$ 480)

dense membrane to the underlying connective tissue and finer fibrils connecting it to the half desmosomes of the adjacent basal cells. The observations of HACKEMANN *et al.* (1968) confirm the presence of physical connections between the basal cells and the underlying stroma via the electron-dense lamina densa.

ASHWORTH *et al.* (1961) have shown that, although the electron-dense lamina densa is too thin to be seen by light microscopy, a comparable but thicker lamina can be demonstrated by histochemical procedures designed to identify acid mucopolysaccharides. Thus a PAS stain combined with alcian blue, or colloidal iron, shows a distinct and continuous lamina in normal cervical squamous epithelium (Fig. 1.13.). According to LAMB *et al.* (1960) this mucopolysaccharide lamina is the basement membrane of the light microscopist. Using a variety of stains they have shown that, whereas a continuous membrane can be seen under certain epithelia, such as the sweat glands of the vulva, it is often thin, absent or discontinuous under the squamous epithelium of the ectocervix and the glandular epithelium of the endocervix. WARREN *et al.* (1966) also found the membrane to be discontinuous. As a result of careful histochemical investigations PUNDEL (1966) and PUNDEL *et al.* (1967) regard the lamina as scleroprotein rather than mucopolysaccharide.

d) The Histochemistry of the Squamous Epithelium of the Cervix Uteri

The histochemistry of cervical squamous epithelium will be considered under three main headings: (1) the chemical components of the cell such as glycogen, nucleic acid, mucopolysaccharides, lipids and keratin, (2) the enzyme systems and (3) the relationship between the enzyme systems and the cellular organelles.

Nucleic acid. There is a direct relation between the amount of RNA in the cytoplasm of cells and their growth potential. DE ROBERTIS *et al.* (1966) and WISLOCKI *et al.* (1950) have shown that the cytoplasmic basophilia of the basal and parabasal cells of the cervix reflect their content of RNA, and SANDRITTER (1953) and VENDRELY and VENDRELY (1959) have shown that in the vaginal epithelium (and presumably also in the cervical) there is a progressive decline in nuclear DNA and cytoplasmic RNA with cellular maturation. These changes parallel the apparent diminution in the number of ribosomes and their complete lack in the upper layers of the cervical epithelium.

Glycogen is present in the upper layers of the squamous epithelium of the cervix (Fig. 1.14.). Histochemically it can be demonstrated by Best's carmine stain or the PAS reaction, controlled by examining diastase-treated sections in parallel. In the vagina HEROVICI (1960a) found traces of glycogen in the parabasal layer, abundant glycogen in the intermediate layer and somewhat less in the superficial layer. SCHRÖDER (1925) found that the vaginal secretion contained 2 to 4 % of glycogen and LAPAN and FRIEDMAN (1950) found 3.3 to 4.7 % in the vaginal mucus of pregnant women but a smaller quantity, 1.9 to 2.6 % in non-pregnant women. It is of interest to note that adult skin also contains glycogen but to a much smaller extent (WEBER 1964).

The glycogen content of the cervical and vaginal squamous epithelium varies with age, the phase of the ovarian cycle and as a result of pregnancy. Glycogen deposition starts with the differentation of the sinus epithelium into the definitive vaginal epithelium at about 140 to 160 mm foetal length (GRAGERT 1926 and FOIX and BURR 1955). The cervix and vagina are rich in glycogen in the newborn but with the postnatal fall in oestrogen level there is marked desquamation of the squamous epithelium, resulting in a thin, glycogen-poor epithelium. With the onset of sexual development, usually before the first menstruation, the glycogen content of the cervical epithelium increases. After the climacteric glycogen diminishes and in old age almost disappears from the epithelium. Experimental studies on women (COTTE *et al.* 1937) have shown a close correlation between the oestrogen level and the glycogen content of the vaginal epithelium. Since the oestrogen level normally reaches a maximum at the time of ovulation, it is not surprising that the glycogen level of vaginal epithelium reaches a maximum in the middle of the menstrual cycle (BERNSTINE and RAKOFF 1953). On the contrary, HEROVICI (1960a) found the maximum quantity of glycogen in the vaginal epithelium in the pre- and post-menstrual periods, and a minimum at the time of ovulation. However, according to PUNDEL (1952) there is no close correlation

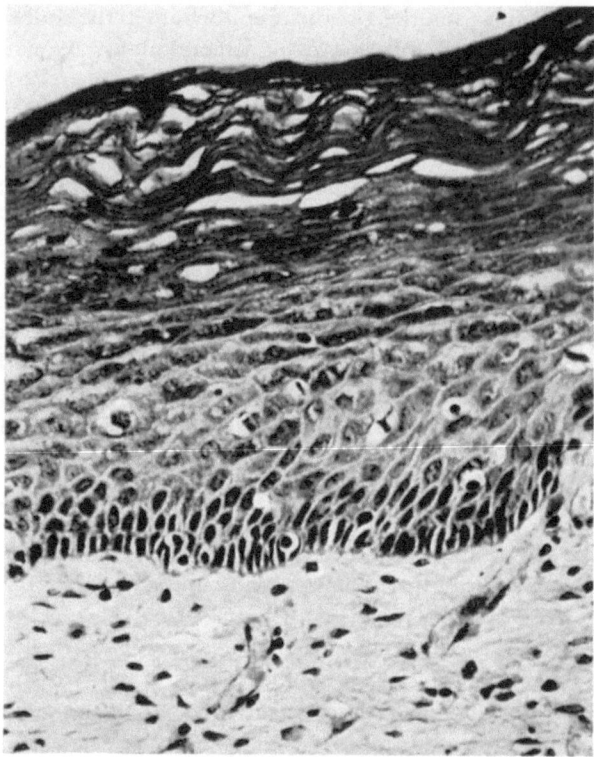

Fig. 1.14. A "basket-weave" type of squamous epithelium stained for glycogen. Notice the granular distribution of glycogen in the intermediate layer and the intense staining of the superficial layer. (Best's carmine × 300)

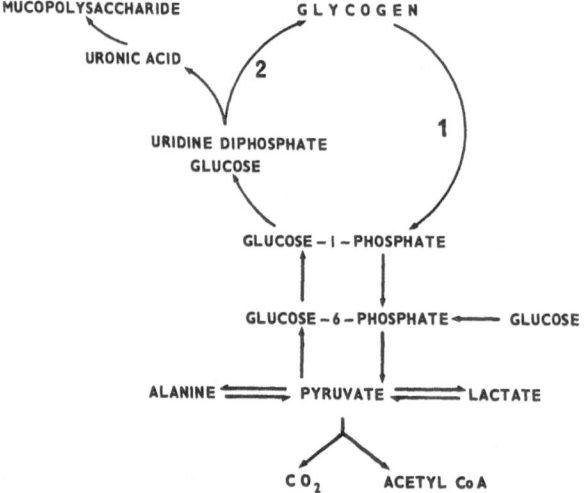

Fig 1.15. The metabolim of glycogen (after FREINKEL, 1964, but modified). Some of the enzymes involved are: in pathway 1, amylophosphorylase: and in pathway 2, glycogen synthetase (UDFG-glycogen transglucosylase) and amylo-1,4-1,6-transglucosidase

between hormone activity and glycogen content but rather with epithelial proliferation.

The synthesis and catabolism of glycogen occur by different pathways which are summarized in Fig. 1.15. Glycogen metabolism is closely related to other metabolic processes, for example, through pyruvate and acetyl-Co-A to the citric acid cycle. It is of interest that uridine diphosphate glucose is the substrate for a dehydrogenase which oxidises it to uronic acid from which mucopolysaccharides can be formed.

Mucopolysaccharides. After diastase treatment, sections of vagina and cervix still give a positive PAS reaction in the superficial layer, which is indicative of the presence of neutral mucopolysaccharide. This has been studied by SANI (1953) and BOTELLA *et al.* (1958) among others. Most of the investigations have been made on vaginal rather than cervical epithelium. BOTELLA *et al.* (1958) have shown that oestrogens increase the thickness of the glycogenic layer and the intracellular content of glycogen. Progesterone increases the mucopolysaccharide content of the superficial layer but does not increase the glycogenic layer. Androgens behave like oestrogens but with a less marked effect. Cyclical changes occur in menstruating women. In the first half of the cycle most of the PAS-positive material in the vaginal epithelium is glycogen whilst mucopolysaccharides increase in the second half.

Using Hale's colloidial iron stain, MATTER (1958) has shown the presence of acid mucopolysaccharides in the cells of the parabasal, intermediate and superficial strata of the vaginal epithelium. The finding is relatively constant in the stratum spinosum but less so in the other layers. The staining is clearly reduced after the action of testicular hyaluronidase but is not completely negative. PEARSE (1968) points out that this method is not specific for acid mucopolysaccharides and that nucleo-proteins and other proteins may also be stained. Cyclic changes in Hale-positive material cannot be demonstrated but it diminishes after the menopause.

Lipid. ZWILLENBERG (1959), using the Sudan-black reaction, has found lipid granules in the basal cells and in the Verdichtungszone of Stemshorn. Using Baker's acid haematein method, he also demonstrated lipid in the desmosomes, confirming Wislocki's previous observations. Lipids revealed by these histochemical techniques constitute only part of the lipid content of cells; much is "masked", forming the membranes of intracellular organelles. In the upper layers of the squamous epithelium these organelles are destroyed and thus liberate "unmasked" lipid of phospholipid type. Apart from forming cellular and intracellular membranes, lipids are an efficient means of storing energy.

Keratin and keratinization. In a previous section we discussed some of the morphological changes in keratinization. Here the chemical basis will be considered. KLIGMAN (1964) has pointed out that the term keratinization literally means the synthesis of a peculiar fibrous protein by cutaneous and mucocutaneous epithelia and the term is not a synonym for the formation of a horny layer. He indicates that much conceptual mischief flows from this error. For example, it is often said that vaginal and oral mucous membranes are nonkeratinizing. What is really meant is that these do not ordinarily form a stratum corneum although the vagina and cervix may develop such a stratum in women with procidentia. In the mouth and vagina, keratinized cells slough individually without being cemented together into a membrane as in the skin. In the mouth there are various morphological patterns of keratinization and these are closely similar to those seen in vaginal and cervical epithelium (MEYER and

MEDAK 1961; ZELICKSON and HARTMAN 1962). The absence of a genuine stratum corneum is the specific reason for the high permeability of the oral mucosa of which advantage is taken when drugs are administered as tablets for dissolution in the mouth.

Whilst bearing in mind the proper chemical meaning of the term keratinization, it must be conceded that, histologically, keratinization in squamous epithelium is recognized by the formation of a superficial acidophilic stratum. One of the principal chemical changes occuring in the process of keratinization is the oxidation of -SH groups in the lower strata to -SS- in the upper layers. SH bonds characterize amino acids present in pre-keratin, and -SS- bonds amino acids in keratin. HEROVICI (1960a), using the ferricyanide method of Chevremont and Frédricq, detected -SH groups in the intermediate and superficial strata of vaginal epithelium. The coloration reached a maximum at about the fourteenth day of the cycle. FORAKER and WINGO (1956) found sulphhydryl groups in all viable squamous cells, whether in the normal portio vaginalis or in intraepithelial carcinoma, and these were found in regions of neoplastic and non-neoplastic keratinization. Disulphide groups were found in keratinizing surface cells, in epithelial pearls of squamous carcinoma and keratinizing neoplastic cells.

e) The Enzymes of the Squamous Epithelium of the Cervix

Numerous histochemical studies have been made of the enzymes present in the squamous epithelium of the cervix, usually in order to detect differences which might distinguish normal from neoplastic epithelium. It would probably be more valuable to approach this aspect of cervical histochemistry from a more fundamental point of view, to determine the localization of the various metabolic pathways involved in the growth and differentation of a tissue, and to see how these pathways are modified by endogenous and exogenous factors. Unfortunately a number of workers have failed to state very precisely the localization of the enzymes they have studied and, when they have, the reports are often contradictory. Table 1.2. lists the cytoplasmic enzymes which are well documented and about which there is general agreement. The table also indicates the strata in which the enzymes are found and the metabolic pathways involved.

Much information is lacking about the metabolism of normal cervical squamous epithelium. Nevertheless an overall pattern is discernible. Anaerobic glycolysis, using lactic dehydrogenase as a marker, and aerobic carbohydrate metabolism, indicated by the Krebs-cycle enzymes, occur in the basal, parabasal and intermediate strata, corresponding to the distribution of mitochondria (MORICARD and CARTIER 1964; HACKEMANN et al. 1968) in the matrices of which the Krebs-cycle enzymes are located (DE ROBERTIS et al. 1966). The pentose shunt, an alternative to the Embden-Meyerhof anaerobic pathway, is also present in the basal, parabasal and intermediate layers. Glycogen metabolism occurs in the parabasal and intermediate layers and glycogenolysis is probably associated with the endoplasmic reticulum (DE ROBERTIS et al. 1966). FORAKER and MARINO (1961) and FIENBERG and COHEN (1968) found amylo-1, 6-glucosidase and amylophosphorylase in the parabasal and intermediate layers where presumably glycogen is formed, but the enzymes are less evident in the superficial layers where most glycogen is concentrated. The superficial layer is metabolically relatively inactive, although β-glucuronidase (FISHMAN et al. 1963) and acid

Table 1.2. The presumptive location of enzymes in the normal squamous epithelium of the human cervix and vagina

	Basal	Parabasal	Intermediate	Superficial	Reference
Mitochondria					
Krebs' cycle enzymes					
Malic DH	Marked in all zones except keratinized layer				[6]
Isocitric DH	++	+	+—	+——	[9]
	+	+	+	++	[8]
	Low except in the keratinized layer				[6]
Respiratory enzymes					
NAD diaphorase	+	+	+	+	[4]
	++	+	+—	+——	[9]
NADP diaphorase	++	+	+—	+——	[9]
Succinic DH	++	+	+—	—	[1, 2, 3, 6, 9]
	+/+—	+/+—	—	—	[8, 10]
Microsomes					
Glycogen synthetase	—	—	+	—	[12]
Amylophosphorylase	+	+	+	—	[3, 12]
Amylo-1,4-1,6 transglucosidase	+	+	+	—	[3, 12]
Lysosomes					
Acid DNA ase	+				[5, 7]
Acid phosphatase	+—	+—	+	+	[1]
	+	+	+	+	[9]
	+	+—	+—	++	[8]
β-glucuronidase	+	—	—	+	[1]
	Very little if any				[9]
Organelles not specified					
α-glycerophosphate DH	Moderate in deeper layers diminishing superficially				[6]
β-hydroxybutyric DH	++	+	+—	—	[9]
	+—	+—	+—	+	[8]
	Slight in subcornified layer, low elsewhere				[6]
Glucose-6-phosphate DH	+	+	+	+	[10]
	++	+	+	+—	[12]
	Low or moderate activity except superficial zone where activity is high				[6, 8]
6-phosphogluconate DH	++	+	+	+—	[9]
Glutamic DH	Moderately intense in basal zone diminishing superficially				[6]
Lactic DH	++	+	+—	—	[6, 8, 9, 10]
Monamino oxidase	Absent or present in low amount				[9]
Alkaline phosphatase	Absent or very little				[8, 9]
Aminopeptidase	Absent or very little				[8]
	+—/+	—	—	—	[11]
Non-specific esterase	Absent or every little				[8, 9]
ATP ase	Only in dendritic cells				[8]
5-nucleotidase	+	—	—	—	[8]
Phosphoamidase	Mostly basal diminishing superficially				[2]

DH is dehydrogenase.

[1] FISHMAN and MITCHELL (1959).
[2] HOPMAN (1960).
[3] FORAKER (1962).
[4] FISHMAN et al. (1963).
[5] WARONSKI (1964).
[6] ISHIHARA et al. (1964).
[7] JONEK et al. (1966).
[8] THIERY and WILLINGHAGEN (1966).
[9] DAWSON and FILIPE (1967).
[10] WIDY and KIERSKI (1967).
[11] ISHIHARA et al. (1968).
[12] FIENBERG and COHEN (1968).

phosphatase (FISHMAN and MITCHELL 1959) have been found in this site. The metabolic pathway for keratin formation is obscure.

f) The Cell Kinetics of Squamous Epithelium

Although only a little work has been done on the kinetics of cervical epithelium, the importance of this topic in relation to epithelial abnormalities renders some general discussion appropriate. Thus, FIELD (1968) has written, "an understanding of the normal regulatory mechanisms and feedback systems is a prerequisite to an understanding of those failures of control of tissue proliferation that result in neoplasia".

The cells composing the squamous epithelium of the cervix form a *renewing population* (DE ROBERTIS *et al.* 1966) in which a continuous loss of cells from the surface is balanced by a corresponding production of cells elsewhere in the tissue. Cell-renewing populations pass through four main phases (BERTALANFFY 1963): (1) cell formation

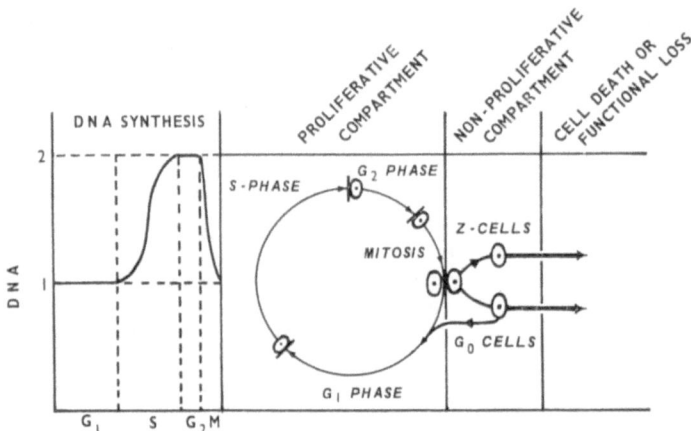

Fig. 1.16. The cell cycle

by mitotic division, usually of less differentiated cells such as basal or reserve cells; (2) cell differentiation which often involves the transformation of cells by a change in size or shape or the development of cilia; (3) a period that can be designated the functional or metabolic phase when the cells perform their task of secretion, absorption or protection; and (4) senescence with desquamation. The period required for all cells of a tissue to pass once through these four phases is known as the renewal or turnover time of the tissue.

The process of cell replication is subdivided into four phases (BRESCIANI 1968) during which an orderly progression of biochemical events occurs, culminating in the birth of two new cells (Fig. 1.16.). G_1 is the post-mitotic phase, S the period of DNA synthesis, G_2 the pre-mitotic phase when the nucleus contains twice as much DNA as in G_1, and M the mitotic phase. After mitosis the new cells may enter a new replication cycle or go into a condition of non-proliferation which is generally associated with differentiation and functional activity. This transition to the non-proliferative state can be irreversible giving rise to the Z cells or, after a period of rest from proliferation, some cells may replicate again, these are the G_0 cells. If T_c is the duration of the cell cycle, from one mitosis to the next, T_m the time in mitosis, T_{g1} the time in the G_1 phase, T_s the time in the S phase, and T_{g2} the time in the G_2 phase,

$$T_c = T_m + T_{g1} + T_s + T_{g2}$$

If the tissue is exposed to radioactive thymidine then the nuclei in the DNA synthetic phase will incorporate the radioactive material and this can be visualized by autoradiography. Fig. 1.17 shows a section of human cervix grown for twelve hours in a

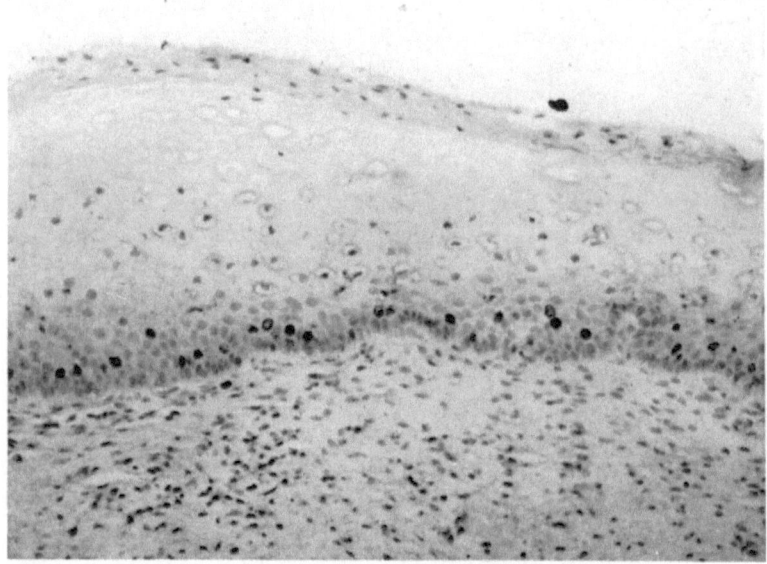

Fig. 1.17. An autoradiograph of human cervical squamous epithelium grown in medium 199 containing radioactive thymidine for 12 hours. The darkly stained nuclei in the parabasal layer have taken up the radioactive thymidine whilst in the synthetic phase of the cycle. ($\times$ 120)

culture medium containing radioactive thymidine. The section has been coated with photographic emulsion and left to develop in the dark for four weeks. The nuclei containing radioactive thymidine are visible as clusters of silver granules in the photographic emulsion and can now be counted. It is readily seen that there are more nuclei in the synthetic phase in the parabasal cells than in the basal cells. The labelling index is the fraction of the total population labelled after a brief exposure to radioactive thymidine. It can be shown (CLEAVER 1967) that:

$$\text{Labelling index} = \frac{\text{duration of S phase}}{\text{duration of cell cycle}} = \frac{T_s}{T_c}$$

It is difficult to estimate the duration of the DNA synthetic phase in the human subject, hence most workers have assumed a value of 6 hours given by JOHNSON and BOND (1961). Table 1.3. summarizes some of the reported values. All the workers, except AVERETTE et al. (1970), have used a similar technique of exposing explants of cervix to tritiated thymidine in culture media. Some of the variations in results are

Table 1.3. The duration of the cell cycle in the normal squamous epithelium of the cervix uteri

		Mean labelling index (%)	Cell cycle time (hr.)
RICHART (1963)		4.6	130
FETTIG and SIEVERS (1966)		6.25	96
FEIT and STANIČEK (1967)		6.4	75
KURY et al. (1967)			
Non-pregnant		2.50— 9.6	240—263
Pregnant		5.13—10.3	108—157
SCHELLHAS (1969)			
Basal		0.37	
Parabasal		18.0	
AVERETTE et al. (1970)			
Normal ovarian function	Basal	1.14	789
	Parabasal	14.25	63
Post menopausal	Basal	1.4	643
	Parabasal	10.5	86
Post menopausal	Basal	3.30	273
(oestrogen stimulated)	Parabasal	22.00	41
EDWARDS and LANGLEY (1971)			
Parabasal		3.0—18.0	200—233

no doubt due to differences in length of exposure time, but only KURY et al. (1967) and EDWARDS and LANGLEY (1971) make the point that the labelling index varies from case to case whilst REID and COPPLESON (1964) have shown that there is an irregular distribution of mitoses along the length of the epithelium, suggesting that at any one time there is rapid growth at one point and complete rest at another.

AVERETTE et al. (1970) injected tritiated thymidine into marked sites in the cervix and vagina and serial biopsies were taken at 24 hour intervals. They determined the labelling index and the mitotic index (i. e., the proportion of cells in mitosis) in each biopsy, and from these figures they were able to estimate T_s, T_{g1}, T_{g2}, T_m and T_c. They found the DNA synthetic phase to be 9 hours and not the 6 hours used in the previous calculations. Although in both the basal and parabasal cells T_{g2} was 5.4 hours and the mitotic phase ten minutes, T_{g1} was 643 hours in the basal layer and 63 hours in the parabasal layer. Similarly REID and COPPELSON (1964), FETTIG and SIEVERS (1966), SCHELLHAS (1966) and EDWARDS and LANGLEY (1971) noted a much lower labelling index in the basal cells than in the parabasal cells. AVERETTE et al. (1970) concluded, that three distinct compartments are normally present in the cervix: (1) the relatively inactive proliferative compartment consisting of the single layer of basal cells, (2) the active proliferative compartment composed of the lowest two or three parabasal layers and (3) the totally inactive differentiated compartment which includes cells in the intermediate and superficial layers. These upper layers can be subdivided again into the functional compartment and the compartment of dead cells about to exfoliate.

g) The Migration of Cells out of the Generative Compartment

BERTALANFFY (1963) has discussed the movement of cells from the basal to the superficial layer. He regards the cell as incapable of active motility. When a cell divides, the daughter cells occupy twice as much volume as the mother cell. They thus exert considerable pressure on the nearby basal cells forcing one to move upward and out of the layer because the basement membrane precludes movement downward and the tightly packed arrangement of the basal cells renders lateral movement impossible. GLÜCKSMANN (1964a) has criticized these views on the grounds that epithelial cells can be actively motile and movement of cells sometimes precedes mitosis. For a further valuable discussion of these views, the letters by BERTALANFFY (1964) and GLÜCKSMANN (1964b) should be consulted.

The extrusion of cells from the basal layer is clearly a complex process since the attachment of the cells to the basement membrane must be broken and attachment to other cells established. However, MISHIMA and PINKUS (1986) have shown that in the skin, under certain conditions, intercellular connections can be readily lost and desmosomes reformed.

Turnover, or transit time, is the period taken by a cell to migrate from the proliferative compartment until it is finally desquamated. AVERETTE *et al.* (1970) in their study of the kinetics of human genital tissues found the minimum transit time for cervical squamous epithelium to be 96 hours. Although this period is less than the generation time of cells in the basal layer, it is somewhat greater than the generation time of cells in the parabasal layer. The transit time is independent of the degree of oestrogen stimulation and for this AVERETTE *et al.* offer two possible explanations: (1) although oestrogen reduces the generation time of the parabasal cells, it also increases the thickness of the epithelium, thus the cells in the stimulated epithelium will have further to travel; or (2) since individual cells probably have different transit times, the effect of changing the mean transit time would not be reflected in their figures, which are an estimate of the minimum transit time.

h) The Action of Extrinsic Factors on Cervical Squamous Epithelium

Oestrogens and allied substances. DE BRUX (1958) has analysed the possible mechanisms through which oestrogens affect the squamous epithelium of the cervix and vagina. He concluded that *in vitro* they operate by stimulating or inhibiting certain enzymes but *in vivo* their action may be more complex, accomplished, at least in part, by the agency of the autonomic nervous system. *In vitro* oestrogens affect cell (1) proliferation, (2) metabolism and (3) differentiation.

AVERETTE *et al.* (1970) found that in postmenopausal women stimulated with exogenous oestrogen there was an increase in the labelling of cells with tritiated thymidine in both the basal and parabasal layers and a decrease in the length of the G_1 phase. The changes were more marked in the basal than in the parabasal strata. SCHELLHAS (1969) found that sequential contraceptives did not produce a significant difference in the pattern of proliferation. In pregnancy the pattern of the labelled cells at the squamo-columnar junction was similar to that of the transitional zone of the normal cervix but more rows of cells were involved. However, in the more distal parts of the stratified epithelium of the cervix the pattern of labelling was similar to that of the non-pregnant woman.

Fairly extensive investigations have been made of the effects of oestrogen and progesterone on the enzyme systems of the vagina of the rat (ROSA and VELARDO 1959) but these studies are hardly applicable to the human subject since the structure and kinetics of the rodent vagina differs from that of woman. FISHMAN (1951) has shown that in women oestrogen raises the β-glucuronidase level of the genital tract, and KERR et al. (1947) have shown that oestrogens increase the level of alkaline phosphatase. On the contrary, oestrogens reduce the level of vaginal esterase and inhibit cytochrome oxidase. One of the more pertinent observations is probably that of WEINSTEIN et al. (1968) who showed the in vitro conversion of oestrone to 17 β-oestradiol in the human vaginal mucosa. In contrast, in neonatal foreskin and abdominal skin the reaction is in the opposite direction. However, the addition of pyridine nucleotides to incubation mixtures enhances the oxidation of oestradiol by vaginal mucosa.

In women oestrogens induce nuclear pyknosis and the production of keratohyaline granules in vaginal epithelium (DEBRUX 1958). The nuclei may disappear from the superficial cells and keratinization, recognized by the presence of a superficial layer of acidophilic material, may occur. GENET et al. (1962) have reported that 16 α-hydroxyoestrone and oestrone have a keratinizing effect on the vagina twenty times greater than that of oestriol. KAHN (1959) was able to produce keratinization in explanted vaginae of rats grown in a chemically defined medium by the addition of 17 β-oestradiol to the medium. EDWARDS and LANGLEY (1971) cultured explants of human cervix in medium 199 and found that oestrogens (oestradiol, oestrone or oestriol) and progesterone accelerated the process of keratinization that normally occurs under such conditions.

Other exogenous substances. Vitamins and other hormones circulating in the blood may affect cervical epithelium but the only well substantiated in vivo effect is that caused by folic acid deficiency (VAN NIEKERK 1966). EDWARDS and LANGLEY (1971) were unable to recognize any consistent effect of adding folinic acids or vitamin B_{12} to cultured explants of cervical epithelium. Although vitamin A inhibits the keratinization of chick-embryo skin grown in tissue culture (FELL 1964), we were unable to detect any similar effect of adding vitamin A to the medium culturing explants of human cervical squamous epithelium.

i) The Control of Epithelium by Intrinsic Factors

The effect of the micro-environment on the development and differentation of cells and tissues has been discussed at a number of recent symposia (see, for example, DEFENDI and STOKER, 1967, and FLEISCHMAJER and BILLINGHAM, 1968). Much of the work which has been reported is not directly relevant to the cervix. Nevertheless, some of the principles and concepts which have emerged merit attention in relation to epithelial abnormalities of the cervix.

FELL (1964) has summarized experimental work on the relationship between dermis and epidermis. If the epidermis of a chick-embryo limb bud is removed from the dermis it survives in organ culture only a few days, but if it is recombined with limb bud mesoderm it grows and keratinizes well. Moreover, isolated epidermis will grow on a Millipore filter interposed between dermis and epidermis. If the dermis is killed by repeated freezing and thawing, epidermis will spread over the dead tissue and differentiate both keratinizing and forming a basement membrane. The material, or factor, in the dermis which is thus necessary to the epidermis is trypsin- and heat-labile. Similarly, EDWARDS and LANGLEY (1971) have shown that mesenchyme is necessary for the survival of explants of human cervix grown in culture media. They attempted to grow cervical epithelium in the absence of connective tissue and found that it rapidly degenerated, whereas in the presence of mesenchyme it survived and grew. FELL suggests that, in addition to the production of growth-promoting factor, mesenchyme provides a scaffold which enables the basal cells to achieve polarity. It is uncertain how far these *in vitro* observations are applicable to cervical tissue *in situ*.

LIPPMAN (1968) has investigated the effects of glycosaminoglycans on cell division. These substances may arise from two sources: first, the glycocalyx, or mucopolysaccharide coating of epithelial cells (BENNETT 1963); second, the electron-dense basement lamella formed by a confluence of materials derived from both epithelial and connective tissue components (PIERCE *et al.* 1964; PIERCE 1966; HAY and REVEL 1963; ROSS and GRANT 1968). LIPPMAN showed that sulphated glycosaminoglycans, such as chondroitin sulphate, heparin and keratan sulphate, inhibited cell division in mouse L-cells when grown in culture and those substances which were most effective *in vitro* also inhibited mouse ascites tumour *in vivo*. In contrast, chondroitin sulphate and keratan sulphate covalently linked to protein produced a marked stimulation of growth rate *in vivo* and *in vitro*. Chemical and histochemical tests showed that the polymers were bound to the cells surfaces. LIPPMAN suggests that the synthesis of large amounts of a differentiated cell product, glycoprotein in the case of epithelial cells, and glycosaminoglycans in the case of mesenchymal cells, may play a role in DNA synthesis by controlling nucleotide pool utilization. While nucleotide intermediates are being poured into RNA and carbohydrate synthesis, the amount of nucleotide available for DNA synthesis is limited. She suggests that the normal feedback inhibition turns off synthesis of carbohydrate polymers and turns on DNA synthesis. The cell coatings are catabolized in the G_2 period, resulting in prophase initiation.

HAMBRICK *et al.* (1966) have grown epidermis in organ culture, using the Trowell technique. They found that the addition of heparin sodium to the medium resulted in a densely packed, non-parakeratotic stratum corneum accompanied by a distinct granular layer which was absent in control explants. They think this effect may be the result of antimitotic activity. EDWARDS and LANGLEY (1971) added heparin sodium to medium 199 but failed to find any significant effect on the culture of cervical epithelium. Their experiments were not extensive and no firm conclusion can yet be drawn from them.

BULLOUGH *et al.* (1967) have shown that extracts of vertebrate epidermis contain an antimitotic chemical messenger, the epidermal chalone, which seems to be important in the control of epidermal mitosis. Epidermal chalone is tissue-specific but it is neither species nor class-specific. Extracts from human skin have been found to be active on mouse epidermis, and IVERSEN (1968) has shown that chalone extracted from mouse and pig skin depressed the mitotic rate of human skin in culture. No studies of the effect of epidermal chalone on cervical epithelium have yet been reported.

This brief, and incomplete survey indicates that growth and differentation of squamous epithelium is controlled by a wide variety of factors. The importance of each factor in respect of each type of squamous epithelium is not known since the experiments have been performed on a wide variety of preparations. It is probable that many, if not all, these factors play a role in the human cervix uteri and it is possible that disturbances of the relationship of these factors to each other may cause changes in the morphology of the epithelium.

3. The Columnar Epithelium of the Endocervix

a) The Histological Pattern

The columnar epithelium of the endocervix has not been as extensively studied as the squamous epithelium and it is not easy to draw comparisons with other types of columnar epithelium because of differences in structure and function.

The division between the corpus uteri and the endocervix is of importance, both in discussion of the lower uterine segment in obstetrics and, as will be seen later, in consideration of the development of cervical erosions or ectopy. Aschoff (1905, 1908) regarded the isthmus as that part of the uterus which lies between the anatomical internal os, which marks the lower boundary of the corpus uteri, and the histological internal os which corresponds to the junction of the mucosa of the isthmus and the endocervix. Schröder (1930) has discussed the difficulties of defining the limits of the isthmus and Danforth (1947, 1954) has cast doubt on the classical description. The lower end of the endocervical canal is defined anatomically by the external os and histologically by the squamo-columnar junction. These two points do not necessarily coincide although they generally lie fairly close together. Before puberty and after the menopause the squamo-columnar junction may lie above the external os, whereas in the newborn and in the childbearing period it may lie outside the external os.

The mucosa lining the isthmus is a modified type of endometrium (Schröder 1930) and is followed by an abrupt transition to endocervical epithelium. The transition from endocervical epithelium to squamous epithelium at the lower end of the canal may be abrupt but often there is a small transitional region of squamous metaplasia (Fluhmann 1964).

The columnar epithelium is thrown into folds and crypts as it lines the endocervical canal, thus greatly increasing the surface area of the canal lining. These folds and crypts are generally regarded as forming branching tubular glands and, in common pathological parlance, we emphasize this by speaking of carcinoma *in situ* showing "gland involvement". However, Fluhmann (1961, 1964) has shown that there are no tubular compound racemose glands in the cervix. The basic epithelial structure of the endocervical mucosa is a cleft or groove. A cleft may run in an oblique, transverse or longitudinal direction; it may bifurcate but it never crosses another cleft. The larger clefts correspond to the grooves between the plicae palmatae. Fig. 1.18 shows the general arrangement of these clefts as seen in section. The clefts may undergo modification, for example, as a result of inflammation. Serial reconstructions reveal three modifications: (1) tunnel-like extensions, (2) exophytic processes and (3) secondary clefts which may also form tunnels. Tunnels are formed by occlusion of part of a cleft so that an area becomes pinched off and continues as a blind tube

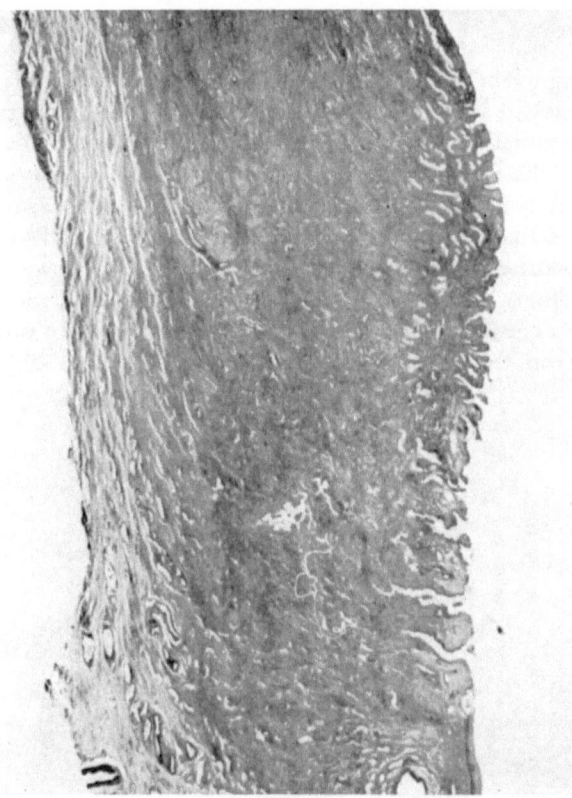

Fig. 1.18. A low power view of the whole thickness of the endocervix to show the clefts lined by columnar epithelium. (H. & E. × 5)

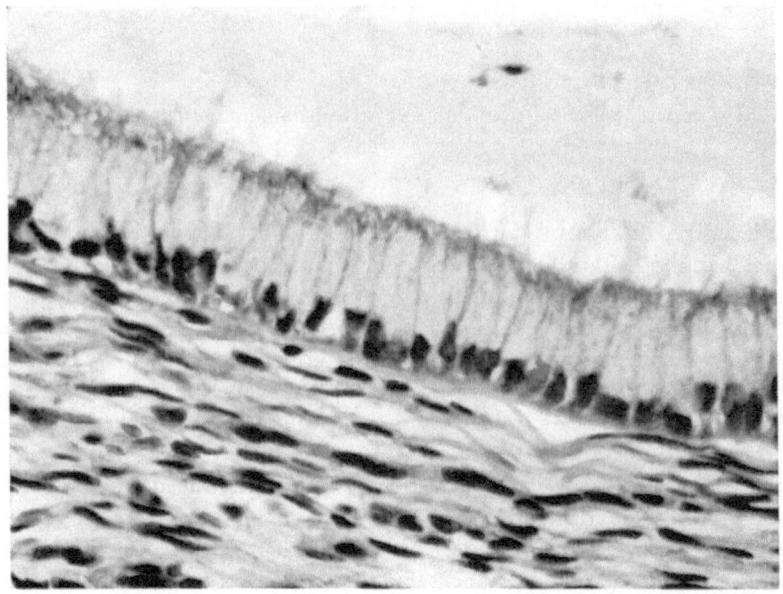

Fig. 1.19. Typical picket arrangement of the columnar cells of the endocervix. (H. & E. × 480)

whose only opening to the surface is through the parent cleft. If this opening to the original cleft is sealed off a retention cyst, or Nabothian follicle, is formed.

The columnar epithelium lining the clefts is similar to the surface epithelium and is not specialized. The epithelium of the endocervix is not of one uniform type. The great majority of the cells are columnar with pale cytoplasm, 30 to 40 μ in height and arranged like an old-fashioned picket fence (Fig. 1.19.). The nuclei are often vesicular but the chromatin may be condensed and they vary in position, the nucleus often being near the base and sometimes even pressed by the mucinous secretory globules into a crescent against the basement membrane. In other cells the nucleus is separated from the base by a sub-nuclear vacuole (Fig. 1.20.). The cytoplasm

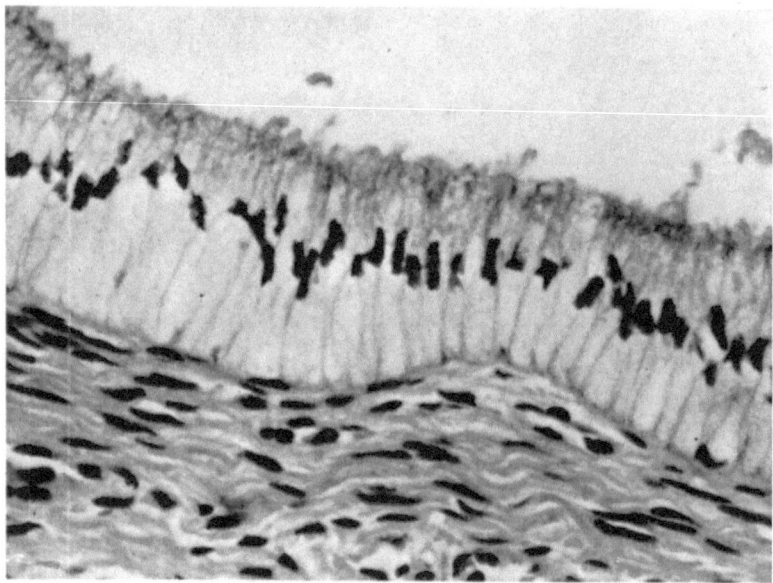

Fig. 1.20. Endocervical columnar cells with somewhat pyknotic centrally placed nuclei. (H. & E. × 480)

may be lace-like, the luminal surface of the cell being slightly irregular and having a parallel band of slightly denser cytoplasm just beneath the border. When the nucleus lies centrally the supranuclear cytoplasm is often less vesicular and more dense. Sometimes ciliated cells can be seen but they are scarce, often occurring in groups lying between rows of the more common vesicular cells (Fig. 1.21.). Their cytoplasm is often acidophilic, and a terminal transverse bar can be seen under the cilia. In smear preparations stained by the Papanicolaou method, the cilia stain red in contrast to the cyanophilic cytoplasm of the cell. According to DOUGHERTY (1960), electron microscopy shows that these fibers are indeed true cilia in that each is composed of nine peripheral and two central filaments. DOUGHERTY (1960) regards the secretory and ciliated appearances as two different phases of the same cell on the following grounds: (1) ciliated and secretory cells are found in the same specimen arranged in long rows of one or other form rather than alternately placed in small

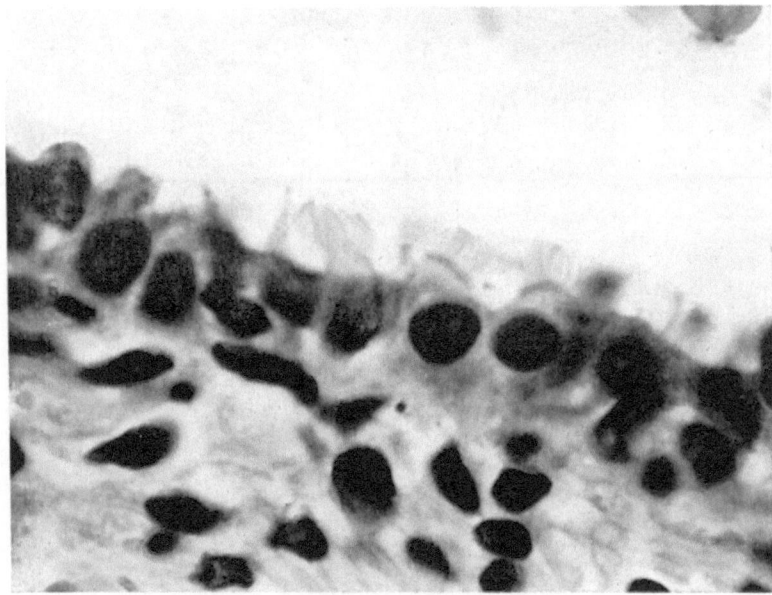

Fig. 1.21. Ciliated endocervical cells showing terminal transverse bar. (H. & E. × 1,200)

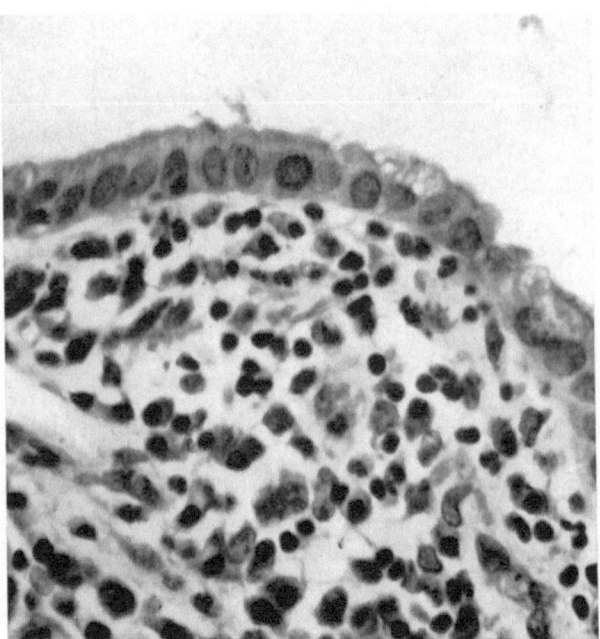

Fig. 1.22. Low columnar cells from the endocervix. They have mostly lost their mucin and the cytoplasm stains strongly for RNA. (H. & E. × 480)

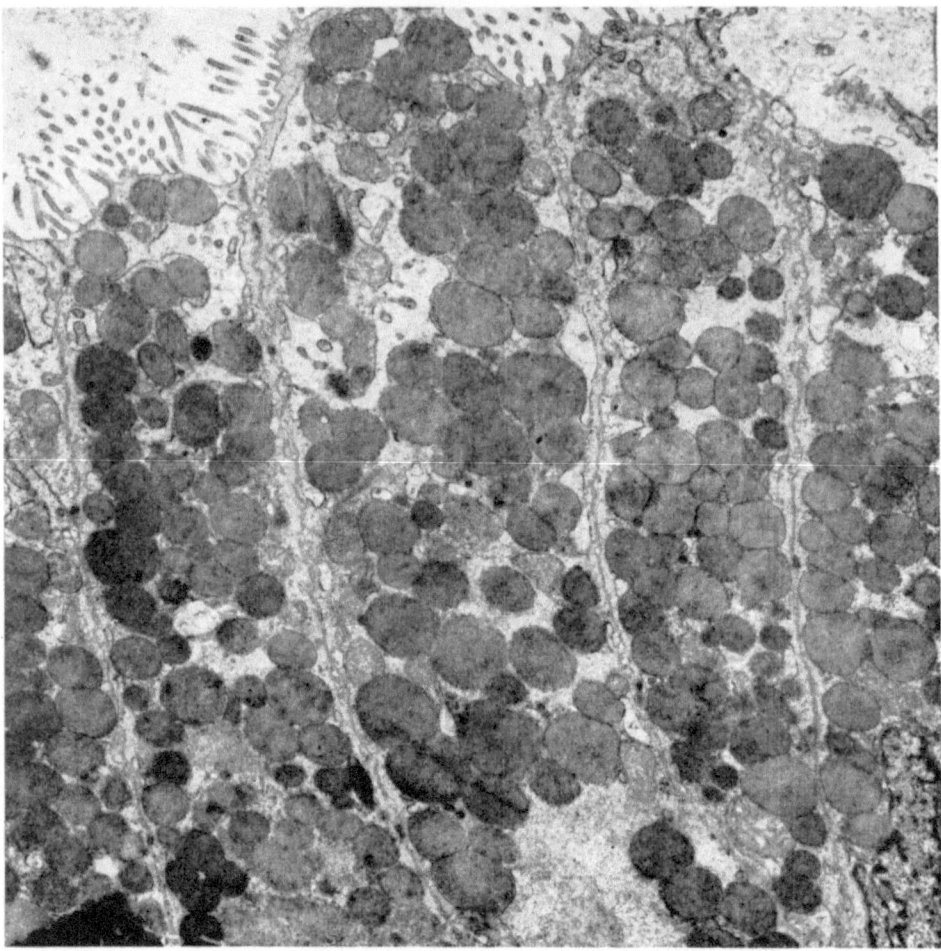

Fig. 1.23. An electron photomicrograph of endocervical columnar cells. Note the microvilli of the luminal border and the desmosomes at the points of contact of the cells. The spherical and ovoid bodies are droplets of mucin. (× 8,000)

groups as in the Fallopian tube. (2) Ciliated cells may contain globules of mucinous material aggregated beneath or distal to the nucleus. (3) Secretory cells possessing cilia have been seen. A third type of endocervical cell usually seen on the surface is low columnar, with a small dense nucleus and acidophilic cytoplasm (Fig. 1.22.). These cells may or may not possess cilia and give the impression of inactive cells which have discharged the secretion but the cytoplasm is markedly pyronophilic, indicating the presence of abundant RNA. DOUGHERTY and LOW (1958) considered that a basement membrane is present between the endocervical columnar epithelium and the stroma but the careful studies of LAMB et al. (1960) appear to show that this membrane is discontinuous.

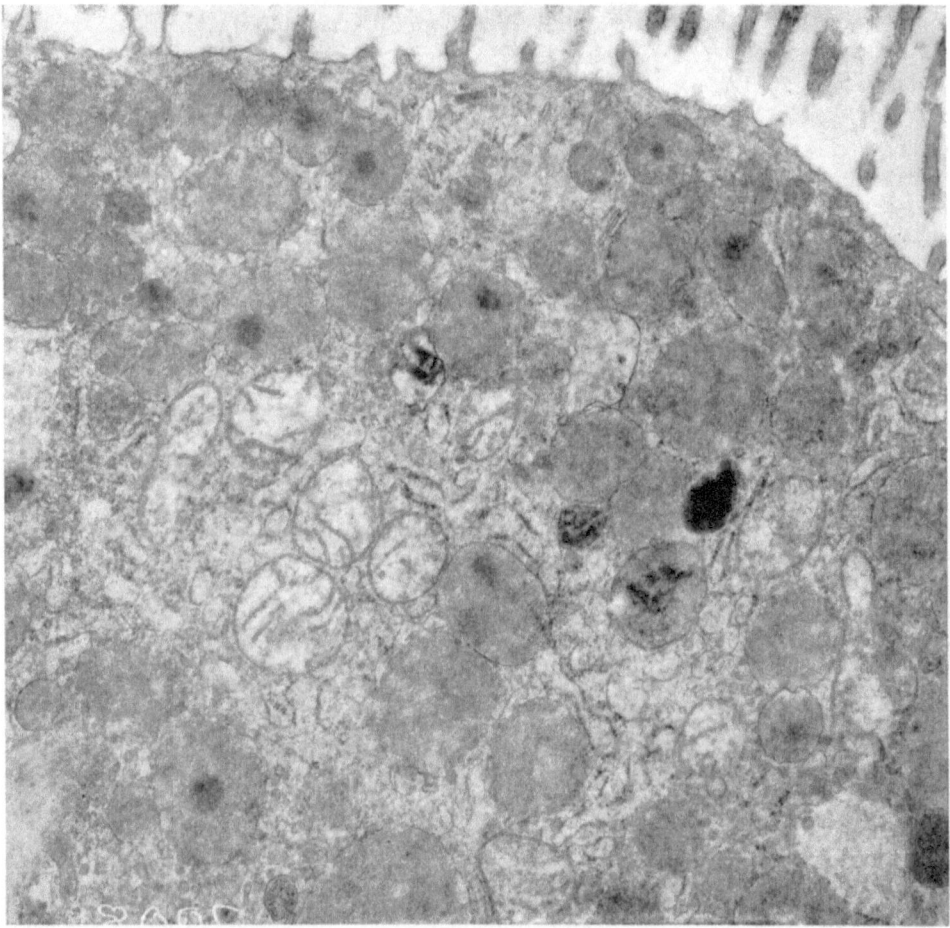

Fig. 1.24. An electron photomicrograph at greater magnification. The globules of mucin have sharp margins and many show a central condensation of electrondense material. Mitochondria are fairly numerous. (× 25,000)

b) The Fine Structure of Cervical Columnar Epithelium

The electron microscopic picture of the columnar cells of the endocervix has been described by a number of authors (HASHIMOTO and YORISATO 1959; GOMPEL 1963; MORICARD and CARTIER 1964; CHAPMAN et al. 1964; LAGUENS et al. 1967). The nucleus shows variations in structure, similar to those seen under the light microscope. It is frequently lobulated or deeply cleft by intrusions of cytoplasm, some nuclei are of low and some of high electron density and many have a large peripherally located nucleolus (Fig. 1.23.). Much of the cytoplasm is occupied by spherical droplets of mucus of varying size. In many droplets there is a central core of high electron density which in high resolution micrographs is seen to be finely granular, whilst the remaining secretion surrounding the core forms a finely reticular meshwork (Fig. 1.24.). Most of the cytoplasmic organelles are located in the infranuclear area. Mitochondria are scarce, the endoplasmic reticulum is poorly developed and of rough type. A curious feature described by GOMPEL (1963) and MORICARD and CARTIER (1964) is a special fibrillary system surrounded by a thin membrane; the nature of this organelle is unknown. Between the plasma membranes of adjacent cells there is an intercellular space, 300 to 400 Å in average width, and desmosomes can readily be seen. The apical plasma membrane may be broken or show extruding secretory droplets. Microvilli can be seen on this border and microfilaments project from them producing a "fuzzy" appearance which in some way resembles the borders of absorbing cells as described by FAWCETT (1965). Cilia project from the free borders of some cells but not, according to LAGUENS *et al.* (1967) from mucus-secreting cells; this contrasts with the opinion of DOUGHERTY (*vide supra*).

c) The Histochemistry of Cervical Columnar Epithelium

The histochemistry of endocervical cells has been studied by a number of workers including FORAKER *et al.* (1954); FORAKER and MARINO (1956); HEROVICI (1960b); BERTALANFFY and BERTALANFFY (1960) and MORICARD and CARTIER (1964). The cytoplasm of the cells contains RNA which is more conspicuous when the cells are "active" as in an erosion (endocervical ectopy). They contain no glycogen but mucopolysaccharides can be demonstrated by the PAS reaction and by alcian blue. SIEGEL (1967) reported an extensive investigation of the mucous substances in the cervix uteri. He found neutral and acid mucous substances present in varying mixtures in both the deeper (i.e. glandular) and more superficial columnar cells. Less frequently he found glandular tubules containing exclusively either neutral or acid mucin and only rarely did he see glandular cells which contained no mucin. ROBERTS and GUPTA (1965) have shown that the mucin of the bovine cervix is heterogeneous and that this is probably related to the mode of linkage of the sialic acid moiety.

Endocervical cells give a strong tetrazolium reaction for reductases. We have found a positive reaction for alkaline phosphatase near the apical borders of the cells but we failed to demonstrate acid phosphatase activity. HEDBERG (1950) found an increase in alkaline phosphatase during the oestrogenic phase of the menstrual cycle and a diminution during the luteal phase.

d) The Kinetics of Cervical Columnar Epithelium

A slow rate of DNA synthesis in the columnar epithelium of the endocervix was noted by REID (1962, 1964a) and KURY *et al.* (1967). REID found labelled cells, after exposure to radioactive thymidine, confined to the superficial areas, whereas SCHELLHAS (1969) found labelling both of the superficial columnar epithelium and of that in the gland clefts but the superficial areas appeared to be more active. He found that severe infection stimulated DNA synthesis of columnar cells and suggested that this is a result of enhanced desquamation.

e) Cyclical Changes in Endocervical Epithelium

After the menopause the glands or clefts progressively atrophy, probably because of an associated atrophy of the stroma and the epithelium becomes low and nonsecretory. The changes which occur in the endocervix with the menstrual cycle are ill-defined. SCHRÖDER (1930), TOPKINS (1949) and DUPERROY (1951) deny that such cyclical changes occur. WOLLNER (1938) described proliferative, secretory and des-quamative phases synchronous with those of the endometrium but, whilst SJÖVAL (1938) found a secretory phase, he could not recognise exfoliation. TOPKINS (1949) found wide individual variations which were independent of the phase of the cycle. These differing and often contradictory results probably arise from the variety and unsatisfactory nature of the material used—cadaveric, biopsy and total hysterectomy specimens. HARTMANN (1962) has described convincing evidence of cyclical changes in the endocervix of the monkey.

4. The Stroma of the Cervix

a) The Histological Pattern

DANFORTH (1947) and DANFORTH and CHAPMAN (1950) have shown that the stroma of the cervix is predominantly composed of fibrous connective tissue but smooth muscle and elastic tissue are also present, although in smaller amounts than had previously been supposed. The transition from the fibrous tissue of the cervix to the muscular tissue of the corpus is usually abrupt but sometimes it is gradual. The elastic tissue of the cervix is mostly seen in the blood vessels. KRANTZ and PHILLIPS (1962) have described the smooth muscle in some detail.

DEMETRAKOPOULOS and GREENE (1958) have shown that true lymphoid follicles occur in the cervix. They found them in almost half of serially blocked specimens except in the foetal cervix. They are well-circumscribed, round or oval, with reticular and reticuloendothelial cells and lymphocytes. Blood vessels enter near the hilum and leave at the periphery of the follicle. Small afferent and efferent lymphatics are sometimes seen. The follicles may be seen immediately under the cervical epithelium or deeper in the stroma.

b) The Normal Vascular Pattern of the Cervix Uteri

The subepithelial capillaries reflect changes in the overlying epithelium and surrounding stroma, whether these are benign, inflammatory or associated with malign epithelia. The colposcope allows the *in vivo* visualization of these superficial stromal vessels. They can be seen through the intervening cervical epithelium at a magnification of 16 to 25 diameters and the interposition of a green filter, originally suggested by KRAATZ (1939) as a way of enhancing the appearance of cervical atypia, accentuates the vessel outlines. GANSE (1958) emphasized the value of orthochromatic photography and he also used mercury-vapour illumination. MAJEWSKI's test (1960), which simply involves the topical application of a dilute non-adrenaline solution, will increase vessel filling. An excellent monograph which contains some of the best published montage colpophotographs of the cervical vessels was produced by KOLLER in 1963.

Apart from direct observation, cervical vessels have been studied in uteri removed at operation. ZINSER and ROSENBAUER (1960) injected the vessels with coloured gelatine and then cleared the specimens. Beautiful preparations of the capillary patterns were obtained in normal squamous and columnar epithelium and in various atypical epithelia. Kos (1960) used Indian ink in gelatine to study the vessel changes in females from the age of eleven years upwards and he also performed a comparative study on human and ape uteri (Kos 1961).

The relatively large amounts of alkaline phosphatase in the endothelial cells lining the cervical capillaries and pre-capillaries enables these vessels to be clearly delineated by the use of an azo-coupling technique. This was the method used by Kos (1962) and Štafl et al. (1963) to study cervical vessels in benign and malign conditions. Štafl et al. also compared the vascular and colposcopic with the histological appearances.

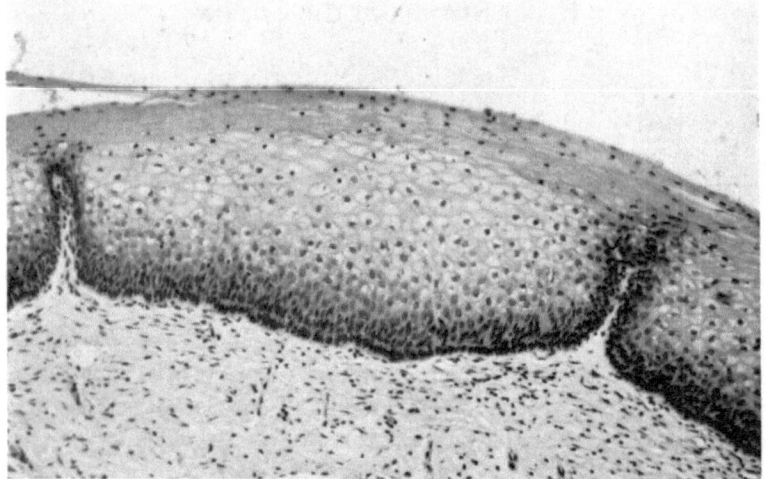

Fig. 1.25. Papillae of stroma project upwards into the squamous epithelium of the ectocervix and carry capillaries with them. (H. & E. × 120)

Colposcopically two capillary patterns are observed in the original epithelium (non-metaplastic squamous epithelium): (1) Stromal papillae project upwards into the squamous epithelium so that only three or four layers of cells intervene between the tops of capillary loops and the surface (Fig. 1.25.). (2) A subepithelial network is also present though this can only be seen clearly when the epithelium is reduced in thickness, as in senile atrophy.

It is characteristic of normal squamous epithelium that the stromal papillae are relatively infrequent. KOLLER (1963) found that these loops were 0.1 to 0.2 mm apart and tended to lie obliquely inclined towards the surface and in rows arranged radially from the squamo-columnar junction. The subepithelial network seen characteristically in older women has a mesh size of 0.05 to 0.2 mm (Kos 1961). Premenstrually, during pregnancy and especially in the presence of inflammation, the capillaries are often more dilated and appear more numerous. Spiral and "double-crested" vessels are then seen, the latter especially in trichomoniasis. Nevertheless, the vessels possess a regularity which distinguishes them from those in areas of malign change. The vessel changes in the malign epithelia are discussed in Chapter 3.

Chapter 2

Bland Epithelial Abnormalities of the Cervix Uteri

The term bland epithelial abnormality includes a number of conditions, such as squamous metaplasia and cervical "erosion", which are closely interrelated and which are not necessarily pathological since they may occur normally in infancy and pregnancy.

1. Bland Abnormalities of Squamous Epithelium

The bland abnormalities of squamous epithelium have been listed by GOVAN *et al.* (1966, 1969) as follows:

Squamous hyperplasia
(a) Reactive hyperplasia
(b) Basal cell hyperplasia
Reserve cell proliferation
Metaplasia
(a) Incomplete
(b) Complete.

a) Reactive Hyperplasia

This is seen in some irritative conditions and particularly in association with uterine prolapse. The whole epithelium is thickened, hyperkeratosis and parakeratosis frequently occur and often there is exaggeration of the rete pegs. The cells are orderly in their arrangement and there are no cytological abnormalities.

b) Basal Cell Hyperactivity or Hyperplasia

The basal layer and adjacent part of the parabasal layer form an unusually well-defined stratum which is increased in thickness and is conspicuous because of the marked basophilia of the cytoplasm. The cells tend to be arranged at right angles to the surface. Above this stratum the cells are mature and stratified (Fig. 2.1.).

c) Reserve Cell Proliferation and Hyperplasia

The terms reserve cell proliferation and hyperplasia are used to describe a proliferation of cells between the columnar cells of the endocervical epithelium and the basement membrane. This proliferation may occur on the surface of the cervix,

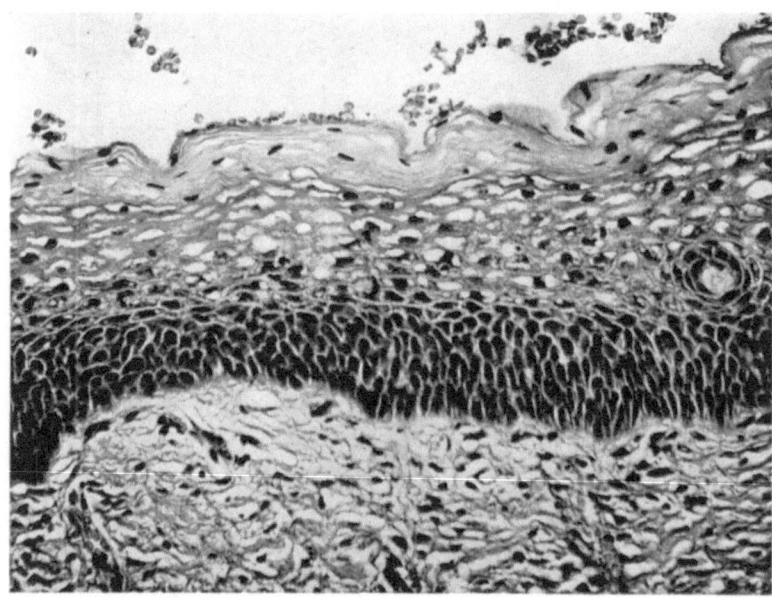

Fig. 2.1. Basal cell hyperplasia. The cells in the parabasal layer are hyperactive and form a zone which is fairly sharply demarcated from the intermediate layer. (H. & E. × 360) (From GOVAN *et al.* 1969, J. clin. Path. **22**, 383)

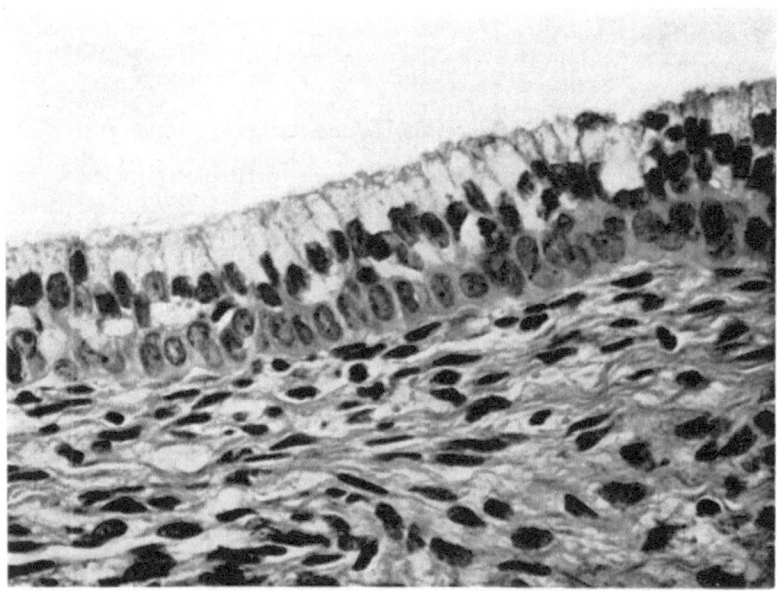

Fig. 2.2. Reserve cell proliferation. A conspicuous row of orderly arranged cells (the reserve cells) lies beneath the endocervical columnar cells. (H. & E. × 720)

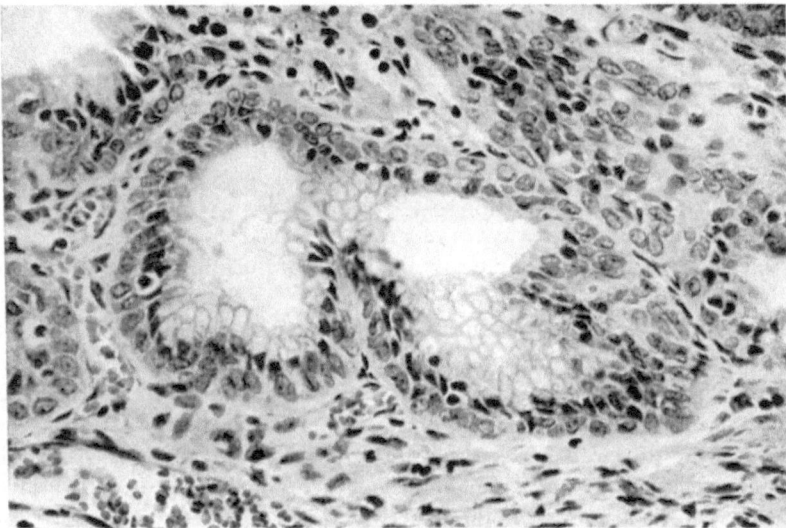

Fig. 2.3. Reserve cell proliferation. A conspicuous row of reserve cells lies between the columnar cells lining the endocervical gland and the surrounding stroma. (H. & E. × 360)

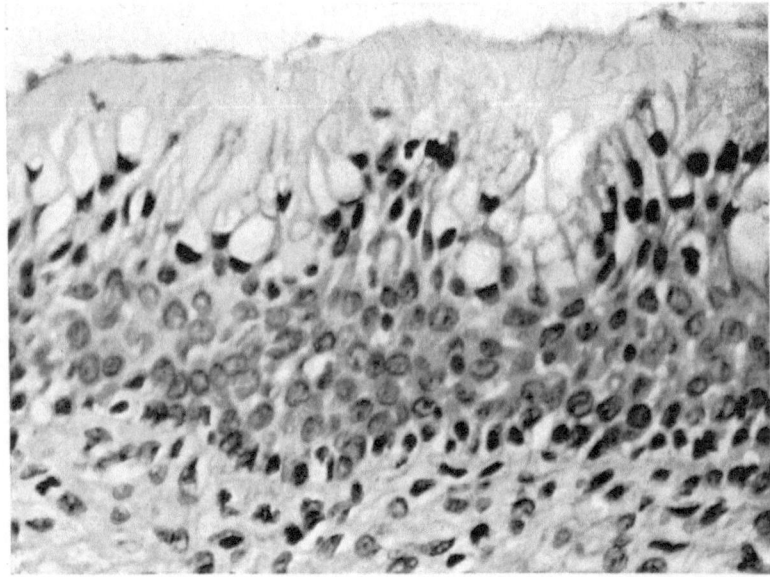

Fig. 2.4. Reserve cell hyperplasia. Several rows of reserve cells lie between the endocervical columnar cells and the underlying stroma. The nuclei of the reserve cells are large and vesicular but the nuclei of the lowest row of cells are already smaller and denser than those above and these cells appear to be beginning to form the stratum germinativum of the fully developed metaplastic epithelium. (H. & E. × 720)

as in an erosion (Fig. 2.2.), or around endocervical glands (Fig. 2.3.). In the early stages of reserve cell proliferation the epithelium may consist of a row of columnar cells lying on a single or a double row of cells. When there are more than three rows of reserve cells the term reserve cell hyperplasia may be used. Reserve cells at first show no specific characteristics; they are polyhedral or cuboidal, having a slightly basophilic, slightly vacuolated cytoplasm and relatively large round or oval nuclei in which the chromatin is evenly dispersed; mitoses are rarely seen. VON HAAM and OLD (1964) have described three types of reserve cells. (1) Non-hyperplastic reserve cells. These usually appear as a single row in an area of inflammation and they do not contain glycogen or mucin. (2) Hyperplastic reserve cells in the absence of meta-plasia; these cells are similar to the non-hyperplastic cells although they sometimes possess a large amount of cytoplasm (Fig. 2.4.). The columnar cells overlying patches of reserve cell hyperplasia may be normal or show evidence of degeneration. (3) Atypical reserve cells. These show changes in cell size and alterations in the nuclei. The nuclei are large with dark and clumpy chromatin and a recognizable nucleolus. The cells are more crowded and the layers of cells more irregular. Atypical reserve cell hyperplasia may be coincidental with carcinoma *in situ*. It is probably best regarded as a form of dysplasia and will be discussed later under this heading.

d) Metaplasia

The term metaplasia means changed form (Greek *meta*—a prefix implying change of position, order, shape or kind, *plassein* — to mould). WILLIS (1958) defines meta-plasia as "the transformation of an adult or fully differentiated tissue of one kind into a differentiated tissue of another kind in response to abnormal circumstances. It is an acquired condition and must be distinguished from *developmental heterotopia*

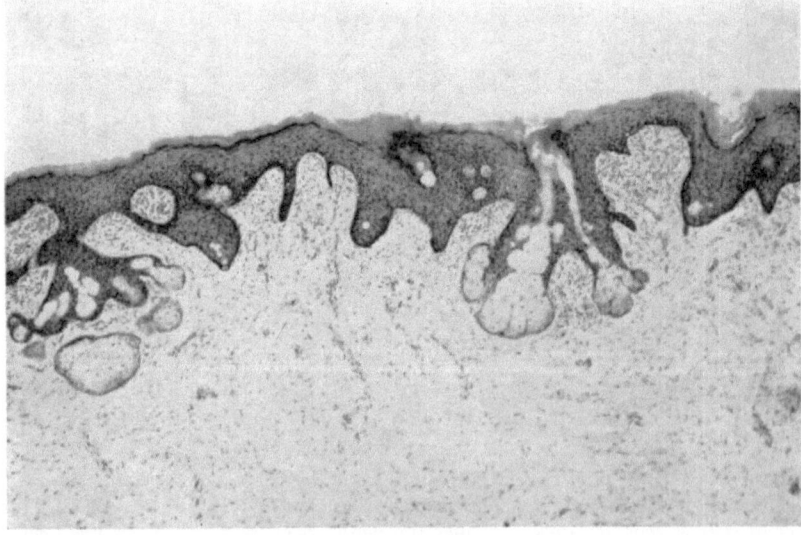

Fig. 2.5. Epidermal metaplasia of the squamous epithelium of the cervix. The epithelium is keratinized and well formed sebaceous glands are present. (H. & E. × 50)

or *heteroplasia*, in which the tissue abnormal for the part has always been present as a primary error of differentiation". Squamous metaplasia is common in the cervix; in this form columnar epithelium is replaced by stratified squamous epithelium. Sometimes squamous metaplasia may give rise to an epithelium which is not only epidermoid but truly epidermal; hair follicles, sweat and sebaceous glands and melanin may be present. NICHOLSON, in 1919, found several sebaceous glands in a section of cervix removed from a patient with squamous cell carcinoma of the cervix. DOUGHERTY *et al.* (1962) encountered a single sebaceous gland in a cervix on two occasions. We have seen a single example of epidermal metaplasia kindly sent to us by a colleague (Fig. 2.5.). WILLIS (1958) has reviewed and illustrated several other cases.

e) Squamous Metaplasia

The terms "epidermalization" and "epidermoidalization" were coined by German pathologists towards the end of the nineteenth centry to describe the transformation of cervical columnar epithelium into squamous epithelium. Many other synonyms are used such as epidermidization and epidermization. FLUHMANN (1961) has pointed out that any term which implies a relationship with the epidermis is incorrect and objectionable while most of the other terms refer to specific theories which have been advanced to account for the cellular transformation. He uses the term "prosoplasia", in accordance with his own beliefs in the matter. He writes, "the word prosoplasia is derived from two Greek words meaning "forward" and "to form" and seems appropriate since it refers not to an isolated pathologic change but to the whole process from its earliest stage to its final appearance as normal mature squamous epithelium".

In its simplest form squamous metaplasia can be regarded as a continuation of reserve cell hyperplasia with maturation of the nuclei and differentiation of the cytoplasm. Intercellular bridges are formed, and whilst the lower cells become orientated at right angles to the basement membrane, the upper cells become arranged parallel to the surface. Complex patterns may develop in cervical epithelium in the course of this transformation. The change is described by GOVAN *et al.* (1966) under two headings:

α) Incomplete Metaplasia

This consists of a partial replacement of columnar epithelium by squamous epithelium. The multilayered proliferating reserve cells are surmounted by a more or less continuous row of mucous cells which may be well preserved but more frequently are degenerate, or they may persist as a row of short peg-shaped cells without obvious mucous secretion. As the process develops the mucous cells become submerged in the wave of proliferating reserve cells and a haphazard mixture of mucus-secreting and squamoid cells results. The mucous cells often appear bloated, distorted or disrupted sometimes being represented only by small rounded spaces in the depths of the epithelium (Fig. 2.6.). Frequently these spaces contain polymorphonuclear leucocytes. FLUHMANN (1961) regards prosoplastic basal cells (reserve cells) as bipotent in that they may evolve into either squamous or columnar epithelium. Some of them consequently secrete mucus and become vacuolated. We prefer to regard these intra-epithelial mucinous foci as arising from residual endocervical cells.

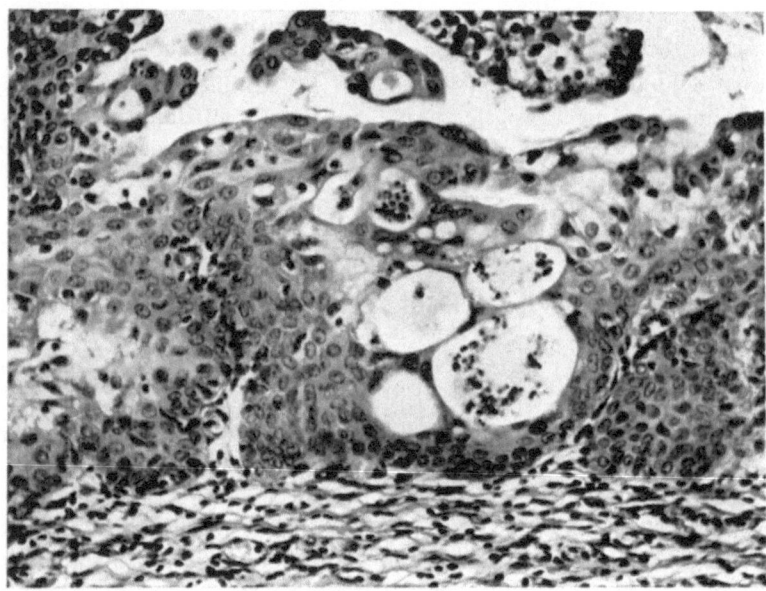

Fig. 2.6. Bloated and distorted cells in metaplastic epithelium. Some have fused to form cysts which include leucocytes and nuclear débris. (H. & E. × 360)

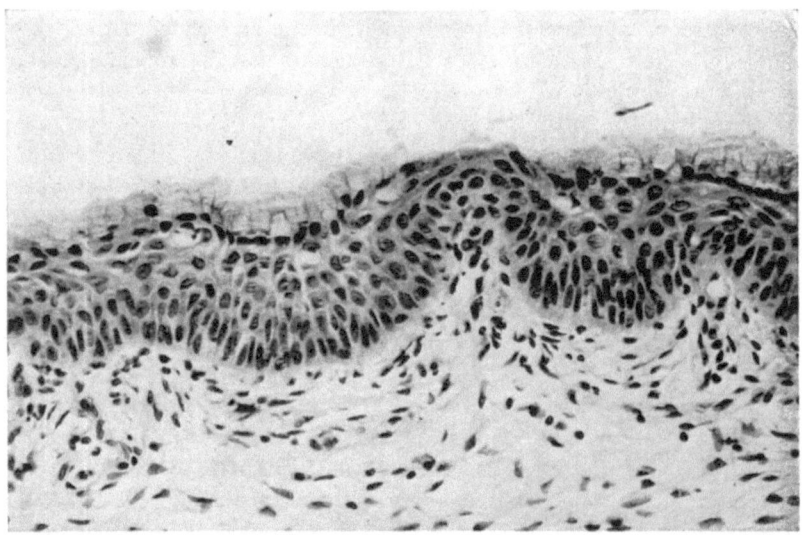

Fig. 2.7. Metaplasia. A sheet of squamoid epithelium lies under the columnar epithelium which itself is beginning to disappear above the stromal papilla. (H. & E. × 360)

Large spaces may sometimes be seen lined by columnar cells, giving the epithelium a fenestrated pattern. The resulting complex patterns may cause difficulty in interpretation and at times the appearances may be mistaken for those of carcinoma *in situ*. However, the proliferating reserve cells show a uniformity of distribution and

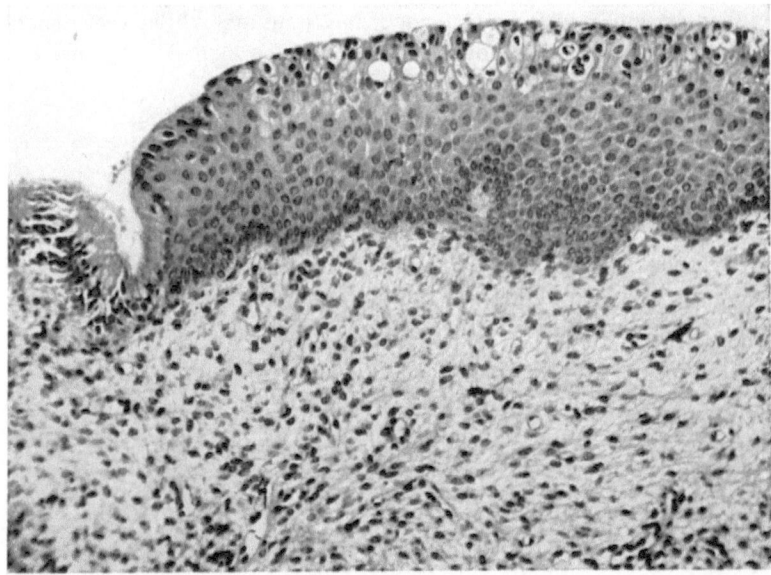

Fig. 2.8. In this metaplastic epithelium the stratification of the later mature epithelium is not yet developed but the lowest layer of cells forms a well defined germinative layer. Vacuoles are present in the upper part of the epithelium representing residual columnar cells which have been included in the newly formed squamoid epithelium. (H. & E. × 180)

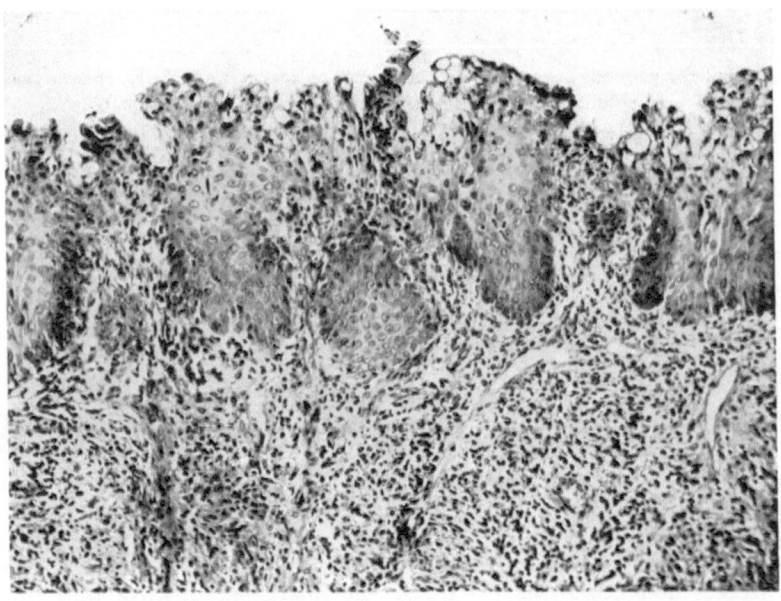

Fig. 2.9. Metaplastic epithelium showing a complex pattern. Groups of residual columnar cells can be seen in the upper part of the squamoid epithelium. (H. & E. × 180)

morphology, including nuclear size, shape and staining, whilst the degenerating mucous cells are quite irregular but they can be identified by the use of special stains such as mucicarmine (Figs. 2.7. to 2.9.).

β) Complete Squamous Metaplasia

This is present when there is a total replacement of columnar cells by squamoid epithelium. The new epithelium forms irregular plaques of squamous cells but with incomplete stratification. The process can be very extensive or patchy. It may occur both on the surface epithelium and in the crypts (Figs. 2.10., 2.11. and 2.12.).

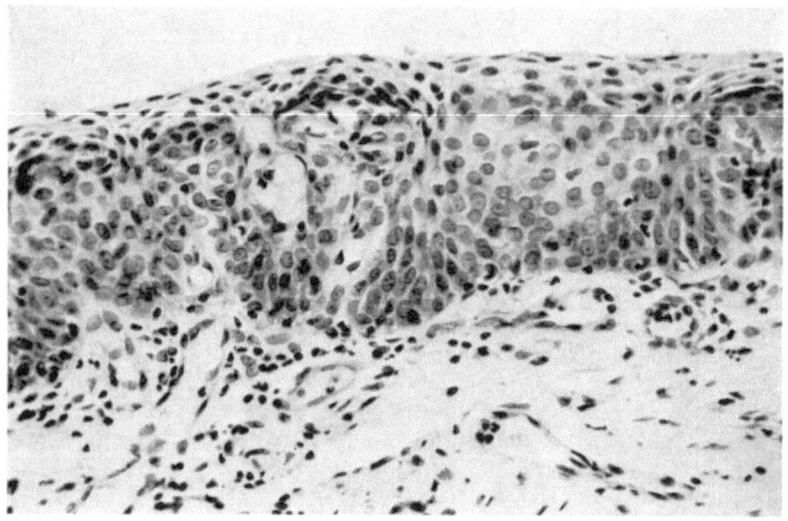

Fig. 2.10. Complete squamous metaplasia. The columnar cells have been totally replaced by squamoid epithelium which shows some stratification. (H. & E. × 360)

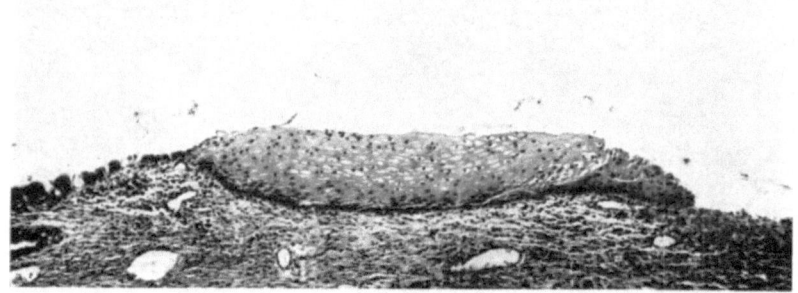

Fig. 2.11. An isolated plaque of metaplastic squamous epithelium. (H. & E. × 60)

The terms complete and incomplete metaplasia refer to the maturity of the metaplastic process and not to its extent. In the final stage of metaplasia the normal strata of well-differentiated epithelium can be seen. At this stage preceding metaplasia can be recognised by a waviness of the base, pegs of epithelium dipping

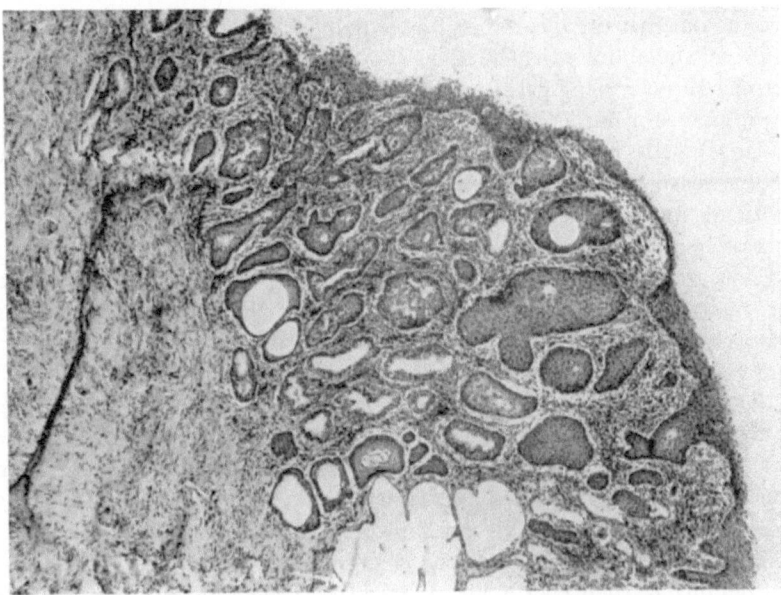

Fig. 2.12. Squamous metaplasia involving endocervical glands and forming a complex pattern not to be confused with invasive carcinoma. (H. & E. × 50)

down into the connective tissue, and by the frequent presence of underlying endocervical glands.

f) The Mechanism of Squamous Metaplasia and the Origin of Reserve Cells

Many hypotheses have been put forward to explain the origin of reserve cells and the mechanism of squamous metaplasia. For the most part these hypotheses are speculative and the evidence adduced is not well substantiated. A critical account of the current views is given by FLUHMANN (1961, 1964) but a proper understanding of the process probably awaits experimental studies. Three hypotheses will be examined here.

MEYER (1910a and b) believed that primitive endodermal cells with the potency to develop into squamous elements could be present in the columnar epithelium. EICHHOLZ (1902) thought that embryonic undifferentiated cells could persist as inclusions. These cells were thought to retain the potentiality of developing into either columnar or squamous epithelium. This possibility has been discussed by GELLER (1923), CARMICHAEL and JEAFFRESON (1939, 1941), AUERBACH and PUND (1945), TOPKINS (1949), HOWARD et al. (1951) and ROSENTHAL and HELLMAN (1952). It was in the course of these studies that the term "reserve cell" was introduced by HOWARD et al. (1951) for the subcolumnar epithelial cells in the cervix, although the term had been employed previously for similar cells in other organs (WOMAK and GRAHAM 1941).

FLUHMANN (1961) objects to MEYER's hypothesis on a number of grounds. (1) Since reserve cells have been found in a very high proportion of all cervices it is more likely that they are a normal tissue component than abnormally included cells.

(2) He points out that there is no assurance that such embryonic cells would always lead to normal squamous epithelium. However, as others have shown, reserve cells do sometimes show cytological abnormalities and HOWARD *et al.* (1951) regard them as a starting point for intraepithelial carcinoma. (3) FLUHMANN regards it as unlikely that cellular remnants could persist for forty or sixty years and even into old age and then become reactivated. However, reserve cells are found in the cervices of many young patients and the fact that reserve cell proliferation or hyperplasia is found in the cervix of an elderly woman does not mean that such changes have only recently occurred since they may have commenced earlier in her life. (4) FLUHMANN's strongest argument against this hypothesis is probably that reserve cell proliferation and squamous metaplasia can occur after extensive cauterization which presumably would destroy any previously existing inclusions of cells.

The concept of squamous prosoplasia was introduced by FLUHMANN (1954). It assumes that the prosoplastic subcolumnar basal cells are derived directly from the columnar cells and they have the potentiality of developing into either columnar or squamous epithelium. FLUHMANN also considers that squamous basal cells have the same property. Thus these cells are bipotential and probably have a common embryonic origin in the endodermal urogenital sinus. VON HAAM and OLD (1964), without prejudice to their origin, also regard reserve cells as bipotential. FLUHMANN regards squamous prosoplasia as an orderly, progressive and physiological change which is a constantly recurring process amply demonstrated by the part it plays in the transitional zone found in most cervices at the squamo-columnar junction. He thinks the stratified columnar epithelium seen in the duct of BARTHOLIN's gland and in the urethra is also prosoplastic.

SONG (1964) has suggested that reserve cells are derived directly by transformation of the stromal cells of the endocervix. He bases his hypothesis on observations of foetal uteri. Prior to thirty weeks' gestation a single layer of reserve cells can frequently be seen in the cervices of foetuses but this assumes a multilayered appearance in the cervices of newborn infants and of children. In the course of development many stromal cells appear to cross the preformed epithelial-stromal junction (the so-called basement membrane) and enter the lower part of the newly formed glandular epithelium, beneath the columnar cells. HOWARD *et al.* (1951) discussing the histogenesis of squamous metaplasia in the adult, wrote: "Often nothing that can be called a basement membrane is seen, as the reserve cells appear to fade gradually into the stromal tissues." GESCHICKTER and FERNANDEZ (1962) also regard reserve cells as derivatives of stromal cells; they state that frequently the basement membrane between the reserve cells and stroma is discontinuous and they note that DARDIN (1955) had made similar observations on metaplasia in a cystic Bartholin's gland.

SONG's electronmicroscopic studies reveal similarities between reserve cells of the foetal cervix and stromal cells. Thus, the cytoplasm of the reserve cells in the foetal cervix occasionally contains a large lamellated body, well demarcated by a thin surrounding membrane associated with which are lipid droplets. A similar, though much smaller type of lamellated structure, presumably of collagen material, is also seen in stromal fibroblasts.

From this review of the theories of histogenesis of reserve cells and squamous metaplasia it can readily be seen that we are still in the dark as to the origin of reserve cells. The hypotheses of FLUHMANN and SONG probably lie nearer the truth than the older suggestions. Song's concept has the added merit of being consistent with and perhaps an extension of Gruenwald's (1959) hypothesis that the uterine stroma and epithelium have a common origin in Müllerian epithelium and that transformation of stroma into epithelium is a constantly recurring process in the endometrium. However, experimental observation is needed to support this contention.

Reid (1964a) and Reid et al. (1967) have described experiments on the human cervix indicating that, following biopsy or electrocauterization, regeneration of squamous epithelium and columnar epithelium occurs by differentiation of cells in the underlying stroma. They suggest the unlikely and unsubstantiated hypothesis that these stromal cells are blood mononuclear cells which have migrated into the site of the lesion. Their experiments suggest that an alkaline environment favours the development of a mucin-producing epithelium and a more acid environment a keratin-producing epithelium.

g) Cyto- and Histochemistry of Reserve Cells and Squamous Metaplasia

The literature on the histochemistry of abnormal epithelium is rather confused because of (1) the differing terminologies used in describing the lesions and (2) indifferent descriptions and illustrations often making it difficult to determine the particular cells or zones of epithelium which are being described. The immature basal cells of squamous epithelium and of prosoplastic epithelium are very similar (see Chapter I, Table 1.2); both show an increase in the RNA content of the cytoplasm and of non-specific esterase, acid phosphatase, phosphoamidase, dehydrogenases and β-glucuronidase (Fluhmann, 1961; Foraker et al., 1954; Foraker 1962; Berger 1961b; Bertalanffy et al., 1961). This chemical pattern occurs in other immature epithelia and is probably an indication of proliferative activity. On the other hand, substances associated with cytoplasmic differentiation, for example, glycogen and polysaccharides, are absent from these immature cells (Fluhmann, 1961; Song, 1964). However, in later stages of prosoplasia Fluhmann described the presence of vacuolated cells which take up the periodic acid Schiff stain. This he regards as evidence of the bipotentiality of reserve cells. In metaplastic foci, Moricard and Cartier (1964) describe cells or cell residues which stain with alcian blue. These they regard as columnar cells which have lost their polarity and, in support, point out that under the electron microscope the cytoplasm of these cells contains granules of secretion intermingled with endoplasmic reticulum, mitochondria, Golgi membranes and clear or dark vacuoles. Foraker and Wingo (1956) have shown that metaplastic squamous cells may become keratinized under certain conditions. In this process the sulphydril group of cystein is oxidized to the disulphide bond of cystine. This process of keratinization is accompanied by a marked increase in cytoplasmic mass, which can be observed by interference microscopy and by soft X-rays (Fitzgerald et al. 1959).

h) The Prevalence and Significance of Reserve Cell Hyperplasia and Squamous Metaplasia

Carmichael and Jeaffreson (1939) examined longitudinal sections of the anterior and posterior lips of 200 cervices; reserve cell proliferation and hyperplasia was found in 95% of specimens and the ages of the patients ranged from infancy to the eighth decade. They also found squamous metaplasia in 41% of 334 cervices removed surgically. VON HAAM and OLD (1964) have described a very extensive study of reserve cell hyperplasia and squamous metaplasia. They found reserve cells in 83.6% of 1,000 consecutive cervical specimens; reserve cell hyperplasia was found in 25.2%, incomplete squamous metaplasia in 24.2% and complete squamous metaplasia in 10.3%.

In the human cervix reserve cell proliferation and hyperplasia can occur at any age but the age of maximum prevalence is uncertain. DAVIES and KUSAMA (1962), using the term "clear cell", stated that islands of clear cells were observed sporadically along the length of the basement membrane of the foetal cervical mucosa, which remained intact at all points. From their illustrations it is evident that these "clear cells" were reserve cells. SONG (1964) found multiple areas of reserve cells in the cervices of newborn infants and children, illustrating this with a photomicrograph of the cervix of a three-year-old child. GESCHICKTER and FERNANDEZ (1962) show a chart indicating that the maximum prevalence of endocervical epidermidization in their material was in the age group 30—39 years. This probably reflects both the age group of the sample as well as the prevalence of the condition. VON HAAM and OLD (1964) found a more complicated pattern. Although both incomplete and complete squamous metaplasia were most prevalent in the 30—39 years age group, incomplete squamous metaplasia was least prevalent in the next age bracket (40 to 49 years) and rose to 25.0% in the over 60 years group, but complete squamous metaplasia progressively declined in frequency.

VON HAAM and OLD (1964) have reviewed the relationship between inflammatory diseases of the cervix and both reserve cell hyperplasia and metaplasia and have found it extremely difficult to affirm or deny any association since only rarely is an adult cervix free from inflammation. They found a frequent association of uterine leiomyomas and adenomyosis with reserve cell hyperplasia and metaplasia. There is an extensive literature suggesting that hormones affect the prevalence and degree of reserve cell hyperplasia and metaplasia. This has been reviewed by VON HAAM and OLD (1964) and by SONG (1964). There is, however, little clear evidence to implicate direct hormonal effects in the human cervix. The age distribution of these lesions suggests that they cannot play a dominant role. Much of the evidence in favour of the view that hormones such as oestrogens or progesterone cause squamous metaplasia is based on animal experiments, particularly rats, mice and rabbits. Because the anatomy of the rodent genital tract differs from that of woman, the results cannot be applied directly to the human situation. However, the cervix of the monkey is morphologically similar to that of woman, and OVERHOLZER and ALLEN (1935) have shown in these animals that metaplasia of the epithelium of the cervical glands can be produced in 60—90 days by the daily administration of oestrogen. According to HISAW and LENDRUM (1936) the administration of progesterone with oestrogen prevents metaplasia in the monkey cervix. In 1939 WOLLNER noted marked squamous metaplasia in the cervices of castrated women receiving oestrone; this disappeared after cessation of the hormone therapy. Similarly, FUNK-BRENTANO et al. (1951) found a high degree of squamous metaplasia in menopausal women following the administration of oestrogens. ROSENTHAL and HELLMAN (1952) and HELLMAN et al. (1954) demonstrated a striking similarity between the changes which occur in the cervix of the pregnant adult and those in the newborn infant. These changes were thought to be reversible and are at least circumstantial evidence relating high hormone levels at these periods to changes in the cervix.

EDWARDS (1971) has investigated the effect of 17 β-oestradiol on explants of endocervical tissue cultured in a chemically defined medium. After 4 hours *in vitro* the columnar cells assumed a rather squat appearance and a single layer of small cuboidal cells with centrally located nuclei and perinuclear vacuoles appeared between

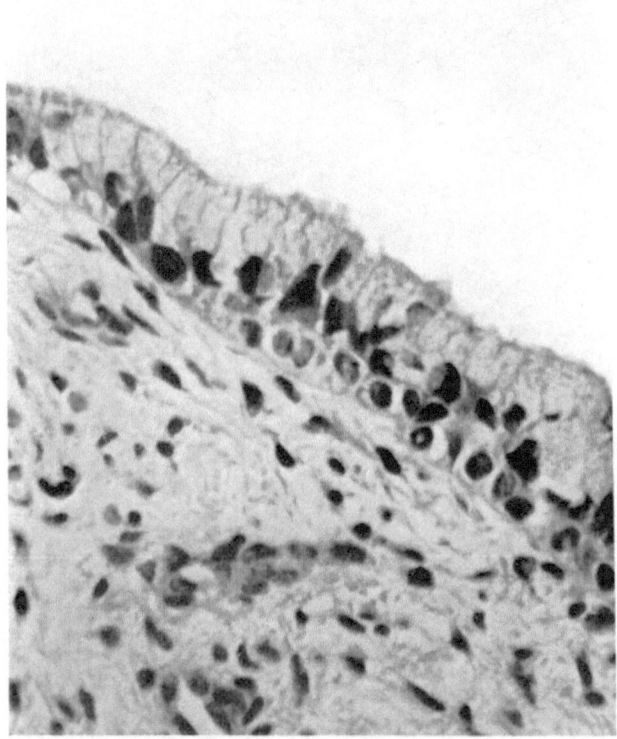

Fig. 2.13. Endocervical tissue which has been cultured for 4 hours in medium 199 supplemented with oestradiol. There is reserve cell proliferation which was absent in the control section. (H. & E. × 480)

the columnar cells and the stroma. The epithelium of surface explants which had been cultured for 6 hours consisted of two or three layers of cells, whilst that lining the more deep seated glands was double layered (Figs. 2.13. and 2.14.). After 24 hours the epithelia in both sites comprised two or three layers. The newly formed cells bore a close resemblance to reserve cells. In addition a positively stained basement membrane could not be identified and the 3 day cultures showed an increase in the population of stromal cells. In view of this time relationship it is unlikely that the newly formed sub-columnar epithelial cells originated in the stroma but further studies will be necessary to confirm this, although these experiments do suggest that oestrogens may have a direct effect on columnar epithelium causing reserve cell hyperplasia.

Reserve cell hyperplasia is not peculiar to the cervix. As long ago as 1894 ASCHOFF described changes in the prostate of newborn male infants that might be interpreted as reserve cell hyperplasia. GERE *et al.* (1962) recorded typical reserve cell hyperplasia in the bronchial epithelium of infants and children. Various toxic agents can cause reserve cell hyperplasia in the bronchial epithelium of animals, e.g., ozonized gasoline

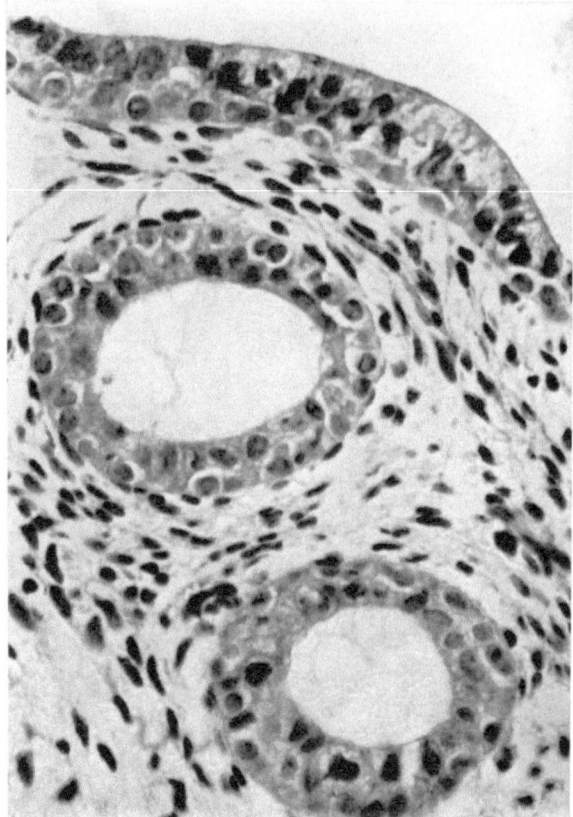

Fig. 2.14. From the same case as 2.13. The tissue has been cultured for 6 hours in medium 199 supplemented by oestradiol. Reserve cell proliferation is present round an endocervical gland. (H. & E. × 480)

and cigarette smoke in mice (KOTIN *et al.* 1958; LEUCHENBERGER *et al.* 1958) and tobacco tar in dogs (ROCKNEY *et al.* 1958).

Perhaps it may be concluded that reserve cell hyperplasia and squamous metaplasia are not peculiar to the cervix but in this site the changes are probably physiological and, to some extent, influenced by steroid hormones.

Earlier in this chapter it was noted that VON HAAM and OLD (1964) described an atypical reserve cell hyperplasia. Since it is difficult in the adult to determine the biological potential of atypical reserve cell hyperplasia, we regard this as a form of dysplasia. However, HELLMAN *et al.* (1954) observed atypical reserve cell hyperplasia in 5% of newborn cervices. SONG (1964) records focal cellular atypia, shown by variation in nuclear size and shape, disarray and crowding of the nuclei, nuclear hyperchromasia and mitoses, in four foetuses aged from 34 weeks' gestation to term. One premature infant was of particular interest. It was born at 32 weeks' gestation to a 21-year-old mother with suspicious cytological smears which led to a cone biopsy. In the mother a diagnosis of severe cervical atypia and, or, carcinoma *in situ* was made. The infant died two days after delivery and its cervix showed similar atypia to those of her mother but to a less degree. From observations such as these it follows that epithelial abnormalities which are bland may occur in the cervices of foetuses and the newborn which in the non-pregnant adult would be regarded as malignant. Similarly, FORD *et al.* (1961) have described atypical metaplasia in the bronchi in men and women dying of diseases other than carcinoma of the bronchus.

2. Cervical Erosion or Ectopy

Until recently, it has been a generally accepted opinion that mucous glands may be found on the surface of the portio vaginalis of the uterine cervix in two conditions. First, eversion as a result of laceration of the cervix in childbirth or continued traction from progressive prolapse or an outward expansion of the endocervical canal as a result of swelling and oedema when inflamed. Second, as a result of a localized loss of squamous epithelium (*erosio vera*) the denuded tissue may be covered by endocervical epithelium giving rise to the so-called glandular erosion. This view of the nature of a cervical erosion is based on the studies of ROBERT MEYER (1910a and b) and the supposed mode of evolution has been well summarized by FRANK (1931) and by HAMPERL and KAUFMANN (1959). If the denuded area is near the squamo-columnar junction then the columnar epithelium may spread downwards to cover it, but if the denuded area is further away endocervical glands may burrow through the cervical stroma until they come into contact with the raw area which they then cover with mucus-secreting epithelium. Fig. 2.15 shows the degeneration of squamous epithelium adjacent to cervical glands but whether the damage to the squamous epithelium has stimulated these glands to proliferate is perhaps an open question. If the loss of squamous epithelium is extensive, the surface of the cervix may be covered by small papillae clothed with columnar epithelium. Such a typically papillary erosion is seen in Fig. 2.16. The columnar cells on the surface may be eosinophilic in contrast to those lining the glands; this change has been called eosinophilic metamorphosis by DE BRUX and DUPRÉ-FROMENT (1960). Multi-nucleated cells may also occur in the columnar epithelium. These slightly abnormal cells may be seen in cervical and vaginal smears. According to FRANK (1931) the later stages of healing of a cervical erosion consist in the replacement of the columnar epithelium by squamous epithelium which grows in from the sides or regenerates from islets of squamous epithelium which were left behind in the initial stages of erosion.

The Meyerian view of the mechanism of evolution of a cervical erosion has been severely criticized by two groups of German workers at Bonn and Cologne, and their observations and conclusions have been summarized by HAMPERL and KAUFMANN

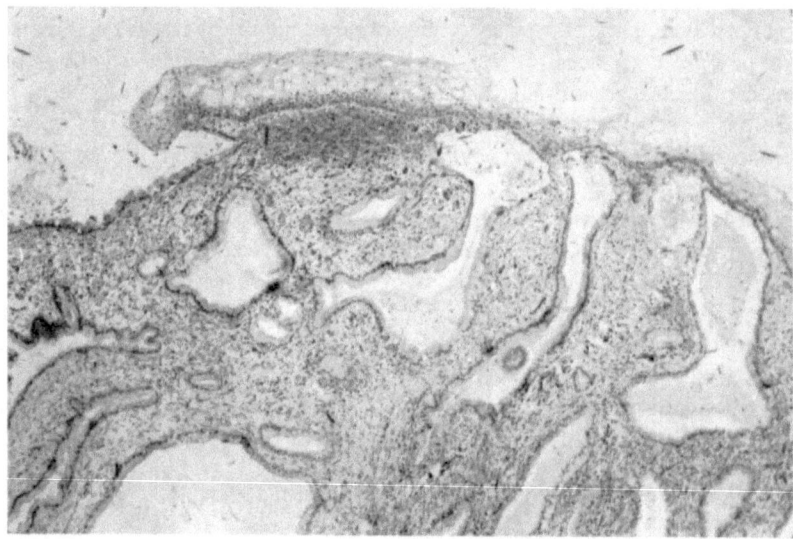

Fig. 2.15. Degenerating squamous epithelium overlying endocervical glands. Loss of this squamous epithelium would result in a surface covered by papillae clothed in columnar epithelium, i.e., a papillary cervical "erosion" in the Meyerian sense. (H. & E. × 50)

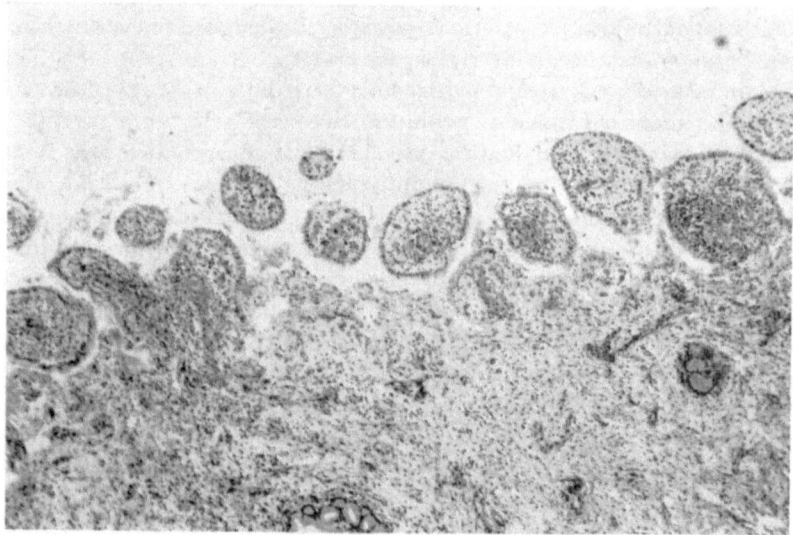

Fig. 2.16. A papillary cervical "erosion". (H. & E. × 50)

(1959). They were unable to find in their material the supposed primary defect in the squamous epithelium (*erosio vera*). They therefore attempted to produce it artificially by scraping the epithelium near the external os. In the process of healing the raw area was covered by squamous epithelium rather than by columnar epithelium as would be expected on the Meyerian hypothesis. Moreover, they regard the sprouting of glands which then burrow through the cervical stroma as highly improbable. From a study of 853 unselected uteri the Bonn-Cologne group of workers were able to establish the patterns of behaviour of squamous and columnar epithelium at their junction. They concluded that when the volume of the cervical wall increases, as in inflammation or pregnancy, the lips of the cervix protrude carrying with them the endocervical mucosa on to the portio vaginalis (eversion, ectropion), whilst at the same time the upper limit of the endocervical epithelium moves down. This concept they regard as applicable to the evolution of the so-called glandular erosion which should therefore be more properly called endocervical ectopy. In the neonate endocervical epithelium may be found on the portio vaginalis due to relative swelling of the cervical stroma under the influence of the maternal hormones; as the hormone level diminishes the cervical stroma shrinks, causing the squamous epithelium to be drawn into the endocervical canal until puberty approaches. During the childbearing period the endocervical glands often extend on to the portio vaginalis and, if squamous metaplasia occurs, they may be covered with newly formed squamous epithelium constituting the transformation zone. After the menopause the cervix once more shrinks and the glands together with the newly formed squamous epithelium may be drawn again into the endocervical canal.

This description oversimplifies the relationship between the pattern of the epithelia and the age of the patient. Thus, GRUENAGEL (1957) has shown that in 26% of newborn infants and 53% of girls, from nurslings to 9 years of age, the squamo-columnar junction lies outside the external os on the portio vaginalis. A survey by COPPLESON and REID (1967) confirms and extends these findings. They examined 7,474 women attending a cancer detection clinic and found the ectocervix covered with native ectocervical squamous epithelium in 18.2%, ectopic columnar epithelium in 8.4% and a typical transformation zone (metaplastic squamous epi-

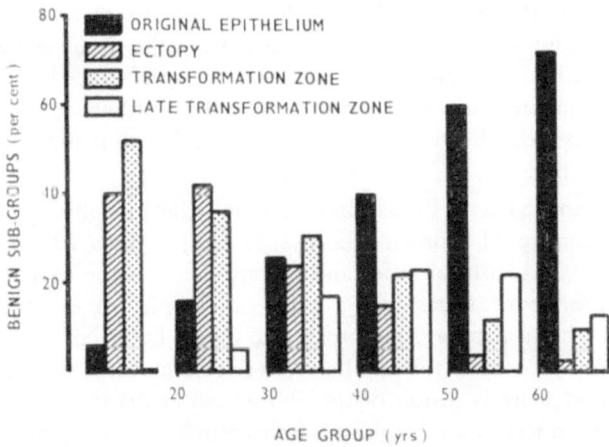

Fig. 2.17. A histogram showing the distribution of the various benign types of colposcopic appearance in each age group. Thus, in the 15—20 year group just over 50% of girls had a well developed transformation zone, 40% showed an ectopy and in only a few was the ectocervix covered by original epithelium. In contrast in the over 50 and over 60 year age groups the ectocervix was usually covered by original squamous epithelium — in part due to shrinkage of the cervical stroma. (CROMPTON 1971)

thelium) in 65.7% of women. The remainder of the women exhibited an abnormal transformation zone or some other lesion such as a cervical polyp. CROMPTON (1971) has studied the distribution of these conditions in the cervices of women attending a colposcopic clinic in our own hospital. The distribution of benign changes at different ages is illustrated in Fig. 2.17.

The red appearance of the ectopy is due to the ease with which vessels can be seen in the stromal papillae of the ectopic "Träubchen" (or villi) as the covering epithelium is usually only one cell layer thick. Kos and LANÉ (1963) described the vessels in their Träubchen as almost like hair-needle loops mainly with simple afferent and efferent arms. In fatter Träubchen the capillary network was much richer but in both types the thickness of the individual capillaries was practically the same and the vessel walls were smooth without out-pouchings.

3. The Benign Transformation Zone

Three types of epithelium can be distinguished in the cervix, the two "original" epithelia—glandular and squamous—and a "third" metaplastic squamous epithelium which lies between the original epithelia and constitutes the transformation zone of the colposcopist. The epithelium of the typical transformation zone is usually benign but it may undergo malignant alterations in the atypical transformation zone.

The colposcopic appearances of this zone depend on: (a) the underlying capillary angio-architecture, (b) the colour and opacity of the epithelium and (c) the contour of the epithelium. These, in turn, depend on the morphological arrangement of the metaplastic epithelium in relation to the glands and other structures. In the benign transformation zone the new squamous epithelium is associated with some vessel changes. There is often an increase in the papillary loops and the presence of Nabothian follicles, gland mouths and underlying residual columnar epithelium produces a more complex vascular pattern. Nevertheless there is a regularity in calibre and in the tree-like branching of the vessels which marks out the tissue as benign. Even on naked eye observation, the transformation zone can sometimes be distinguished by its violaceous colour in distinction from the original epithelium which is pink and the ectopy which is red. The vessel patterns associated with malign cervical epithelia are detailed in Chapter 3.

LINHARTOVA and ŠTAFL (1965a) have studied the morphology of the normal transformation zone in 11 women whose ages ranged from 22 to 37 years. Serial sections were prepared from biopsies and the structure of the tissues reconstructed. The transformation zone starts in a region of ectopic, or everted, endocervical epithelium which has a papillary structure, the crypts between the papillae opening freely on the surface. Some of the papillae adhere to each other. COPPLESON and REID (1967) suggest that there is fusion of the epithelium at the tips of adjacent papillae. This epithelium undergoes metaplastic transformation to squamous epithelium. Meanwhile, according to LINHARTOVA and ŠTAFL (1965a), there is a new formation of connective tissue in the walls and at the bases of the crypts. Thus the crypts between the papillae are partially or completely closed and they are ultimately converted into canalicular structures or they disappear. Some of the canaliculi retain continuity with the surface, others are closed off to form Nabothian follicles. These changes are illustrated in Figs. 2.18. and 2.19.. A well-developed transformation zone usually shows a combination of areas of metaplastic squamous epithelium and ectopic islands of columnar epithelium.

COPPLESON and REID (1967) have investigated the effect of parity on the incidence of typical transformation zones. They found typical transformation zones in 49% of symptomless nulliparae, in 61% of women who have had one confinement and in

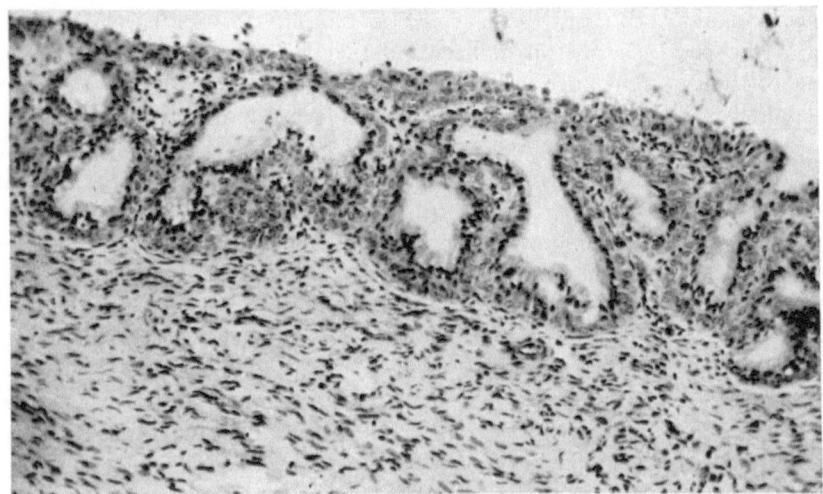

Fig. 2.18. With the proliferation of reserve cells under the endocervical epithelium the papillae which covered the area of "erosion", or ectopy, are becoming agglutinated and fused together. (H. & E. × 120)

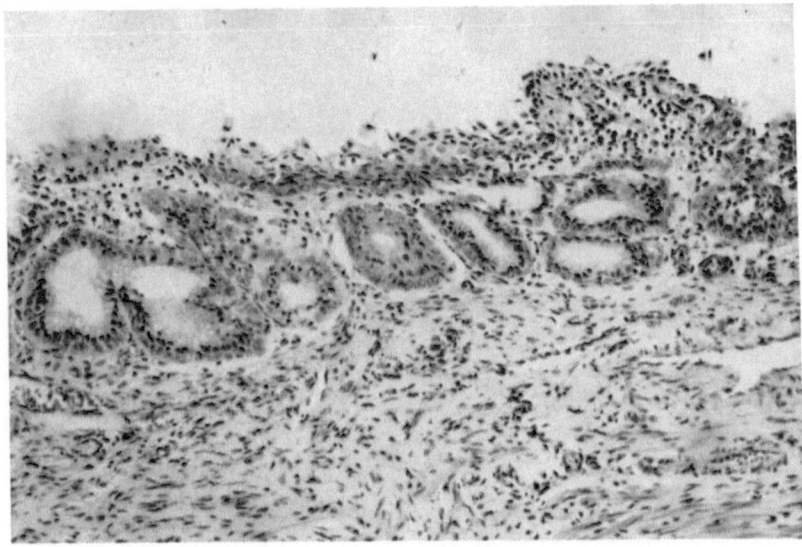

Fig. 2.19. From the same cervix as Fig. 2.18. The process of fusion has proceeded further and the surface epithelium has taken on a squamoid appearance whilst a loose fibrous stroma separates it from the underlying residual glands. (H. & E. × 120)

68% of women with two or more confinements. The effects of pregnancy on the cervix seem to be twofold: (1) often there is marked hyperplasia of the columnar epithelium (EPPERSON *et al.* 1951; FLUHMANN 1959) with consequent prolapse of the vaginal portion of the cervix and thus displacement of the squamo-columnar junction, and (2) there is a softening of the cervical collagen and ground substance (DANFORTH *et al.* 1960; BUCKINGHAM *et al.* 1962). Whilst the cervices of most women undergo these changes in their first pregnancy, a few primigravidae are unaffected.

COPPLESON and REID (1967) have suggested that HUGHESDON's (1952) anatomical studies of the cervix afford an explanation for the observation that subsequent pregnancies after the first have little effect on the extent of the transformation zone. HUGHESDON described the muscle of the cervix forming an outer investment continuous with the corporeal muscle above and the vaginal muscle below and an intrinsic musculature derived from muscle bundles which branch off the ensheathing layer and arch over the fornix. This intrinsic musculature runs in all directions and, together with the collagen bundles which accompany it, forms a diaphragm which is characteristically present in the primigravid cervix. The integrity of this diaphragm is lost in the first labour, and as a result the lips of the cervix diverge and the endocervical epithelium may be everted but no further eversion can arise from this cause in subsequent pregnancies.

It follows from the above discussion that the presence of columnar epithelium, often with an associated transformation zone, on the portio vaginalis of the cervix is common at all ages and must be regarded as physiological and that pregnancy may cause extension of the ectopic epithelium. Thus the presence of ectopic columnar epithelium, which forms a red zone round the cervical os, in women attending gynaecological clinics, may well be coincidental to their complaints and should not be regarded as necessarily pathological.

Chapter 3

The Definition and Diagnosis of Malign Lesions of the Cervix Uteri.

GOVAN *et al.* (1966, 1969) have divided epithelial abnormalities of the cervix into bland and malign lesions. Bland lesions include squamous hyperplasia, reserve cell proliferation and squamous metaplasia. The malign lesions include dysplasia, carcinoma *in situ* and microcarcinoma but not frankly invasive carcinoma which is truly malignant. It is this malign group which will be defined and discussed in this chapter. In order that the natural history and malignant potential of these conditions may be assessed objectively, it is necessary to define them in clear morphological terms without prejudice to their possible biological significance. The attempt to identify morphological entities and relate them to their biological potential is not simply an academic exercise. Failure to recognize potentially malignant epithelium may lead to women with early carcinoma of the cervix slipping through the therapeutic net at a curable stage of the disease; whereas too ready diagnosis of carcinoma *in situ* may cause women in the child-bearing period to lose their uteri unnecessarily. Moreover, precise diagnostic concepts are a necessary preliminary for the comparison of studies by various authors.

1. Diagnostic Criteria

a) The Conceptual Basis of *in situ* Carcinoma

The basic concept of carcinoma *in situ* is that the epithelium of the cervix, or indeed of any other site in the body, has undergone an irreversible malignant change but the malignant epithelium has not yet broken through its normal boundaries. The concept stated in such terms is essentially simple but the recognition of the irreversible change presents many difficulties. When malignancy is associated with invasion or metastasis little attention may be paid to subtle changes in tissue pattern or to cytological abnormalities, but when there is no invasion such changes become all important. In any tumour, the changes in the cells may be degenerative or neoplastic. Cells showing degenerative changes have, generally speaking, reached the end of their active life and will not proliferate. Such cells are frequently bizarre showing, for example, individual cell keratinization and karyorrhexis. Neoplastic cells necessarily retain their ability to proliferate and, although they may have a high nucleo-cytoplasmic ratio and show nuclear hyperchromasia in the cervix, they are not usually very bizarre. This distinction was brought out by GLÜCKSMANN's (1947) work on the radio-sensitivity of cervical carcinoma. Tumours which retained a high proportion of "resting cells" after radiation had a worse prognosis than tumours in which there was a lower proportion of such cells, whilst the occurrence of many differentiated or degenerate cells was a good prognostic sign. Because degenerate cells are often large and bizarre they may appear to cause more disorder in the epithelial pattern than the malignant but more uniform proliferating cells. Further, degenerative changes may be produced in cervical epithelium by exogenous factors, the effects of which are reversible when the stimuli are removed. It is thus of prime importance to be able to distinguish between the reversible and the irreversible morphological changes that can occur in the cervix. Unfortunately, it is difficult to make this distinction with precision in women although under experimental conditions in animals more clear-cut differences can be recognized. The morphological definition of carcinoma *in situ* may, in the present state of our knowledge, appear to be based on arbitrary criteria. It is thought that a large, but indeterminate number of cases diagnosed as carcinoma *in situ* would become invasive carcinomas if left untreated but some of these abnormal epithelia would probably revert to normal. Some, but a lower proportion, of malign lesions showing less severe changes might also become malignant and a larger proportion of these would revert to normal. These less abnormal epithelia are termed dysplastic.

b) An Historical Note

It is necessary, at this point, to outline the historical development of the concept of *in-situ* carcinoma in order to explain the otherwise apparently arbitrary diagnostic criteria used. In the Harveian lecture for 1886 WILLIAMS illustrated a symptomless early carcinoma of the cervix. GORE and HERTIG (1964) think that much of the tumour must have been *in situ* and they consider this to be the first case recorded in the literature. CULLEN (1900), SCHAUENSTEIN (1908) and RUBIN (1910) described structural changes in the epithelium at the margin of invasive carcinomas. RUBIN argued that these changes were fundamentally cancerous and that this alteration preceded the stage of invasion. He introduced the term "carcinoma *in situ*" but this was not a generally accepted term until after Broders' paper in 1932. GLATTHAAR (1950) distinguished four types of epithelial abnormality in the cervix: (1) abnormal epithelium, (2) "unruhiges Epithel", (3) atypical epithelium and (4) cancer stage 0. These terms described progressively severer lesions and the classification was supported by the experience of the Zurich workers between 1945 and 1948 (HAEFELI 1950). The first three conditions might be regarded as dysplasia and only the last as carcinoma *in situ*.

c) Carcinoma *in situ* (Synonym: Intraepithelial Carcinoma)

In 1952 a committee of pathologists in Paris formulated the following criteria for the diagnosis of carcinoma *in situ* (GRICOUROFF 1952):

(1) Cellular anomalies
  (a) Anaplasia—variation in cell form, basophilic cytoplasm, lack of glycogen, increased nucleo-cytoplasmic ratio.
  (b) Abnormal nuclei—e.g., multiple or multilobed nuclei.

(c) Abnormalities of proliferation—frequent mitoses, atypical mitoses (e.g., three-group metaphase) or mitoses in epithelial cells near the surface.

(2) Structural abnormalities
   (a) A sharp boundary between the normal and the pathological epithelium.
   (b) Disorder of epithelial structure.

GUSBERG and MOORE in the following year (1953) proposed useful criteria in which stress was laid upon the occurrence of the changes throughout the whole thickness of the epithelium.
   (1) Loss of normal stratification and polarity.
   (2) Squamous cells vary in size and shape, increased nucleo-cytoplasmic ratio.
   (3) Frequent mitotic figures, often bizarre.
   (4) Absent or incomplete differentiation.
   (5) The whole thickness of the epithelium is affected.

An International Committee on Histological Definitions which met in Vienna (1961) also laid stress on the importance of the changes involving the whole thickness of the epithelium:

"Only those cases should be classified as carcinoma *in situ* which, in the absence of invasion, show as surface lining an epithelium in which, throughout the whole thickness, no differentiation takes place. The process may involve the lining of the cervical glands without thereby creating a new group. It is recognised that the cells of the uppermost layers may show some slight flattening. The very rare case of an otherwise characteristic carcinoma *in situ* that shows a greater degree of differentiation belongs to the exceptions for which no classification can provide."

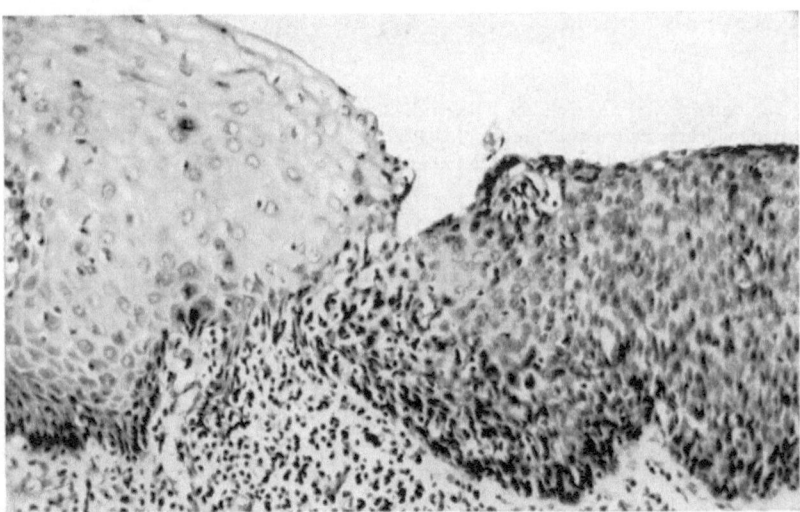

Fig. 3.1. The normal squamous epithelium of the cervix on the left is separated from the abnormal epithelium (carcinoma *in situ*) on the right by a sharply defined oblique line. Note the cellularity of the abnormal epithelium and the lack of stratification. (H. & E. × 120)

Epithelial abnormalities of the cervix show a spectrum of changes and so the committee, having defined as an upper limit of change "absence of invasion", defined a lower limit in these terms:

"All other disturbances of differentiation of the squamous epithelial lining of surface and glands are to be classified as dysplasia. They may be characterised as of high or low degree, terms which are preferable to suspicious and non-suspicious, as the proposed terms describe the histological appearance and do not express an opinion."

GOVAN *et al.* (1966) have laid stress on three morphological changes which characterize carcinoma *in situ*: (a) complete loss of stratification; the undifferentiated

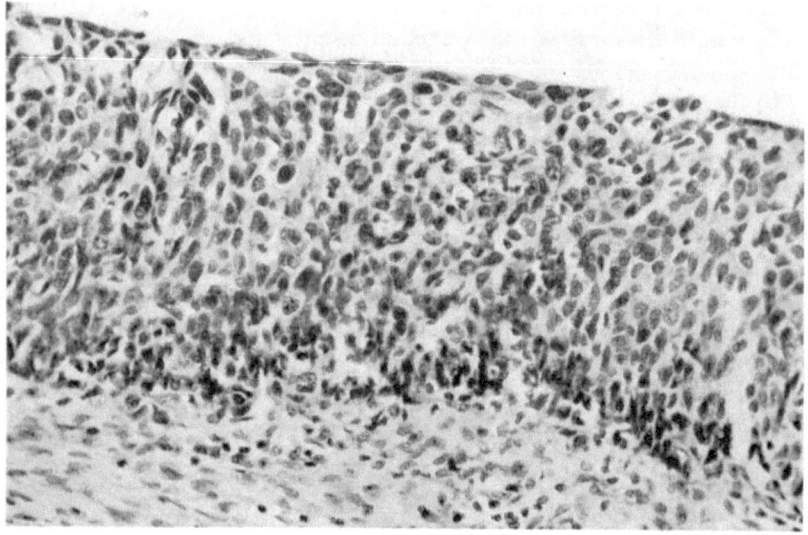

Fig. 3.2. Carcinoma *in situ* of the cervix. The epithelium is cellular, the cytoplasm is scanty and there is variation in nuclear size. The cells are irregularly arranged and stratification is absent but the surface layer of cells is flattened. (H. & E. × 180)

and immature cells constituting the lesion usually extend throughout the whole thickness of the epithelium, (b) loss of cytoplasmic differentiation and (c) nuclear abnormalities. This is the definition of carcinoma *in situ* employed in this text and it is illustrated in Figs. 3.1., 3.2. and 3.3..

COPPLESON and REID (1967) believe that the term carcinoma *in situ* as traditionally defined is both ill-advised and often unwarranted. They quote the view of DE BRUX and WENNER-MANGEN (1961): "Some authors rejected the term carcinoma *in situ* which is heavily loaded with consequence, not only theoretical but clinical and therapeutic." COPPLESON and REID agree with GRAY (1964) that the term carcinoma *in situ* should be abandoned and replaced by the designation "pre-cancer". It seems to us that this term is as open to objection as carcinoma *in situ*.

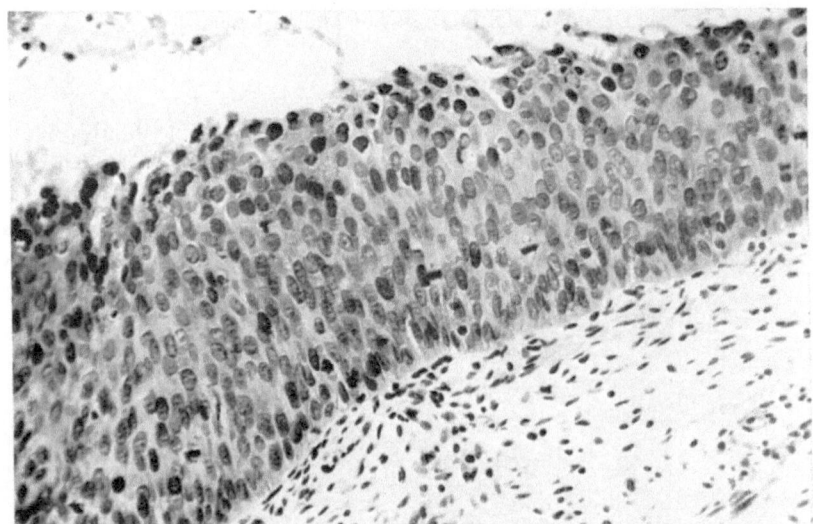

Fig. 3.3. Carcinoma *in situ*. The cells are more regular in their arrangement than in Fig. 3.2 and the nuclei are somewhat more dense near the surface than elsewhere. Mitoses are fairly numerous in the deeper parts of the epithelium and many are abnormal. (H. & E. × 180)

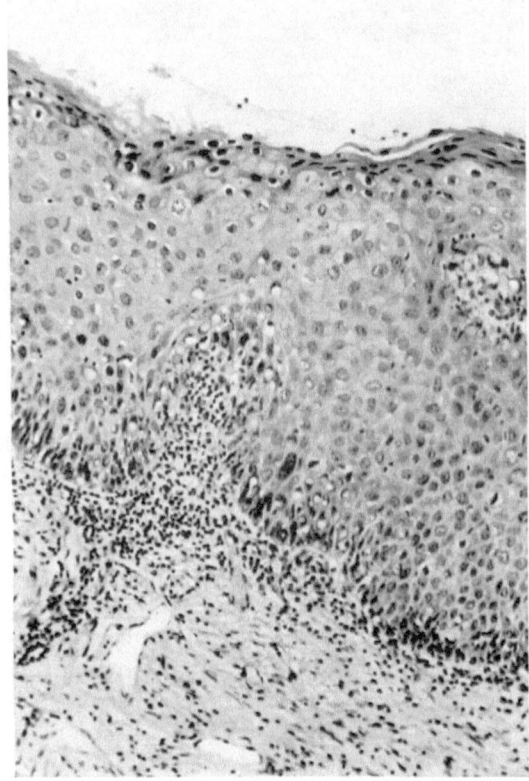

Fig. 3.4. Mild dysplasia. Occasionally an abnormally large, hyperchromatic nucleus is present but maturation of cells is fairly orderly and stratification is maintained. (H. & E. × 180)

d) Dysplasia

This term was introduced by REAGAN *et al.* (1953, 1955, 1956b). He writes (1964): "This designation has been applied to certain reactions which involve the stratified squamous or the squamous-like (metaplastic) epithelium of the uterine cervix. Fundamentally the cells making up these lesions are characterized by varying degrees of cytoplasmic maturation while their nuclei are abnormally large even at

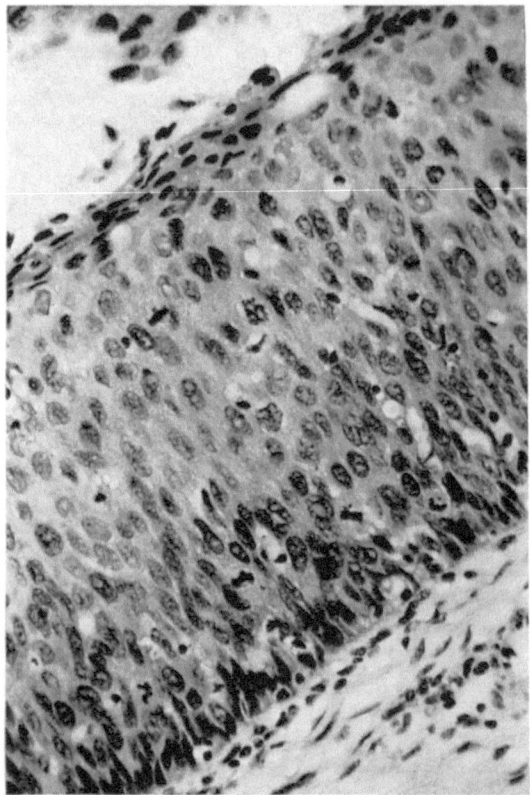

Fig. 3.5. Severe dysplasia. The general architecture of this epithelium is similar to that of Fig. 3.4. but mitoses extend into the upper third of the epithelium. (H. & E. × 360)

high levels in the altered epithelium. The disordered growth is manifested by a premature keratinization of the cells and by an abnormal differentiation of the most superficial cell layers." Epithelium showing these changes is thus distiguished from bland epithelial abnormalities, on the one hand, and carcinoma *in situ*, on the other. As indicated above, the International Committee on Histological Definitions found it convenient to use the term dysplasia to describe a histological appearance of less marked abnormality than carcinoma *in situ*. The abnormal epithelium, unquiet epithelium and atypical epithelium of GLATTHAAR (1950) and BAJARDI (1961a) are included in this category of dysplasia. REAGAN (1964) lists a number of terms

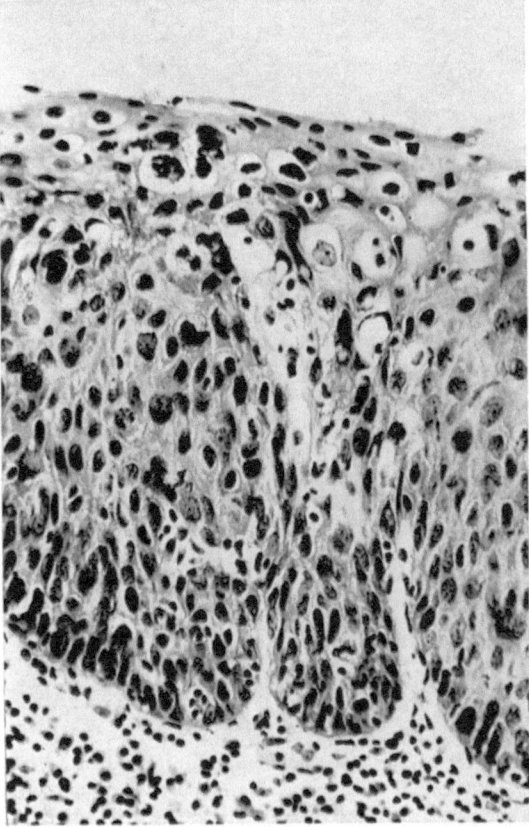

Fig. 3.6. Severe dysplasia. The cells exhibit severe pleomorphism with variable nucleo-cytoplasmic ratio but there is some maturation as the surface is approached. A number of nuclei near the surface show karyorrhexis and some cells show perinuclear haloes, both these changes are to be regarded as degenerative. (H. & E. × 360)

which are probably synonymous. GOVAN *et al.* (1966) use the term dysplasia for a disorder in the arrangement, morphology and activity of the epithelial cells less marked than those of carcinoma *in situ*. They divide it into two grades, mild and severe. Their definition is illustrated in Figs. 3.4. to 3.9.

e) Microcarcinoma

The term microcarcinoma was introduced by MESTWERDT (1953). GLÜCKSMANN and CHERRY (1964) distinguish three types of early invasion or microcarcinoma of the cervix: (1) carcinoma *in situ* with early or questionable invasion of the cervical stroma, (2) carcinoma *in situ* with definite invasion of the stroma but lacking ability to grow in xenotopic sites and (3) the massive invasion without clinical (i.e. macroscopic) symptoms, clinical occult carcinoma. GLÜCKSMANN and CHERRY consider the first two conditions resemble carcinoma *in situ* as regards inability of xenotopic

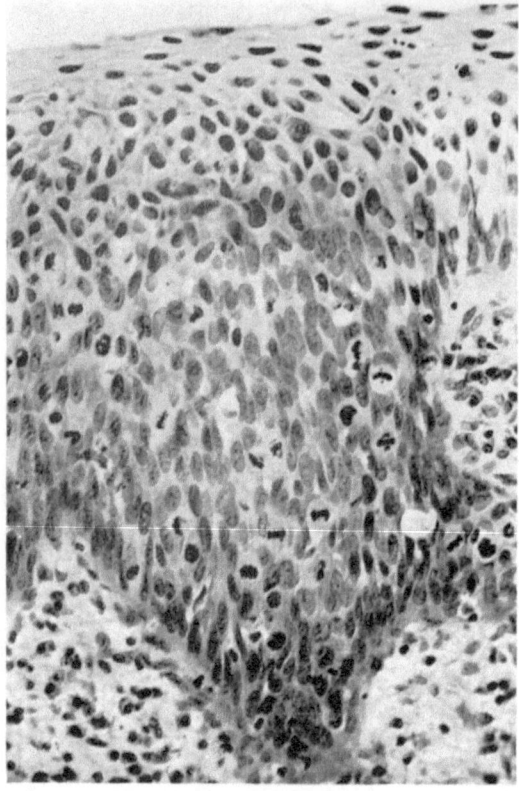

Fig. 3.7. Moderately severe dysplasia. The parabasal and intermediate layers are unusually cellular but fairly regularly arranged. Mitoses in these zones are unusually numerous and most are abnormal showing the picture of "three-group metaphase". (H. & E. × 360)

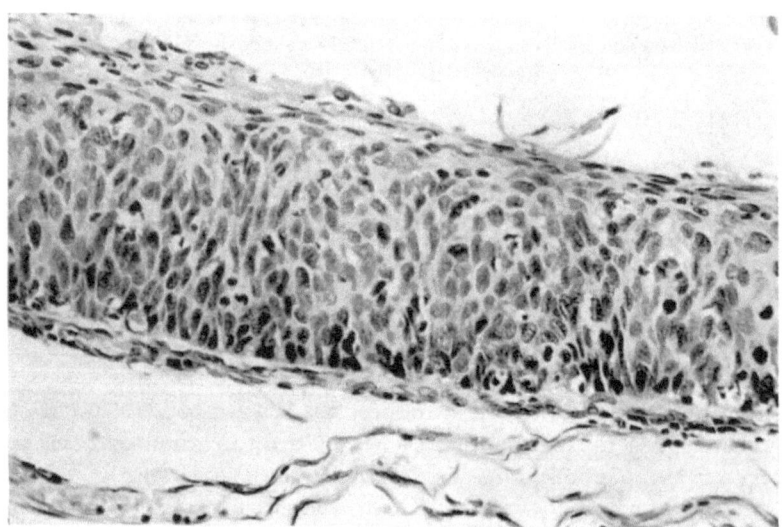

Fig. 3.8. Severe dysplasia bordering on carcinoma *in situ*. Immature cells are present throughout the epithelium, except in a few surface layers, and mitoses are frequent. (H. & E. × 180)

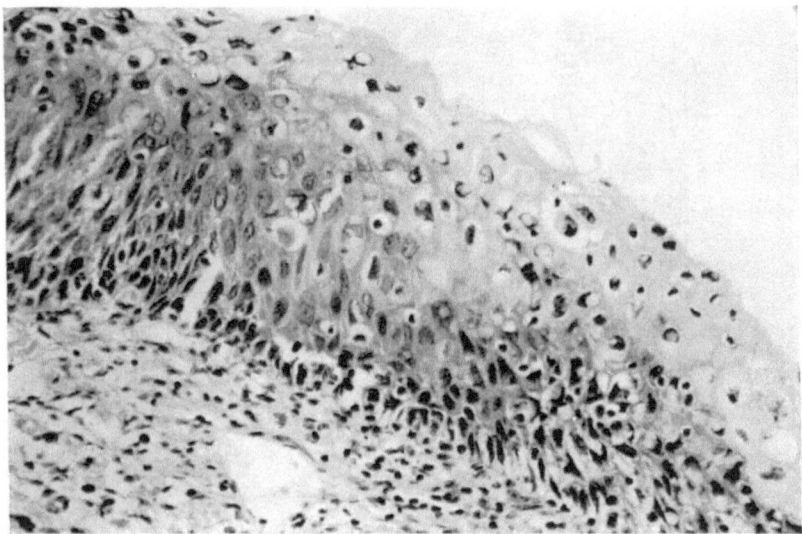

Fig. 3.9. Severe dysplasia. The cells exhibit severe pleomorphism with increased nucleo-cytoplasmic ratio, but there is some maturation of the surface so that the appearances are those of dysplasia rather than of carcinoma *in situ* (GOVAN *et al.* 1966. J. Obstet. Gynaec. Brit. Cwlth. **73**, 883). (H. & E. × 180)

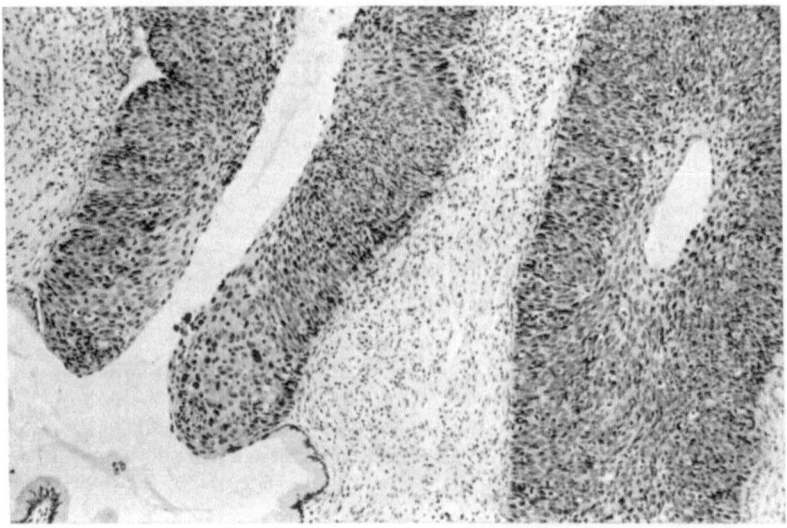

Fig. 3.10. Endocervical gland involvement. Carcinoma *in situ* involves the mouth of a mucous gland but the process remains intraepithelial (GOVAN *et al.* 1966. J. Obstet. Gynaec. Brit. Cwlth. **73**, 883). H. & E. × 120)

growth but not with regard to invasiveness. It is the ability of tumour cells to grow in a foreign environment that renders a tumour malignant. However, it is difficult to determine in a section whether or not infiltrating tumour cells have this ability. KOTTMEIER *et al.* (1959) state, "Experience has clearly shown that the criteria for

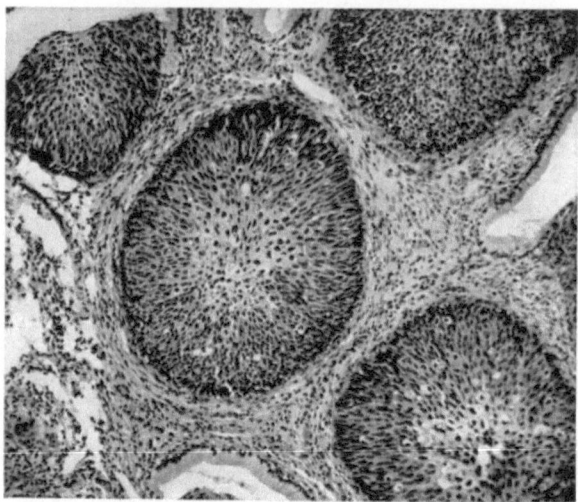

Fig. 3.11. Gland involvement. Malign epithelium fills and distends gland crypts. The contour and symmetry of the crypts is preserved and such glandular involvement should not be mistaken for carcinomatous invasion (GOVAN *et al.* 1966. J. Obstet. Gynaec. Brit. Cwlth. **73**, 883). (H. & E. × 120)

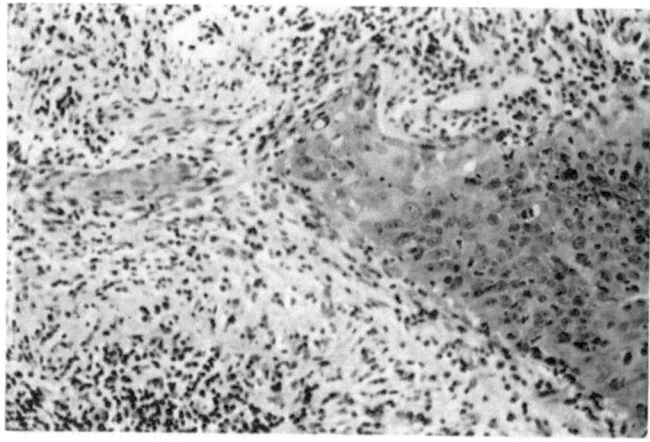

Fig. 3.12. Microcarcinoma. The tip of this downgrowth of abnormal epithelium has lost its rounded contour and become spiky, simultaneously the cells have acquired a more differentiated appearance. A group of isolated cells lies to the left of this spike. (H. & E. × 180)

early invasive carcinoma vary among different pathologists." GLÜCKSMANN and CHERRY stress the rupture of the basement membrane by invading tumour cells. HAMPERL (1959) considers that in the early stages ("early stromal invasion") the advancing tumour cells may push the basement membrane before them and even incite a new formation of the membrane, and indeed the basement membrane may be present in unquestionable cancers. GOVAN *et al.* (1966) suspect microcarcinoma when there are prolongations of abnormal epithelium into the stroma and when apparently discrete clusters of abnormal epithelial cells are seen in the stroma.

In microcarcinoma there is usually an irregular spikiness of the cell mass with fraying of the periphery and sometimes there is condensation of the collagen (Figs. 3.10. 3.12.). The invading tumour cells are often more differentiated than the rest of the epithelium.

f) The Problem of Diagnostic Consistency

It is clear from the above account that the morphological distinctions which pathologists make between the different categories of malign lesion have evolved over a period of time. Nevertheless, because the basic concept of carcinoma *in situ* is biological and not morphological, all pathologists are not agreed about the definitions. Thus, HAMPERL (1959) in a discussion on carcinoma *in situ* states, "We are not convinced that the complete lack of stratification is absolutely necessary for the diagnosis." Other workers (FLUHMANN 1961; Koss 1968; DE BRUX and DUPRÉ-FROMENT 1965; OLD *et al.* 1965) also extend the definition of carcinoma *in situ* to include lesions with surface differentiation. Not only does uncertainty with regard to the behaviour of these lesions render definition difficult but also the similarity between the cytological patterns seen in cervical smears in dysplasia and in invasive carcinoma makes some workers hesitate to draw too fine a distinction. Thus, GRUBB and JANOTA (1967) compared both the histological pattern and cytological appearances in the cervical smear in cases of severe dysplasia and invasive carcinoma and concluded that severe dysplasia should be regarded as differentiated carcinoma *in situ*. The differences in diagnostic criteria have been confirmed by SIEGLER (1956) and KIRKLAND (1963) both of whom sent sections of cervical lesions to competent histopathologists and found considerable and disturbing differences in diagnosis.

Variation in diagnostic criteria probably accounts for the wide differences in the assessment made by various workers of the proportion of malign lesions which regress. ASHLEY (1966a) has stated that the changes of carcinoma *in situ* can be identified with certainty and with a low degree of observer error by any competent histopathologist, although there may be a consistent slight variation between observers. On this assumption he compared results from different centres in his study of the biological status of carcinoma *in situ*.

ASHLEY's (1966a) contention assumes, not only that all pathologists are agreed on the histological criteria on which the diagnosis of carcinoma *in situ* is made, but also that pathologists use these criteria consistently. This second assumption has been examined by COCKER *et al.* (1968). The assessment of visual appearances, which is the basis of diagnostic histology, is rarely objective and quantitative but usually subjective and qualitative. This renders comparison between different observers difficult and between the same observers on different occasions variable. The difficulty is not peculiar to histology. The same sort of problem occurs in the comparison of radiographic changes in miners' lungs and has been discussed by FLETCHER and OLDHAM (1949, 1951), and a modification of their analytical technique was used by COCKER *et al.* (1968). Sections of the cervix were examined by a group of experienced pathologists, all working in the same laboratory and all applying the same diagnostic criteria. The lesions were graded according to the diagnostic code of Table 3.1. This code does not imply that the categories are regarded as a sequence of changes which take place in the development of carcinoma of the cervix but only that 5 is a more serious lesion than 6, and 4 more serious than 5 and so on. Two series of cases were examined. The first consisted of 28 cases, selected from the laboratory files by an independent worker, about half of which were originally diagnosed as carcinoma *in situ* and most of the others as dysplasia or borderline between dysplasia and carcinoma *in situ*. Some of the specimens were from simple cervical biopsies and others from full cone biopsies with 12 to 14 blocks cut serially.

Table 3.1. Diagnostic code

Code	Diagnosis
1.	Invasive squamous carcinoma
2.	Borderline invasion
3.	Carcinoma *in situ*
4.	Borderline carcinoma *in situ*
5.	Dysplasia
6.	Epithelial changes not amounting to dysplasia, e.g. reserve cell hyperplasia, metaplasia

These were examined by three pathologists A, B and C. The inconsistencies in diagnosis, both in comparison with the original diagnosis and between the three pathologists, were surprising, hence a simpler test based on a second series of slides was made two years later. For this second series 30 cases were selected by an independent member of the staff but only one section from each case was made available for examination. The selection of cases was more evenly divided between the diagnostic categories than in the first series. In the interval a series of photographs had been prepared of various cervical lesions and by agreement these were available as a standard of reference.

For the purpose of comparison two parameters were used, one of consistency and one of trend. In Fig. 3.13.a the original diagnosis, O, is compared with that of

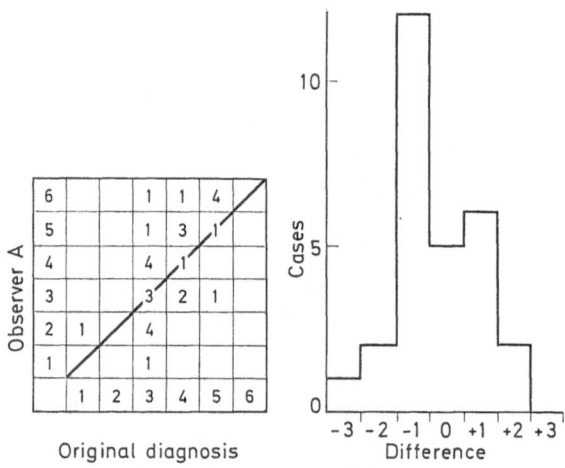

Fig. 3.13. a The numbers along the bottom are the diagnostic codes of the original diagnosis, the numbers on the left-hand side are the codes assigned by observer A, b The differences along the bottom indicate the difference between the diagnostic code originally assigned and that given by observer A. (Cocker *et al.* 1968. J. clin. Path. **21**, 67)

observer A in the first series. Each column, moving from left to right, represents
the diagnostic category originally assigned to the case by O. Similarly each row
represents the category given to the case by observer A. Thus case 1 was diagnosed
as carcinoma *in situ* by O and hence was placed in the column headed 3; similarly,
since A made the same diagnosis, it was placed in row 3. The case was therefore
scored in the square where the row and column intersect. The numbers in the
squares correspond to the numbers of cases scored in this way. If there were complete
agreement between the diagnoses of the two observers, all cases would be scored
along the diagonal. Since there was not complete agreement there is a scatter about
the diagonal. The scatter represents the inconsistency between the two observers.
This is illustrated in another way in Fig. 3.13.b. There were five cases in which O
and A agreed, this is represented by the column zero; twelve cases in which A is
one category less severe than O, this is represented by column —1; six cases in which

Table 3.2. Statistical analysis of the diagnostic comparisons

Series	Comparison	Difference of means	Variance	t	p
1	O, A	— 0.322	1.48	1.36	0.2 > 0.1
1	O, B	— 0.930	1.03	4.82	< 0.001
1	O, C	— 0.360	1.72	1.45	0.2 > 0.1
1	A, B	— 0.608	1.95	2.31	0.05 > 0.025
1	B, C	+ 0.572	2.03	2.19	0.05 > 0.025
1	C, A	+ 0.036	2.08	0.13	0.9 > 0.8
2	A_1/C_1	— 0.167	1.21	0.84	0.5 > 0.4
2	A_2/C_2	+ 0.233	1.15	1.19	0.3 > 0.2
2	A_1/A_2	— 0.267	0.34	2.51	0.02 > 0.01

The subscripts 1 and 2 in series 2 indicate the first and second set of observations by A and C,
separated by a year and a half.

A is more severe than O by one category, this is represented by column +1, and
so on. A typical cocked-hat histogram is formed with a shift to the left of zero.
This shift represents the trend of A's diagnoses compared with O and is measured
by the mean of the histogram. A narrow histogram indicates that A fairly consistently differed from O by an amount equal to the mean; a wider histogram indicates
that A is not so consistent. For the purpose of analysis the categories were regarded
as ranks and the standard deviation calculated as a measure of the width of the
histogram and thus a measure of consistency; the smaller the standard deviation the
greater the consistency, and the greater the standard deviation the less the consistency. Trend was measured by the mean of the differences of the categories
assigned to each case by the two observers, or by one observer at different times
(Table 3.2.), and consistency by the standard deviation of their differences, or more
timply, by their variances. The significance of the trend was determined using the
t-test (MATHER 1943). The results are summarized in the table.
    It can be seen that each of the observers, by and large, gave the lesions a less
serious diagnosis than the original, O. This is indicated by the negative sign of the

mean difference. This is as might be expected since in the test no clinical information
was available and there was thus no bias to regard the lesion more seriously than
was warranted objectively. B was less severe in his diagnosis than O, A or C and the
difference was statistically significant. Subsequently it transpired that at the time
when the test was being carried out B was reading papers by DE BRUX *et al.* (1961)
on the different types of dysplasia and their diagnostic criteria and this probably
influenced his judgement. Nevertheless, as judged by the spread of his histogram
(Fig. 3.14.) he was fairly consistent; indeed, probably more so than A or C.

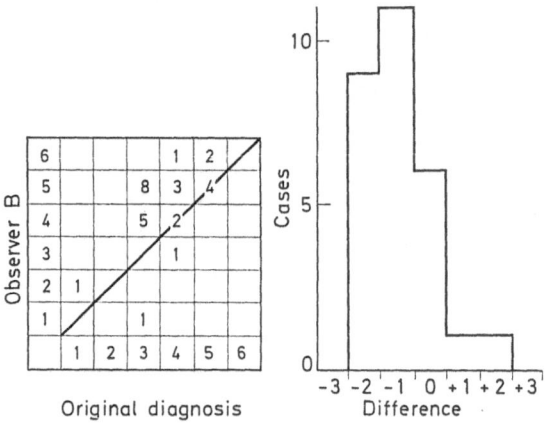

Fig. 3.14. Correlation diagram and histogram comparing the diagnoses assigned by observer B
with those made originally. (COCKER *et al.* 1968. J. clin. Path. **21**, 67)

Observation of the second series of cases was repeated after an interval of a year
and a half. On the first occasion C was less severe than A (indicated by the negative
difference between the means) and on the second occasion he was more severe. On
both occasions the difference was greater than in series 1 but still not statistically
significant. The most interesting observation is the comparison between A on the
two separate occasions. Of the 30 cases, the same diagnosis was made on both
occasions 21 times. On the second examination the diagnosis was one category less
severe in seven cases and two categories less severe in one case; only once was it
more severe. These differences are illustrated in the histogram (Fig. 3.15.). Because
the changes are mostly in one direction the differences in the means of the two series
of observations (the trend) is relatively large but the variance of the difference, as
shown by the width of the histogram, is small. Hence the difference between the two
series becomes significant. This suggests that A's diagnostic criteria had shifted in
the year and a half. This was probably because A had been collaborating with
another group of pathologists during this period in defining more precisely the
diagnostic criteria of epithelial abnormalities of the cervix.

FLETCHER and OLDHAM (1951) used standard radiographs for comparison in
their studies of pneumoconiosis and found that, although they helped the less
experienced person to be consistent, they did not help the more experienced observer.
Probably this is because the more experienced worker has a more clearly defined

mental picture of the condition than his less experienced colleague and therefore does not rely on the standard photographs. In the study of COCKER *et al.* the availability of photographs during the second series of observations did not make agreement closer between A and C, but they were both experienced histopathologists. Nevertheless their mental images of the lesions were not immutable, as illustrated by the shift in A's diagnoses.

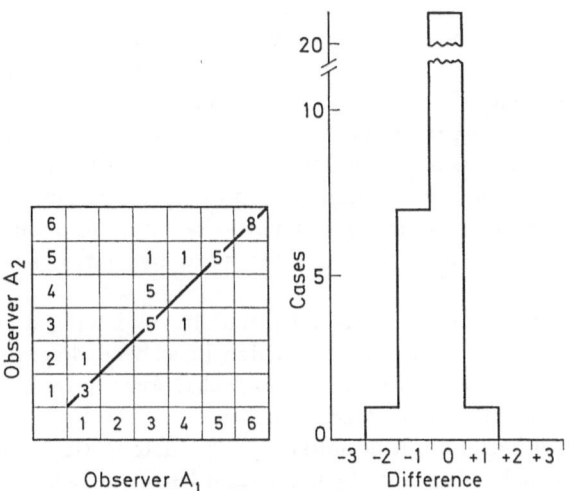

Fig. 3.15. Correlation diagram and histogram comparing the diagnoses assigned to the sections on two occasions, separated by a year and a half, by observer A. (COCKER *et al.* 1968. J. clin. Path. **21**, 67)

This technique of assessing consistency can serve two purposes. First, it can be used as a method of quality control in the training of young histopathologists. Second, it can be used to compare the diagnoses of experienced pathologists with different training backgrounds. Wider use of such a method based on an agreed set of photographs might help to reveal the differences in the usage of the various diagnostic criteria.

2. The Use of Exfoliative Cytology in the Investigation of Epithelial Abnormalities of the Cervix

In the study of cervical lesions exfoliative cytology may be used in three different ways: first, to screen populations of well women both as a prophylactic measure and to investigate the epidemiology of the lesions; second, as an investigative tool combined with colposcopy and colpomicroscopy to study the morphogenesis of these conditions (RICHART 1967); and third, to control the clinical management of the patients with malign cervical lesions. It is with the first two of these purposes that we shall be concerned here. Whilst the histological criteria for the diagnosis of epithelial abnormalities of the cervix have been considered in some detail because they form the basic patterns of reference, the cytological patterns of exfoliated cells will not be considered here. Standard text books on exfoliative cytology adequately describe the changes seen in vaginal and cervical smears although there is often some difference in detail between one authority and another. The account given by PATTEN (1969) is particularly detailed and valuable. It is, however, important to assess the degree of confidence which can be placed on cytological reports.

a) Types of Error

A recent account of the types of error which may occur in cytological diagnosis has been given by BUTLER (1973). She has pointed out that when smears are reported as "positive", "suspicious" or "negative" the *false negative* smear is one which is reported as negative in the presence of a cervical lesion but, when smears are reported in terms of disease processes, any report which underestimates the severity of the lesion is, strictly speaking, a false negative report. Likewise any report which overestimates the severity of the lesion is a *false positive* report. It should be noticed that these definitions are not the same as those used by statisticians (LUSTED 1968; ARMITAGE 1971).

The false negative rate is usually estimated by reviewing a series of cases of carcinoma *in situ* or invasive carcinoma which have been diagnosed histologically and comparing these reports with the cytological reports of the same patients. This method underestimates the error since, if the lesion cannot be seen clinically and the cytological report is negative, it is unlikely that a diagnostic biopsy will be taken. If colposcopy is available the clinically inapparent lesions may be found and biopsied and a truer index of the error rate obtained. A more accurate estimate may be available when the results of a study currently in progress at the Christie Hospital, Manchester, are published (YULE 1971). In this project a proportion of the women taking part in a population screening programme are recalled for a second smear three months after taking the initial smear. Assuming that very few women will have developed a malign lesion in the three-month interval, any positive smears found on the second examinations will be a measure of the false negative rate.

The false positive rate is more easily estimated since any positive smear needs further investigation by repeating the smear, by colposcopic or colpomicroscopic assessment or by biopsy and histological examination. Cytology is a very sensitive, though perhaps not a specific test, and sometimes routine evaluation of a cone biopsy may fail to reveal a lesion although the smear is positive because the atypical focus is extremely small. NICHOLS et al. (1968) found that they were able to recognise 17% more lesions when the cervix was examined by step serial sections. Such a procedure is tedious and not practicable in a routine laboratory.

False negative rates are usually given with respect to the diagnosis of carcinoma *in situ*. The values given by various authors differ surprisingly, from 1.4% (RICHART 1964) to 28% (ACHENBACH et al. 1951) but in most laboratories the range is from 6 to 13%. The low figure recorded by RICHART was derived from a series of patients followed under research conditions by colpomicroscopy. BUTLER (1973) has discussed the various usages of the term false negative and false positive and illustrated them by her experience in St. Mary's Hospital, Manchester, for the year 1969, in a laboratory with a work load of approximately 15,000 smears per annum. If false negative is understood to mean that the smears were completely negative, 2% of smears were negative from 152 cases with histologically proven malign lesions; but if an underestimation of the disease process is included in this category, the false negative rate rises to 13%. In the same way the frequency of false positive reports might be given as 0 or 9.0% depending on whether positive is used in the sense of Papanicolaou Class V or in the sense of overestimation of the severity of the lesion. OSTERGARD and GONDOS (1971) investigated a group of patients with known normal cytological smears but with abnormal colposcopic findings. In each case a biopsy was taken from the most abnormal site and examined histologically. Of 100 patients, 96 were negative both cytologically and histologically, three had mild and one mild to moderate dysplasia. The cytological false negative rate was therefore 4%.

When the results between different centres are compared, it is important to remember that both the cytological and the histological criteria between the centres may vary and, of course, they may vary within one centre from time to time. This is of particular importance in population studies which may extend over more than a decade, since it is probable that there has been a change of personnel making the diagnosis. EVANS (1970) conducted an investigation into the screening error rates between different centres. A batch of 100 cervical smears was sent to each of five leading cytology centres and compared with the assessment made in Cardiff based on all available relevant information including follow-up and histology. The diagnoses were graded in a rather similar manner to that of COCKER *et al.* (1968): normal, atypical (inflammatory), dyskaryotic, suspicious of malignancy and positive. There was considerable variation between the centres; centre 1 agreeing most closely with the Cardiff assessment, and centre 5 agreeing least. In centre 1, there was agreement in 67 cases but 22 were regarded as more severely affected than the Cardiff assessment, indeed four smears were regarded as suspicious or positive although Cardiff regarded them as normal. Eleven cases were regarded as less severely affected than the Cardiff assessment. In centre 5, although there as agreement with Cardiff in 68 cases, 27 were regarded as less severely affected and 10 cases as more severely affected. The estimated false negative rate for centre 1 was 3%, and for centre 5 it was 13%; the false positive rates were 3% and 26% respectively.

In none of the population studies considered in the next chapter is there evidence that an attempt was made to control or assess these errors of interpretation.

Major errors may also be introduced into cytological diagnosis by unsatisfactory methods of collecting specimens and inadequate control of the mode of screening the smears.

b) The Collection of Specimens

A cytological examination may be erroneous or even fruitless if the smear is badly taken or poorly spread. Undoubtedly the best preparations are made when the person taking the smear also examines it. This is rarely possible and a variety of types of people take smears ranging from gynaecologists and family doctors to nurses and midwives. It is important that whoever takes and spreads the smear should be properly trained.

Studies have been made in a number of centres, comparing smears prepared from aspirates of the vaginal fornices and cervical scrapes. MILLER and VON HAAM (1961) examined 361 sets of slides from 238 proven cases of uterine malignancy. The slides were from parallel aspirate and scrape smears. In 30% of these examinations the vaginal aspirate was unsatisfactory, negative or atypical whereas the scraping, taken at the same time, was suspicious or positive. This superiority of the cervical scraping was seen in all types of uterine cancer with the exception of adenocarcinoma of the endometrium where the two techniques were equally accurate. BREDAHL and LEFEVRE (1965) found that of 120 cases in which abnormal cells were demonstrated, 89% showed abnormal cells in the cervical as well as vaginal smears, while 8% had abnormal cells only in the cervical and 3% only in the vaginal smears. They comment that this superiority of the cervical smear is in keeping with the results of others (CUYLER et al. 1951; SLATE et al. 1953; MESSELT 1955 and SONG et al. 1959). MILLER and VON HAAM (1961) pointed out that from a practical point of view factors other than the relative accuracy of the two techniques must be considered. The simplicity and ease of taking a vaginal aspirate make it suitable for use in mass screening, especially by non-medical personnel when the cervix cannot be visualized by the use of a speculum. Contrariwise, under favourable circumstances both vaginal aspirates and cervical scrapes should be examined. FROST (1969) advocates the use of a combined vaginal pool smear, cervical scrape and endocervical aspirate.

Because of the difficulties of collecting smears in some populations, attempts have been made to devise a self-administered test which could be performed at home by the women who would then send the specimen to a central laboratory. Ideally, no further training would be needed for the technician in processing or in interpretation. Two techniques approach this ideal, the Draghi tampon and Davis irrigation smear. The Draghi tampon samples the cells in the vaginal pool and the cervix (BRUNSCHWIG 1954; NIEBURGS 1956; BADER et al. 1957; SCOTT et al. 1957). Although a woman can insert it herself, she has to remove the tampon at a collection centre because it requires immediate processing on removal. RICHART and VAILLANT (1965) have summarized the additional problems that arise. (1) 7% of the women could not insert the tampon unaided. (2) The optimum wearing time was one to two hours which is a rather short time between home insertion and clinic removal. (3) Smears were often difficult to interpret because of a histiocytic response to the tampon or because of cellular degeneration. (4) The false negative rates were approximately 25%, tending to be higher in carcinoma *in situ* and dysplasia than in invasive carcinoma.

The irrigation smear was developed by DAVIS (1962a and b). It utilizes a disposable plastic container and pipette, containing a cell preservative for irrigating the upper vagina and cervix. After ejection into the vagina the fluid is aspirated back into the container and mailed to the laboratory. BREDAHL et al. (1965) compared an irrigation smear taken on the day of admission of the patient with a cervical scraping and vaginal pool smear taken the next day. All the smears were taken by physicians. The irrigation smears were examined in a laboratory where the technicians were familiar with this technique, the other smears were examined in a second laboratory and histological evaluation carried out in a third laboratory. Five hundred and fifty consecutive gynaecological patients were reviewed. Nine cases of *in-situ* carcinoma, 16 cases of invasive carcinoma of the cervix and 6 cases of endometrial carcinoma were found. With the irrigation smear, one invasive cervical carcinoma and one endometrial carcinoma were not recognized. With the cervical scrape, two *in-situ* carcinomas and two endometrial carcinomas were missed. The corresponding figures for the vaginal pool smear were five cases of carcinoma *in situ* missed, one invasive carcinoma and three cases of endometrial carcinoma. Thus the irrigation smear and cervical scrape yielded similar results, both being superior to the aspiration smears.

RICHART and VAILLANT (1965) carried out a valuable study of the use of the irrigation smear. At the end of each clinic visit the patient was handed an irrigation-smear mailing kit together with a sheet of instructions. The instructions directed the patients to complete the identification form and to take the test one week after the next menstrual period had stopped. Two hundred and seventy-four examinations were performed with the irrigation smear, of these only 172 (this is 63%) were adequate for diagnosis. Of the other 37%, five pipettes were cracked and empty, nine were returned without a name, twenty-seven were unsatisfactory because of degenerated cells and in sixty-one the cell population on the slide was too low. In these latter cases the cause was probably the patients' inadequate irrigation technique; many of the pipettes were returned half full without any cellular sediment. The 172 satisfactory smears were reviewed. The false negative rate for presumptive carcinoma *in situ* and occult invasive carcinoma was 50%. For cases in which the diagnosis was histologically proved the false negatives constituted 39%, and for presumptive dysplasia 51%. These figures are difficult to reconcile with the Danish series, see BREDAHL *et al.* (1965). However, it should be remembered that physicians took the Danish smears and the patients themselves those in RICHART's and VAILLANT's series. The poor irrigation results are comparable with those of vaginal-pool aspirations. BREDAHL *et al.* (1965) commented on the different appearances of smears obtained by cervical scraping and by irrigation. In the irrigation smear the abnormal cells often lie singly in contrast to the multicellular strands of such cells in cervical scrapings. There are also some differences in staining. BREDAHL and colleagues recorded that a cytologist having many years of experience in evaluating cervical scrapings but who had not previously seen irrigation smears failed to detect one third of the malignancies presented by this method. It is possible that lack of previous experience of screening irrigation smears might in part account for the different results of RICHART and VAILLANT, who also commented on the differences in appearance of irrigation and conventional smears.

ANDERSON and GUNN (1965) investigated the irrigation smear in an out-patient clinic serving a low social class population in Miami. 57% of women used and returned the kit. The results were not as good as those of scrape smears. DAVIS (1962a) reporting on population screening in Maryland, found the irrigation smear was not as good as the scrape but it compared favourably with the aspiration smear. However in a later study DAVIS and JONES (1969) found irrigation smears as accurate as scrapes.

c) Screening and Checking

At the level of screening and checking quality control exerts a very significant influence. Fundamentally the value of the service is determined by the screeners. They must be carefully trained either in their own laboratory or at a training school. The quality of their work subsequently depends on their continued education by those who check the work, be they other cytotechnologists (checkers), cytologists or pathologists. The quality of this checking procedure may depend on personal relations and certainly on the training the supervisors have received. It is also important that cytology laboratories do not in-breed too much, otherwise errors of interpretation are apt to develop and be perpetuated.

It is customary to check all the suspicious or malignant smears that a screener records. It is more important and more difficult to check the negative smears. KLIONSKY and COHEN (1971) have described a comprehensive method for the random selection of smears which eliminates possible bias by the reviewer.

A detailed consideration of quality control is outside the scope of this monograph, but it must be emphasized that without adequate surveillance of all the stages involved in collecting material, processing it and reading the stained smear the results of population studies are valueless, however large the sample. The basic principles of quality control have been enunciated by WIED (1965), and WEAVER and LA PUENTE (1964) have shown how sequential analysis may be applied to certain aspects of quality control of vaginal cytology.

d) Recall in Cytological Screening

In a cytology screening programme recall of patients is necessary for three reasons: first, in the women's own interest continuous surveillance is desirable throughout the cancer-prone period of life; second, to assess the extent of false negative smears, as discussed above, and third, to determine the incidence of the lesions encountered. The incidence of any condition, as distinct from the prevalence, is the number of new cases occurring in a year. This is estimated (see Chapter 4) by recall of previously screened women.

The structure of the population of women initially screened in a large study often differs significantly from that of the overall population of the region with regard to both social class and age structure. Thus in the Manchester Region, WAKEFIELD (1971) has shown that among the women examined there is an excess of women in the more favoured socio-economic classes and a deficiency of those in the less favoured. Moreover, among women smeared at family planning clinics there is a relative excess of younger women and among those attending local health authority clinics an excess of older women. WAKEFIELD found that about 54% of women responded to postal recall and that the response varied little with social class. The similarity of structure of the initial and recall populations makes estimation of incidence relatively simple in this instance but this comparison of the two groups is necessary in all properly conducted population surveys.

It is interesting and important to note the sort of things that can prevent a patient accepting an invitation to recall: anxiety caused by delay in reporting the first test, an over-hearty brushing off of personal worries and some small disregard of personal dignity on the part of the receptionist. WAKEFIELD has discussed these psychological factors with great lucidity and it can readily be seen how disregard of them may distort an otherwise carefully planned investigation.

3. Colposcopy

In this section an attempt is made to indicate the indispensible value of the colposcope in the study of cervical epithelial abnormalities, especially in relation to morphogenesis. The historical background to the development and early evaluation of colposcopy is well described by NAVRATIL (1964).

The beginnings of colposcopy date back to the time when HINSELMANN was working in the gynaecological clinic of VON FRANQUÉ in Bonn. He had reasoned that the earliest symptomless stages of carcinoma of the cervix were represented by tiny tumours or ulcers which were not usually detected by the clinical methods then in use, namely digital palpation and speculum examination. Starting with a modified head lamp system he went on to devise the colposcope (HINSELMANN 1925) which basically consisted of a binocular stereoscopic low-power microscope with a powerful source of illumination and an object-to-lens distance sufficiently great to enable the instrument to be used several centimetres away from the vulva. Standard colposcopes now in use, e.g. the Zeiss instrument, have magnifications between 6 and 40 diameters, changeable light filters, an object-to-lens distance of 20 centimetres together with facilities for photography and an observer's tube.

HINSELMANN found that although asymptomatic small invasive cancers could be detected earlier than by traditional examination techniques other changes were often present on the cervix which fell short of invasive cancer. He devised a rather complicated numerical coding system (Hinselmann's Rubrics) which correlated the colposcopic findings with the histological appearances.

In the two decades after its introduction, colposcopy was adopted into gynaecological practice in many of the German-speaking areas of Europe, sometimes as a screening technique before cytology had yet made any impact and at a time when potentially malignant epithelial lesions were being investigated and better understood by pathologists. CRAMER (1956), NAVRATIL (1964), MESTWERDT and WESPI (1961) and GANSE (1963) amongst others have published extensively on colposcopy. In France interest is more recent but significant contributions, including a monograph, have been made by BRET and COUPEZ (1960). In the United States RIES (1932) and MARTZLOFF (1932) reported on colposcopy though the latter's long-term experiences were disappointing (1955). A more recent revival of interest is seen in the papers of SCHEFFEY et al. (1955), LANG (1957), BOLTEN (1960), OLSON and NICHOLS (1960, 1961), BELLER (1966), ORTIZ et al. (1969) and TOWNSEND et al. (1970). The work of COPPLESON and his colleagues from Australia is referred to in this volume, and their own books contain a wealth of information on colposcopy and its application to the study of cervical epithelial abnormalities. Colposcopy has been used in some centres in Great Britain but not in any consistent fashion until the last six or seven years.

The *colpomicroscope* is fundamentally different from the colposcope and was developed in Vienna for the examination of cells *in situ* on the surface of the cervix. The work of PICK (1937) and VONWILLER (1947) was taken up by ANTOINE and GRUENBERGER who developed a more practical apparatus which was introduced into gynaecological practice in 1949. In this technique cell nuclei are stained *in situ* by the surface application of toluidine blue and the tissue is then examined at a magnification of about 180 diameters. A variety of physiological and pathological changes are illustrated in ANTOINE and GRUENBERGER's atlas (1956). It is worth noting that though cell nuclei are only stained to a depth of two or three layers, cells from the basal regions are swept up towards the surface at those points where the stromal papillae protrude into the epithelium. The use of the colpomicroscope in studying the process of transformation and the diagnosis of cervical atypia has been discussed by WALZ (1955, 1961), ETON and VINCE (1961) and KAUFMANN et al.

(1962), whilst RICHART (1965, 1966) has found it a valuable tool in studying the distribution of dysplasia and carcinoma *in situ*.

a) Colposcopic Appearances and Terminology

The colposcopist studies the topographical appearances of the cervix which reflect the nuclear richness of the epithelium and the type and arrangement of the underlying vasculature. The former can usually be enhanced by the application of acetic acid (a 2% aqueous solution is adequate) and the latter by the use of a green filter, especially if the cervix is only cleaned with normal saline initially. KOLLER (1963) has made a special study of the vessels and finds that by measuring the inter-capillary distance and noting the type of vessels he can closely correlate the observed changes with the histology of the overlying epithelium. It is usual to combine an initial assessment of the vessels with the enhancement of topographical detail which follows the application of dilute acetic acid. Finally SCHILLER's test is used to judge the degree of glycogenation of the tissues.

Table 3.3. Types of colposcopic appearances

Benign findings (see Fig. 2.17)
Original epithelium (native squamous epithelium)
Ectopy (native columnar epithelium)
Typical transformation zone
Colpitis (vagino-cervicitis)
Unremarkable Schiller-positive zones (inconspicuous iodine non-staining areas)
Polyps
Condyloma acuminatum
Atypical findings (see Fig. 3.16)
Atypical transformation zone
        mosaic patterns: fine and coarse
        ground patterns: fine and papillary
Leukoplakia
Adaptive vascular hypertrophy
Niveau differences
Atypical red area
Erosio vera

In our clinic we have adopted an overall clinical colposcopic grouping. There are four categories: *benign*, e.g. typical transformation zone; *low index* of suspicion, e.g. atypical transformation zone in which the maximum abnormality is fine mosaic patterning; *high index* of suspicion, e.g. an atypical transformation zone with areas of papillary ground and early adaptive vascular hypertrophy; and finally, *cancer* which is used for unequivocal evidence of cervical cancer, e.g. niveau differences, and adaptive vascular hypertrophy. This grouping is used as a guide to the clinician in interpreting the colposcopic reports, so that a low index indicates no more than a mild to moderate degree of dysplasia and high index indicates a diagnosis of severe dysplasia or carcinoma *in situ* (Table 3.3. and Fig. 3.16.).

COPPLESON and REID (1967) divide their cases of atypical transformation zone into three grades: I, II, III. These are also arrived at by a consideration of the epithelial patterns and vascular architecture of the cervix. The grade I cases are those where minor atypia are found, and grades II and III are the cases of more marked dysplasia and carcinoma *in situ*.

Original epithelium is the smooth pink squamous epithelium extending from the vagina to the original squamo-columnar junction and which is well glycogenated in the mature woman. After the menopause the cervical epithelium thins and becomes less glycogenated, though this is not always a uniform process and is often more marked on the posterior lip of the cervix.

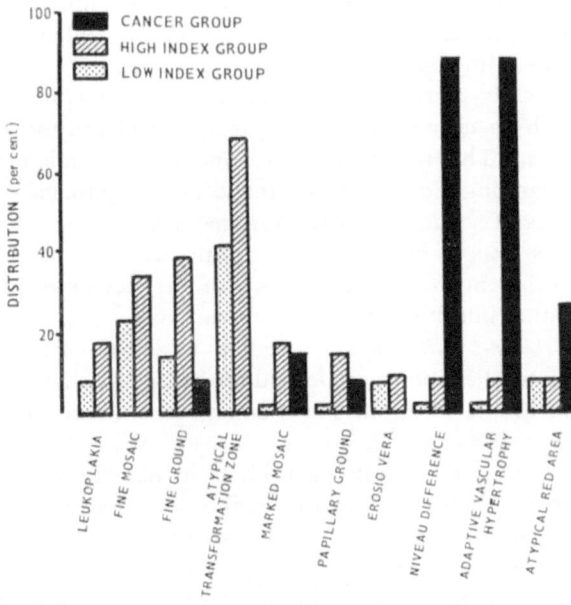

Fig. 3.16. This diagram correlates the colposcopic assessment of malignancy with the various types of colposcopic appearances in cases seen in St. Mary's Hospital, Manchester (CROMPTON, 1971)

Ectopy FLUHMANN (1961) described the complex arrangement of primary and secondary clefts in the endocervix, noting that in the lower half of these areas stromal papillae are present covered by a single layer of columnar cells. When present on the ectocervix they give it a velvety feel and the area looks much redder than squamous epithelium because the blood vessels in the papillae shine through the much thinner cellular covering. As extensive areas of "ectopy" have been noted on the cervix of the foetus, newborn and young adolescent, and during and after pregnancy, it might be argued that "ectopy" is not strictly an accurate term but it is a clearly understood and distinctive word widely used by colposcopists. The red appearance has led to the persistence of ideas of infection associated with the clinical term "erosion", a loosely defined word embracing all red areas on the cervix including "ectopy". NAVRATIL (1964) uses the term erythroplakia in place of erosion. Application of acetic acid causes pallor of the papillae and exaggerates the villous appearance producing the typical "Träubchen" of the German literature.

The typical transformation zone. The changing pH in the vagina was the factor held responsible for precipitating squamous metaplasia by HINSELMANN and this was confirmed by WALZ (1958) and supported by COPPLESON and REID (1967).

The first sign of the formation of the transformation zone is an increased cloudiness and whitening of the "villi" and the next stage is their adherence or clumping. They form agglomerations or, more usually, ridges. Squamous metaplasia occurs on the surface and, though isolated patches of new epithelium are seen, most areas develop or possess a continuity with the periphery. The process of transformation, if it continues, leads to the covering of the previous area of ectopy with squamous epithelium, though small openings may be left leading into persistent columnar-lined spaces. If these become closed off then Nabothian follicles are formed. This new squamous epithelium becomes well glycogenated in the typical transformation zone but can be clearly distinguished from the original epithelium by its more violaceous colour, by a change in vascular pattern and the indicators of residual glandular epithelium. The transformation zone is *the* fundamentally important concept in understanding how most of the cervical epithelial abnormalities are formed. The process of squamous metaplasia may take place quite rapidly and it is possible that at this time of active metaplasia spermatozoa (as suggested by REID 1965), viruses or other micro-organisms may be phagocytosed, producing another kind of transformation but this time at the cellular level.

Unremarkable Schiller-positive zones. This refers to zones which may be just about discernible after the application of acetic acid but stand out sharply after the application of SCHILLER's iodine solution. These zones are not sinister and histologically show mild hyperkeratosis or parakeratosis.

Condyloma acuminatum may look disturbing on naked-eye examination of the cervix but colposcopy shows a regularity in the vessels which, though frequently prominent, differ from those in adaptive vascular hypertrophy.

Atypical transformation zones contain nuclear-rich epithelium which whitens on the application of acetic acid as well as taking up the Schiller's iodine stain only lightly or not at all. The underlying stroma is intimately involved in the development of atypical epithelium and one indicator of this is the way that atypical vessels and atypical vascular arrangements occur. We favour using the term "atypical transformation zone" to embrace those cases in which mosaic, ground and leukoplakic areas occur. These latter terms are sometimes grouped together as the matrix areas. Mosaic patterns are produced by the intercalation of stromal bridges containing prominent vascular networks into the nuclear-rich epithelium. Fine areas of mosaic may show no more than the most minor atypia in squamous metaplastic epithelium. The cobblestone-like appearance of coarse mosaic patterns is often characteristic of severe dysplasia and carcinoma *in situ*. Similarly, ground patterns represent minor atypia in their finer forms and severer epithelial atypia in their coarser or papillary forms. Leukoplakia, in the colposcopic sense, refers to raised whitened areas of hyperkeratosis and, when at all extensive, detachment of this layer often reveals an underlying ground or mosaic pattern. Such areas should be examined histologically.

Erosio vera is a complete lack of surface epithelium and may well be traumatically produced by the insertion of a speculum, especially if a brisk inflammatory reaction or a severe epithelial abnormality is present as such epithelia are rather loosely attached to the underlying stroma. The term *atypical red area* sounds rather imprecise but in practice is a necessary small category. Biopsy usually shows that these areas are due to stromal inflammation.

Niveau differences are changes in the regularity of the surface easily detectable under the stereoscopic view of the colposcope and characteristically seen in invasive cancer and sessile papillomata.

As mentioned earlier, the colposcope enables the direct visualization of the terminal capillaries in the cervical epithelium and this can be enhanced by using a green filter or by MAJEWSKI's test, the surface application of a dilute noradrenaline solution (MAJEWSKI 1960).

b) The Vascular Patterns of Cervical Abnormalities

JOHN HUNTER noted an abnormal and apparently increased vascular pattern in malignant tumours over 150 years ago. THIERSCH described tumour vessels in detail in a monograph in 1865 and there have been numerous studies related to this subject since that time. Tumour capillaries were noted by RIBBERT (1904) and GOLDMANN (1908) to be variable in size and abnormal in that they do not show the regular tree-like branching which characterizes normal vessels. Considerable interest in vascular problems has been shown in Oslo by KREYBERG in 1929 and more recently by KOLLER and KOLSTAD (1962, 1963, 1964). KREYBERG (1929) conducted experiments on white mice using a tar derivative and stressed the changes produced in the vessels (e.g., telangiectasia) as well as an apparent increase in their numbers. More recently KERN and ZANDER (1959) described the vessel changes leading up to the experimental production of tumours when using methylcholanthrene to paint the ears of mice. CLARK and CLARK (1939) found that hypoxia of a particular degree and duration was a principal stimulus to the growth of vascular endothelium.

Thus it can be seen that originally workers were impressed by the abnormal vessels observed within the substance of established tumours. The experimental induction of tumours led to observations on pre-invasive lesions in which vessel changes were found to be prominent. Apart from directly applied chemicals, physiologists have shown that oxygen levels played an important part in stimulating the growth of vascular endothelium. The capillary patterns of the cervix can thus be seen to be important to the colposcopist because vascular as well as epithelial changes reflect abnormalities in a tissue prior to the development of tumours.

Hinselmann's term *adaptive vascular hypertrophy* (1940) describes the newly formed vessels which become visible in association with severe epithelial atypia and which become more marked when early invasion occurs. Examples are cork-screw, hair-needle (GANSE) and giant capillaries (CHIARI). The apparent increase in the vascular supply to a malignant tumour does not prove to be substantiated at the tissue level. Using reconstruction models prepared from the normal cervix and cervical squamous cancer SUGIHARA is reported as showing that, though the tumour stroma contains more blood vessels, the tumour itself contains fewer (1958).

Vessels in the atypical transformation zone. GANSE (1958) described several types of terminal capillary loop in ground patterns. They varied from simple loops in fine ground to glomerular arrangements in papillary ground. In the latter he recognized varicosities and secondary loops leading to a so-called "Knäuel" or ball of wool appearance. Kos (1961) considered the mosaic appearance to be the result of the atypical growth of blood vessels. Detailed work by KOLSTAD (1964) showed that the inter-capillary distance tended to increase as the degree of epithelial atypia increased. There are similarities between the types of vessel change observed colposcopically in the more severe epithelial atypia and those produced experimentally in animals. KOLSTAD showed that the relatively avascular areas in tumours have indeed a lower tissue oxygen tension than neighbouring areas, and COPPLESON and REID (1967) have speculated on the possible importance of similar gradients for immunological factors. The evidence available suggests that the atypia in the vessels is a reflection of the same carcinogenic influence that causes the epithelial abnormality.

c) The Clinical Application of Colposcopy

Colposcopy has been used as a screening technique together with cytology in some centres for over twenty years and, used in this way, it has been shown to increase the "pick-up" rate for cervical atypia when compared with the results achieved with colposcopy or cytology separately (NAVRATIL et al. 1958). COPPLESON and REID (1967) have emphasized that these two techniques are complementary but go on to say that it is debatable which method is the more valuable. As a population screening method colposcopy requires far more specially trained gynaecologists than there appears any likelihood of obtaining in the foreseeable future. We agree with the opinion of COPPLESON and REID (1967) that accurate results with colposcopy are very dependent on the experience of the examiner. Colposcopy is most readily employed in an out-patient clinic set aside for the examination of patients with atypical smears or clinically unusual-looking cervices. Used in this way, it has the following advantages:

  a) It allows accurate localization of the abnormal area.
  b) A good estimate can be made of the histological change present.
  c) Adequate tissue sampling can often be provided by directed (target) biopsies.
  d) Some unnecessary biopsies will be avoided.
  e) Management and further observation can be planned in a more logical fashion.

It is obvious to the colposcopist that his technique allows the ready display of the great majority of transformation zones. The everting effect on the endocervix of opening a vaginal bivalve speculum can be appreciated by any gynaecologist. PRZYBORA and PLUTOWA (1959) examined 100 cervices showing carcinoma in situ and, after allowing for tissue fixation and distortion, they estimated that in only two cases would they have considered that no atypia were visible to the colposcopist. Nevertheless, it must be emphasised that there is a small group of patients in whom the transformation zone and the actual squamo-columnar junction are entirely out of view. This small group includes women who have already had some form of surgical intervention, such as a Manchester repair operation, and some patients after cone biopsy or diathermization of the cervix. Knowing the extent of a lesion will obviously influence management. If there is a large atypical transformation zone with marked mosaic or papillary ground patterns spreading off the cervix on to the vaginal fornices then treatment will be very different from those cases with small areas of fine mosaic or ground restricted to the cervix. ANDERSON and LINTON (1967) compared the diagnostic accuracy of cervical punch biopsy and conization (without using colposcopy) in a series of women with abnormal smears. In 49 of their patients in whom punch biopsy had been benign, 19 (39%) had pre-invasive or invasive carcinoma on cone biopsy. Of 81 patients with a punch biopsy diagnosis of carcinoma *in situ*, 12 had invasive changes. BELLER and KHATAMEE (1966) and BOLTEN (1967), amongst others, have reported that colposcopy and target biopsies provide an accurate assessment of patients with abnormal Ayre's smears. ORTIZ *et al.* (1969) examined 147 patients with no obvious clinical cervical abnormality yet with class III or IV smears. Colposcopically guided biopies followed by cone biopsy or hysterectomy, 4 to 16 weeks later, revealed only 4 patients (3%) with a significantly more advanced lesion than had been predicted initially, and in only one case did this amount to carcinoma *in situ*. No invasive cancers were found. TOWNSEND *et al.* (1970) adopted a rather different approach in examining 76 patients with persistently abnormal smears. They compared colposcopically directed biopsies and endocervical canal curettage with subsequent cone biopsies. If no histological abnormality was found in the endocervical curettings, then colposcopically directed biopsies provided a good assessment compared with cone biopsy, but the presence of any epithelial abnormality on curettage strongly indicated cone biopsy. It has long been routine practice in some colposcopic clinics, e.g. that of NAVRATIL in Graz, to perform outpatient endocervical curettage if the upper limits of an atypical transformation zone cannot be visualized. Though recognizing the place for endocervical curettage, we tend to perform this rather infrequently unless the patient has symptoms, e.g. abnormal bleeding, and, if visualization has not been satisfactory, we prefer diagnostic cone biopsy.

We have found that colposcopy and directed biopsy fail to detect any abnormality in approximately 5% of women with abnormal smears. If no adequate explanation for the abnormal smear is found and further smears remain abnormal, we perform endometrial curettage and diagnostic cone biopsy. A small series of cases from our own clinic are analysed in Table 3.4.

Thus some reduction in the numbers of cone biopsies required for diagnosis can be made by the use of colposcopically directed biopsies, although conization may well be the preferred method of treatment in an individual case. COPPLESON *et al.* (1971) have found also a good correlation between the colposcopic appearances and histology in patients with doubtful cervical smears.

Table 3.4. Comparison of colposcopically directed biopsies and cone biopsies in forty-two patients with abnormal smears

Cone histology	Histology on directed punch biopsy				
	Agreement	Slight over-estimate	Slight under-estimate	Missed diagnosis	Abnormality removed by punch
Benign	3	—	—	—	1
Mild/moderate dysplasia	11	1	3	—	—
Severe dysplasia, carcinoma in situ	18	—	3	2	—
Total	32 (76%)	1 (2.5%)	6 (14%)	2 (5%)	1 (2.5%)

Many cervical appearances which seem clinically to be suspicious can readily be seen colposcopically to be no more than benign changes, e.g. "erosion" is often no more than a benign ectopy or transformation zone, especially when these zones are particularly prominent in patients on the "pill" or during pregnancy. These patients can be spared unnecessary biopsies.

d) Colposcopy and the Management of Patients with Cervical Atypia

Having delineated an epithelial abnormality, assessed its nature and severity, confirmed this by biopsy from the most atypical area, and having taken into account the age, marital status, desire of the patient for further pregnancies and the presence or absence of abnormal bleeding or other genital disease, it becomes possible to plan a logical campaign of treatment. At one end of the spectrum there are slightly atypical transformation zones with changes amounting to no more than minimally atypical squamous metaplasia. In such patients annual follow-up without treatment is adequate and a similar policy may be followed with most cases of mild dysplasia. The patient's age must modify the treatment in cases of severe dysplasia and carcinoma *in situ*. Such changes found in a young nulliparous and possibly promiscuous girl require local therapy with a minimum of residual cervical damage.

Electrocoagulation has been considered to act as prophylaxis against the later development of cancer of the cervix (PEMBERTON and SMITH 1929). BOUDA and DOH-NAL (1965) reviewed 13 series in which 94,072 patients had been subjected to electro-coagulation; in these women only 12 cases of cervical cancer were known to have developed and in 7 of these there was probably already persisting early cancer. They observed that after electrocoagulation the squamo-columnar junction is commonly found within the endocervical canal three to five years earlier than occurs physiologi-cally. Amongst 206 cases of carcinoma of the uterine cervix, 15 of their patients had a past history of cervical cauterization and in most cases the tumour had developed within the canal. They felt that cauterization of the cervix was of much less value in the prevention of carcinoma of the cervix than has been claimed in the literature.

Electrodiathermy can be used in the treatment of cervical epithelial atypia if these areas are small, if their extent is clearly visible colposcopically and if a punch biopsy is first taken for histological control. With very small areas the punch biopsy alone may suffice. RICHART and SCIARRA (1968) consider that electrocoagulation is often an effective treatment for mild to moderate dysplasia, and COPPLESON *et al.* (1971) frequently treat mild dysplasias by electrodiathermy.

Recently TOWNSEND and OSTERGARD (1971) have used cryosurgery as the sole means of therapy in 95 patients with pre-invasive cervical neoplasia, the majority (43) being cases of severe dysplasia or carcinoma *in situ* (19). Preliminary evaluation procedures included cytology, colposcopy, endocervical curettage and colpo-scopically directed biopsies. They considered cryosurgery was effective in 90% of their patients and that its reliability was partly determined by the ability of the surgeon to control the depth of tissue destruction so that deeper-lying gland clefts can be treated. Apart from a heavy watery discharge, morbidity was minimal despite the fact that the technique was used as an out-patient procedure. They warn that the management of pre-invasive cervical neoplasia should only be attempted by those experienced in adequate pre-treatment evaluation techniques.

In the particular problem posed by finding cervical atypia in the young nulliparous woman conservative management should be employed. In those cases where colposcopy and punch biopsy are deemed adequate for diagnosis, electrocoagulation or possible cryotherapy seems to be the proper approach, with the proviso that every effort should be made to maintain an adequate follow-up.

Increasing use of colposcopy will alter the approach to the diagnosis and management of cervical epithelial atypia, and it has been the aim of this section to draw attention to some of the ways in which it may be of practical help to the clinician. The ways in which colposcopy can assist research with the problem of the morphogenesis of these lesions is touched on elsewhere in the text.

Chapter 4

The Natural History of Malign Lesions of the Cervix Uteri

The morphological distinctions which have been drawn between the various cervical lesions just described in chapter 3 will have their ultimate validation if they are shown to correspond to differences in biological behaviour. Up to the present no laboratory test of this behaviour has been devised and thus the final arbiter is a careful correlation of morphology and natural history. However, this correlation presents difficulties and uncertainties some of which will be explored in the following paragraphs.

1. The Model

There is broad general agreement with the concept that invasive carcinoma may be a sequel to carcinoma *in situ* which is itself a sequel to dysplasia, but there is much uncertainty about the details of this sequence. The diagram (Fig. 4.1.) illustrates the current views and indicates some of the diverse possibilities.

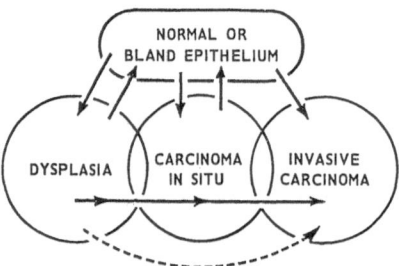

Fig. 4.1. Model illustrating the probable relationships between the various abnormalities of cervical epithelium

Normal squamous epithelium of the cervix or, more probably, epithelium showing bland abnormalities can become dysplastic or proceed directly to carcinoma *in situ* or invasive carcinoma. Dysplasia may progress to carcinoma *in situ* and then to invasive carcinoma but dysplasia or carcinoma *in situ* may regress before invasion occurs, the epithelium returning to "normal". The extent to which regression occurs and the duration of each phase of the sequence is uncertain. It is probable that dysplasia may occasionally progress directly to invasive carcinoma by-passing the carcinoma *in-situ* phase. The overlapping areas in the diagram indicate that two lesions may be present simultaneously.

The evidence in support of the sequential relationship of the phases is briefly as follows.

a) Morphological Evidence

According to McKay (GRAHAM *et al.* 1962) carcinoma *in situ* is found at the margin of invasive cancer of the cervix in 60 to 75% of cases. This is especially so if the neoplasm is small, but when invasion occurs over a wide area the *in-situ* lesion may not be seen. Clearly, all invasive carcinomas must initially be *in-situ* before breaking through the basement membrane but the suggestion is that in the cervix, in a large proportion of cases, the *in-situ* lesion is not just a small focus but covers a relatively large territory. Moreover, a similar association between an *in-situ* lesion and an invasive lesion may sometimes be seen in the vulva (ABEL and GOSLING 1961) and in the bladder (SCHADE and SWINNEY 1968). It is possible, of course, as GRAHAM *et al.* (1962) point out that the invasive tumour may induce the change in the adjacent tissue because occasionally *in-situ* carcinoma is found in the squamous epithelium next to an adenocarcinoma. Dysplasia and carcinoma *in situ* also often co-exist and indeed in one cervix it is sometimes possible to see dysplasia, carcinoma *in situ* and invasive carcinoma.

The atypical non-invasive zones around invasive cervical carcinoma have been discussed by BAJARDI (1961 b) and others in a written symposium. In this symposium TAYLOR (1961) pointed out that the epithelium adjacent to a carcinoma may be normal or show a variety of changes, and it is difficult to be sure whether the changes precede or follow the onset of the carcinoma. He pointed out that in other parts of the body a surface epithelium can show reactionary changes to an underlying or adjacent carcinoma (e.g. Paget's disease of the nipple). BAJARDI listed four possibilities to explain the existence of atypical, non-invasive zones around an invasive carcinoma:

(a) The atypical non-invasive zone exists in the form of carcinoma *in situ* and the invasive tumour evolves from this zone. (b) The carcinoma grows not only invasively into the connective tissue but also superficially towards the normal epithelium which is displaced and destroyed. (c) The tumour cells of the invasive region cause a gradual "cancerization" of the adjacent normal squamous epithelium. (d) The atypical, non-invasive zones arise independently of the invasive carcinoma although probably caused by the same aetiological factors.

Thus some caution must be exercised in interpreting the concomitant occurrences of these abnormalities. The simultaneous occurrence merely indicates the possibility of sequential change. However, this possibility is rendered a probability by the records of a number of patients with carcinoma *in situ* who have been allowed, wittingly or unwittingly, to develop invasive carcinoma. KOTTMEIER (1953) was able to collect from the literature 46 case reports of this transition, although he was not convinced that all showed the change alleged. GRAHAM *et al.* (1962) collected records of 265 cases of untreated carcinoma *in situ* which, when combined, showed a transition in 10% of cases to invasive carcinoma. The objection to this type of evidence is that the original biopsy, on which a diagnosis of *in-situ* carcinoma was made, may have missed a focus of invasive tumour already present. As KNOX (1968) has pointed out, non-invasive lesions cannot be diagnosed as being non-invasive until they have been completely removed.

b) The Temporal Relationships

The temporal relationship of the lesions supports the idea of a sequence. If dysplasia precedes *in-situ* carcinoma and this in turn precedes invasion, patients with dysplasia should, on an average, be younger than those with carcinoma *in situ* who, in turn, should be younger than women with invasive carcinoma. Table 4.1. shows

Table 4.1. The mean age of detection of various types of epithelial abnormality of the cervix uteri

	Dysplasia	Carcinoma in situ	Microinvasive carcinoma	Invasive carcinoma	Source
REAGAN *et al.* (1953)					
(a) Non-white	—	43.2	—	49.7	Cleveland U.S.A.
(b) White	—	39.5	—	46.2	
NIEBURGS *et al.* (1957)	—	39.0	41.6	47.8	Floyd County, Georgia, U. S.A.
LANGLEY (1959)	—	40.6	—	51.0	Manchester, U.K.
HERTIG & GORE (1960)	—	38.0	42.2	51.0	Boston, U.S.A.
GRAHAM *et al.* (1962)	34.9	38.0	42.2	48.5	U.S.A.
BOYES *et al.* (1962)	—	41.1	46.5	52.8	British Columbia, Canada
CHRISTOPHERSON & PARKER (1964)	36.5	39.4	—	50.6	Louisville, U.S.A.
REAGAN (1964)					
(a) Non-white	30.8	—	—	—	Cleveland, U.S.A.
(b) White	38.3	—	—	—	
VILLASANTA (1968)	38.1	37.3	—	50.1	Baltimore, U.S.A. (mostly negro)
JORDAN *et al.* (1969)					
(a) American Indian	36.8	38.8	—	48.6	New Mexico,
(b) Non-Indian	36.5	36.8	—	50.1	U.S.A.
MEISELS (1969)	36.2	40.2	45.7	52.4	Quebec, Canada
KASPER *et al.* (1970)	—	38.0	43.9	49.3	Alberta, Canada

that this relationship is usually but not invariably true. VILLASANTA (1968), in a mostly negro population, found carcinoma *in situ* to occur at an earlier age than dysplasia, and JORDAN *et al.* (1969) similarly found little difference in the ages of women with these two lesions. Likewise, KOTTMEIER (1953) found no difference in age between women with carcinoma *in situ* and those with frankly invasive carcinoma but he regarded his as late cases, many being referred to the Radiumhemmet with questionable stromal invasion.

Many workers have compared the mean ages of women with dysplasia and carcinoma *in situ*, or carcinoma *in situ* and clinically invasive carcinoma to estimate the duration of the pre-clinical lesion (HERTIG and GORE 1960; BOYES *et al.* 1962; MACGREGOR and BAIRD 1963; BRYANS *et al.* 1964; FIDLER *et al.* 1968a). On such a basis it follows from Table 4.1. that the dysplastic phase lasts from two to three years, followed by an *in situ* phase of five to ten years. KNOX (1966) has pointed out that such deductions are fallacious since most authors have not taken into account that one of the conditions has been ascertained on a basis of population screening and the other on a selected basis, or that the mean age in one case represents onsets and in the other discoveries. All that can properly be deduced from the Table is that, generally speaking, dysplasia occurs at an earlier age than carcinoma *in situ* and this lesion occurs earlier than invasive carcinoma; findings which support the hypothesis that these lesions form a sequence. This is further strengthened by the observation of BOYES *et al.* (1962) that the greater the extent of the *in-situ* lesion the older the patient.

c) Regression of Epithelial Abnormalities

KOTTMEIER (1953) reviewed 114 cases with pre-cancerous lesions in the cervix or portio vaginalis. In 59 cases no treatment was carried out except a curettage or small biopsy. During a period of follow-up ranging from 1 to 14 years, 13.6% of these women developed invasive carcinoma. At the time of review no pathological change could be seen in the cervix in 45 cases. In two patients a subtotal hysterectomy was performed for fibroids; a panhysterectomy was carried out in one patient a year after the first examination and in two patients almost 11 years later. In none of these surgically removed uteri were remnants of carcinoma *in situ* found on microscopic examination of sections of the cervix. Thus, whilst invasive carcinoma may develop in patients with carcinoma *in situ*, KOTTMEIER concluded that "it is very probable that atypical epithelial changes in the cervix, so-called carcinoma *in situ*, can spontaneously regress".

In 1955 PETERSEN published a monograph describing his findings in a retrospective study of 212 patients with pre-cancerosis of the cervix uteri. The histological lesions in 124 cases were described as "epithelial hyperplasia with nuclear abnormalities". He considered these appearances to correspond to carcinoma *in situ*. However, examination of his illustrations indicates that they also correspond to dysplasia. Eighty-eight of the lesions were described as "borderline"; these showed the same cytological features as the previous group but one or more sections gave rise to a suspicion of incipient invasion. One hundred and twenty-seven of the patients were untreated during the period of observation. "Untreated" was taken to mean that they did not have any treatment which "reasonably can be assumed to have altered the spontaneous course of the cervical lesion. Irrigations, chemotherapy, painting with silver nitrate, mercurochrome, etc., superficial electrocoagulation leaving no visible cicatrical changes in the cervix and performed only once are not counted as actual treatment". Of the 127 untreated cases, 84 belonged to the group "epithelial hyperplasia with nuclear abnormalities" and 43 to the borderline group. All were followed for a minimum of 3 years, 82% for 5 years, 30% for 10 years and 4% for over 10 years. This study showed that the untreated cases did not invariably develop invasive carcinoma within a follow-up period of 15 years. With an increasing follow-up period there was a regular increase in the cancer cases, but after the ninth year this levelled out asymptotically to between 30 and 40% of the original number of cases. During the first year only 4% of untreated patients develop cervical carcinoma and only a little more than half still showed pre-cancerous changes. Regression was confirmed histologically in 19.7% of these cases. Of those patients still showing pre-cancerous changes at the end of the first year, not more than two thirds would be expected to develop cancer.

In 1963, Koss *et al.* published a careful and beautifully illustrated review of 93 cases of early malignant lesions of the uterine cervix. They concluded that carcinoma *in situ* is beyond doubt a precursor of invasive carcinoma of the cervix. However, they pointed out that carcinoma *in situ* is very fragile and poorly established and may be readily eradicated by a variety of minor procedures. Its course may be profoundly modified by even small biopsies, drugs (for example terramycin applied locally) and possibly by physiological trauma such as delivery. They were satisfied that carcinoma *in situ* does regress but this they regarded as an extraordinarily rare event. Dysplasia behaves similarly but it may develop into carcinoma *in situ* or even invasive carcinoma. If the contention of these workers is true, that local damage to the fragile epithelium may easily eradicate the disease, then PETERSEN's (1955) high rate of regression in his so-called untreated cases might possibly be an artefact. It is difficult to believe that such a sinister condition as intra-epithelial carcinoma (carcinoma *in situ*) can be treated so easily. Since, however, no other human neoplasm which is subject to mild trauma has been so intensively studied this idea cannot be rejected out of hand.

The above investigations all depend on histological examination of biopsy specimens for diagnosis. RICHART (1967) has employed non-destructive methods in diagnosis. He has shown that in his hands diagnostic cytology is an accurate tool in the diagnosis of the different types of malign cervical abnormality and of invasive carcinoma and that the colpomicroscope, although somewhat less accurate, is a useful adjunct. Using these two tools, he has carried out a long term follow-up of 518 patients with dysplasia. His results show that in a significant proportion of patients dysplasia progressed to carcinoma *in situ*. The rate of progression increased with the severity of the dysplasia. Apparently spontaneous regression occurred but, under the conditions of the investigation, it was confined to patients in whom atypical cells in the smear were of superficial or intermediate cell types. On the basis of earlier studies RICHART also considered that carcinoma *in situ* invariably progresses to invasive carcinoma unless there is interference.

d) Invasive Carcinoma of the Cervix without a Prior *in situ* Phase

In two closely argued, but difficult, papers ASHLEY (1966a and b) has postulated that there are two biologically different forms of cervical cancer: a slow-growing type, susceptible to therapy, which may be preceded by carcinoma *in situ*, and a rapidly growing type more resistant to treatment which occurs later in life and is not preceded by carcinoma *in situ*. His evidence is mainly epidemiological, but he advances some histological observations in support of his contention. DAVIS (1967) has severely criticized this argument, pointing out that in the surveys analysed by ASHLEY no allowance has been made for the errors in cytological diagnosis in estimating the prevalance of pre-invasive carcinoma. RICHART (1967) and COPPLESON and REID (1967), among other workers, stress that cervical intra-epithelial neoplasia occurs in areas of "transformation" on the portio, the limits of the transformation zone defining the lower limits of the neoplasia. Squamous cell carcinomas occur in

Table 4.2. Incidence rates of invasive carcinoma of the cervix uteri (cases per 100,000 of population)

Age	Denmark 1943—1957 (CLEMMESEN, 1965)	Birmingham, U.K. 1960—1962 (KNOX, 1966)	Memphis-Shelby County, U.S.A. 1950—1951 (DUNN et al. 1954)	
			White	Negro
15—19	0.2	—	—	—
20—24	2.7	—	—	—
25—29	14.6	1.58 ⎫	15.3	26.9
30—34	34.1	8.44 ⎭		
35—39	54.9	22.58 ⎫	54.1	127.6
40—44	68.0	31.45 ⎭		
45—49	73.0	30.45 ⎫	79.6	126.5
50—54	70.9	28.46 ⎭		
55—59	62.0	34.20 ⎫	101.6	132.5
60—64	54.8	34.27 ⎭		
65—69	47.4	34.12 ⎫	103.9	254.6
70—74	44.5	41.59 ⎭		
75—79	35.3	37.46 ⎫	136.7	28.8
80—84	32.5	36.74 ⎭		
85—89	—	42.37	—	—
Mean incidence:	31.4		37.6	64.1

Table 4.3. Incidence of invasive carcinoma of the cervix in Denmark. Average number of cases per 100,000 population (CLEMMESEN, 1965)

	Denmark	Capital	Capital suburbs	Provincial towns	Rural areas
1943—1947	28.8	44.5	37.6	33.8	16.8
1948—1952	31.1	45.3	29.4	36.5	20.1
1953—1957	34.0	53.0	31.6	37.6	21.8

Table 4.4. Incidence of invasive carcinoma of the cervix (cases per 100,000 of population)

Denmark	1943—1957		31.4	CLEMMESEN (1965)
		White	Non-white	
Tennessee, U.S.A.	1950—1951	37.6	64.1	DUNN et al. (1954)
Kentucky, U.S.A.	1953—1955	40.2	76.0	CHRISTOPHERSON et al. (1970)
	1965—1967	25.5	51.1	

each year added to the pool. Second, it depends on the mortality from the condition; this has been stressed by KNOX (1966). Third, the effect of treatment, whether to cure the patient or only to prolong life, affects the number of women in this pool. Analysis of the prevalence of invasive cervical carcinoma therefore throws little light on the natural history of these lesions. Prevalence and mortality statistics are important, however, in evaluating the effects of early diagnosis and treatment.

HILL and ADELSTEIN (1967) have studied the cohort mortality from carcinoma of the cervix. In England and Wales cervical carcinoma was first coded separately from other uterine causes of death in 1948. Apart from a peak in 1958, when there was an epidemic of influenza which hastened deaths from other causes, the crude death rate for cervical carcinoma has shown a steady decline. A similar downward trend is shown in the standardized mortality ratio. However, when the age-specific death rates are examined, an upward trend is found in the lower age groups. It occurs earliest in the 30—39 year group, later in the 40—49 year group and later still in the 50—59 year group. This suggests a generation, or cohort, pattern of disease affecting especially those born between 1911 and 1926. The same trend is found when all uterine cancer is considered, so it is unlikely to be caused by changes in diagnostic accuracy. It may be that some social process, as postulated by MARTIN (1967) and discussed below, might account for this pattern. For example, disturbance of sexual relationships during the Second World War may have played a part. Although this study by HILL and ADELSTEIN is concerned with death rates, it is implicit in the argument that factors which affect a generation in this way must also operate during the precancerous phase of the disease and affect the numerical analysis of this phase in a similar manner.

b) The Presymptomatic Invasive Carcinoma Pool

When discussing Table 4.2. we point out the mode of diagnosis on which the information is based. Thus in Denmark it was by notification of clinical disease or of disease found at necropsy. It was thus largely symptomatic disease. By use of cervical cytology followed by biopsy it is possible to recognize invasive carcinoma in a pre-symptomatic (or occult) phase. The average duration of this phase can be determined by the ratio of the sum of the unweighted age-specific prevalence rates of pre-clinical invasive carcinoma and those for the incidence of the clinical disease. DUNN (1966) using observations from the Memphis study estimated the duration of this phase as 4.1 years. When making such an estimate, it is assumed that once a neoplasm has become invasive it is irretrievably committed to malignant progression. However, it is possible, as discussed above, that some neoplasms having a histologically micro-invasive structure are not necessarily cancerous. The presymptomatic invasive phase can be subdivided into two parts (a) an *in-situ* phase with microscopic foci of invasion and (b) an occult phase, in which the tumour is frankly invasive histologically, but asymptomatic. BOYES *et al.* (1962) have shown that in British Columbia the mean age of women with *in-situ* carcinoma is 41.4 years, with microinvasive carcinoma 46.5 years, with occult invasive carcinoma 51 years, and clinically invasive carcinoma 52.8 years.

c) The Precancerous, or Malign, Pool

This is made up of two components: carcinoma *in situ* and dysplasia. It is not always possible to be sure whether or not authors have clearly distinguished these two states either conceptually or diagnostically. Thus it is very probable that workers who find a high level of regression of lesions which they designate as carcinoma *in situ* are including lesions which others would call severe, or even moderate, dysplasia. Similarly what some would regard as mild dysplasia others would exclude from the malign pool altogether. These differences in interpretation are increased when the diagnosis is made on cytological rather than histological grounds. In population studies the incidence of new cases of dysplasia or carcinoma *in situ* entering the precancerous pool is usually estimated from the results of a cytological screening programme supported by histological studies. When estimating the incidence of malign lesions, it is necessary to evaluate errors such as those introduced by the "false negative" smear (see Chapter 3) and to bear in mind the preferential selection of certain social strata and groups in the population studied.

DUNN (1966) has pointed out that, in screening for any disease, if the prevalence/incidence ratio is large and if the screening technique has an appreciable false negative error, the first rescreening will provide an inflated estimate of incidence. For example, with a prevalence/incidence ratio of 10:1 and 90% efficiency in discovering

Table 4.5. Number of screenings, cases of carcinoma *in situ* and rates per 1,000 women screened (limiting time up to 3 years between negative and positive smears) (CHRISTOPHERSON, 1966)

Screening	No.	Rate
First	289	3.91
Second	43	1.34
Third	16	1.23
Fourth and over	8	0.91

carcinoma *in situ* cytologically, the incidence rate will be inflated by 80% at the first annual re-examination. Thus, incidence rates should be determined by second and subsequent rescreenings since, when rescreening the cervix cytologically, the first rescreening will pick up an appreciable number of the false negative errors made at the initial screening. A corresponding correction must also be made in the estimate of prevalence. CHRISTOPHERSON's (1966) investigations at Louisville, Kentucky, illustrate the effect of repeated rescreening and provide an estimate of the incidence of carcinoma *in situ* in that city (Table 4.5.). The first screening gives an estimate of the prevalence of carcinoma *in situ*, whilst the fourth screening (i.e. the third rescreening) estimates the incidence of the condition.

It is difficult to be sure in such studies that the rescreened population has the same structure as the initial population. Healthy women who are interested in their wellbeing will return more readily than others who are less interested, and this difference may well have a socio-economic bias (MACGREGOR 1966). BIBBO *et al.* (1971) found in the second and third year of observation relatively constant values for the incidence of carcinoma *in situ*. However, their incidence rates increased in the fourth and fifth years and they suggested that this is due to the heterogeneity of therapeutic measures.

In a rescreening programme women are followed for varying periods of time, and one patient followed for 10 years should have the same risk as 10 patients followed for 1 year. For this reason BOYES *et al.* (1962) have used the number of women developing *in situ* carcinoma per patient-years of risk as the measure of incidence. By the end of 1959 they had a group of 20,424 patients who contributed 39,245 years of risk, equal to 39,245 patients followed for one year. 18 of these patients developed *in situ* carcinoma, representing an annual incidence of 46 cases per 100,000 women. Following more extensive studies these workers (FIDLER *et al.* 1968a) have recalculated the age-specific incidence rates for carcinoma *in situ* of the cervix. These are shown graphically in Fig. 4.3. The overall incidence for women over 20 years is 0.66 cases per 1,000 person years. Thus the occurrence of carcinoma *in situ* is a rare event and, not surprisingly, the shape of the curve corresponds approximately to a Poisson distribution, or a binomial with a small value for p. The curve is skewed, rapidly reaching a maximum of 1.19 cases per 1,000 person-years in the 25—29 quinquennium and thereafter progressively decreasing. DUNN (1966) has compared the earlier Vancouver results with those of San Diego County and Memphis-Shelby County. Broadly the trend is the same, the peak incidence is before the age of 30,

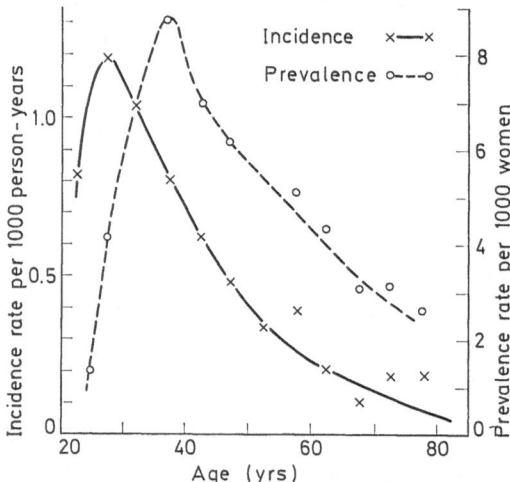

Fig. 4.3. Age-specific incidence and prevalence rates for *in-situ* squamous cell carcinoma of the cervix uteri in British Columbia (FIDLER *et al.*, 1968a)

but in both surveys from the United States the incidence and prevalence rise in the postmenopausal period. Whether or not this rise is real is open to question because cases are few and the number of person-years is small. KASPER *et al.* (1970) noted a similar rise in these indices among women in Alberta. KASHGARIAN and DUNN (1970) suggested that these distributions around the menopause may indicate that at this time host barriers are broken down and intraepithelial carcinoma becomes rapidly invasive. DUNN (1966) suggests that the fact that the peak incidence in the 25—29 age group follows the modal peak of age at marriage by some seven or eight years may have aetiological implications. Table 4.6. shows some recent estimates of the overall incidence of carcinoma *in situ*.

The composition and age structure of the precancerous pool is affected by a number of factors. Ignoring the effects of treatment and death from other causes, the frequency of regression and the type of patient in whom regression occurs will modify the population as will also the rate of growth of the disease. Lesions which progress rapidly from normal epithelium to invasive cancer will only be in the precancerous pool for a short time, whereas slowly progressive lesions will be in the pool for a long time. Hence there is a preponderance of slowly progressive lesions in the pool (DUNN 1966). Invasive tumours with a short *in-situ* phase have been described by FIDLER and BOYD (1960), DE BRUX and DUPRÉ-FROMENT (1965) and LIU (1967). In LIU's study two patients developed invasive carcinoma within a relatively short time. In one case, the interval between the negative smear and the positive smear was only 18 months. She does not think it likely that these two cases represent examples of direct tumourigenesis without either a dysplastic or an *in-situ* phase, but rather a rapid transition through these phases. The ages of these patients are not given, but it remains a possibility that in these patients there was indeed no precancerous phase; they would then fall into ASHLEY's second group (*vide supra*). DUNN and MARTIN (1967) have described four women who developed positive

Table 4.6. Estimates of the overall incidence of *in-situ* carcinoma of the cervix (per 1,000 women)

British Columbia	
BOYES et al. (1962)	0.46
FIDLER et al. (1968a)	0.66
Alberta	
KASPER et al. (1970)	0.58
Memphis, Tennessee	
KASHGARIAN and DUNN (1970)	
White	0.35
Non-white	0.56

smears whilst under observation, each having had at least two previous negative smears, in whom biopsy showed the presence of invasive carcinoma. These they regard as a "component of new disease not having a long *in-situ* phase". They estimate that 10 to 15% of cervical carcinomas become invasive early in their development. If the type of lesion is age-related, for example, if the precancerous phase is longer in younger women than in older women, the proportions of the various types will modify the shape of the age-specific prevalence curve. Similarly, if regression of the lesion is age-related, differences in the proportions of regressing to progressing lesions will also modify this curve.

Estimates of the mean duration of the precancerous phase are fraught with difficulty because the mathematics necessary involves more variables than there are equations to solve. Hence most workers implicitly or explicitly make certain assumptions. MACGREGOR (1966) reports that in North East Scotland, on the basis of a ten-year interval between the first appearance of a positive smear to the development of clinical signs of cancer, the prevalence of positive smears should be 0.5%. If, however, the latent period is 20 years then the positive smear rate should be 1.0%. The detection rate in a group of general practices in Aberdeen was 0.7%, suggesting progression of the lesion over a period of time nearer 20 than 10 years. It is probable that MACGREGOR's estimate includes both the dysplastic and the *in-situ* parts of the precancerous pool. KASHGARIAN and DUNN (1970), on the assumption that the lesion does not regress, used the formula:

$$\text{Duration of the intraepithelial phase} = \frac{\text{sum of age-specific prevalences}}{\text{sum of age-specific incidences}}.$$

They found the average duration of the intraepithelial phase in white women to be 10.7 years and in negro women 8.5 years. They also found that the duration of intraepithelial carcinoma is longest in women 25—35 years of age, when it averaged 16 years. When the lesion begins at a younger or older age the average durations are shorter, being about 10 years before the age of 25, and about 5 years in the 40s and one year about the age of 65 years.

The difficulty in estimating the mean duration of the *in-situ* phase is illustrated by the report of FIDLER *et al.* (1968a). They found the mean incidence of carcinoma *in situ* to be 0.66 per 1,000 person years and the prevalence 4.31 per 1,000 persons. Using the same formula as KASHGARIAN and DUNN they calculated the *in-situ* phase to last 6 years. However, using an "adjusted prevalence" to take account of patients who had previously had minor atypicalities in their smears, the mean prevalence was found to be 5.50 per 1,000 women and the duration of the *in-situ* phase 9.5 years. However, since the mean age of onset of carcinoma *in situ* was 37.5 years in their population of women and the mean age of cases with occult invasive carcinoma was 49.3 years, they concluded that the duration of the *in-situ* phase could be regarded as about 12 years.

Table 4.7. Age of maximum prevalence of carcinoma *in situ* (rate/1,000)

	Rate	Age	
Floyd County Ga. (White)	5.5	41—50	NIEBURGS *et al.* (1957)
Wisconsin (rural) (Mostly white)	5.5	30—34	CALABRESI *et al.* (1958)
Los Angeles, Cal.	6.2	30—39	STERN and NEELY (1963)
Memphis, Tenn,	4.47	40—49	Quoted by KNOX (1966)
San Diego, Cal.	5.6	30—34	DUNN and MARTIN (1967)
British Columbia	6.73	35—39	FIDLER *et al.* (1968a)
Iceland (Reykjavik)	12.63	40—44	THORARINSSEN *et al.* (1969)
Iceland (rural)	12.71	35—39	THORARINSSEN *et al.* (1969)
Alberta	8.2	35—39	KASPER *et al.* (1970)
Chicago, Ill.	6.9	35—39	BIBBO *et al.* (1971)

Table 4.7. shows the maximum prevalence of *in-situ* carcinoma recorded in a number of studies. There is considerable variation not only in the level but also in the age at which this maximum occurs. Both will be determined by the balance of gain from new cases and loss by transfer to the invasive pool or by regression, and each of these will be related to the age structure, socio-economic background and ethnic origin of the population sampled. Differences may also be caused by variations in cytological and histological criteria employed, but these cannot account for the differences in Iceland between the urban population of Reykjavik and that of the rural areas of the rest of the country.

α) Dysplasia

The incidence of dysplasia can be assessed in the same way as that of carcinoma *in situ* by rescreening a returning population of women who previously had negative smears. The same problems of interpretation apply as for carcinoma *in situ*, but it may be more difficult to classify the cellular abnormalities with certainty.

Table 4.8. summarizes the observations of CHRISTOPHERSON and PARKER (1964) in Louisville. The first screening gives a measure of the prevalence of the lesion, and the second and third screenings of women with a previous negative cell study measure the incidence of the lesion. They regard the third screening as a better representation of incidence than the second screening. However, this may be offset by the small number of lesions found. Comparison of the incidence rates of dysplasia and carcinoma *in situ* suggests that only 30 to 36% of cases of dysplasia progress to carcinoma *in situ*.

Table 4.8. Number of screenings, cases of dysplasia and carcinoma *in situ* and rates per 1,000 women screened (CHRISTOPHERSON and PARKER, 1964)

| Screening | Dysplasia | | Carcinoma *in situ* | | Number of |
	No.	Rate	No.	Rate	women
First year	210	3.20	243	3.70	66,043
Second year	57	2.12	17	0.63	26,913
Third year	14	1.47	5	0.53	9,518

The incidence of dysplasia has also been investigated by STERN and NEELY (1963), whose estimates are based on a returning population previously negative for dysplasia and cancer, and by DUNN and MARTIN (1967) who studied a population with two previous negative cytological examinations. Their results are shown in Table 4.9. From the table it follows that there are fairly wide differences in the estimates of the incidence of dysplasia in the State of California: 1.1 per 1,000 women per annum in Los Angeles and 0.78 per 1,000 in San Diego. The San Diego study is about five times larger than the Los Angeles study and to this extent is the more reliable. Differences in the population sampled and diagnostic criteria probably contribute to the differences in incidence.

Table 4.10. shows wide variations in the reported prevalence of dysplasia. The lesion is more common when the diagnosis is made histologically than when made

Table 4.9. Incidence of dysplasia

| Age | STERN et al. (1963) (Los Angeles) | | DUNN et al. (1967) (San Diego) | |
	Cases	Rate/1,000 cases	Cases	Rate/1,000 patient years
20—29	0	—	13	1.34
30—39	4	2.6	18	1.10
40—49	7	2.4	4	0.29
50—59	5	1.7	3	0.44
60—69	7	3.3	1	0.36
70+	2	3.2	1	1.13
All ages	25	2.4	40	0.78
Average annual incidence		1.1 [a]		0.78

[a] The average number of years since the initial examination was 2.17 (STERN, 1969).

Table 4.10. Prevalence of dysplasia

	Cases of dysplasia (%)	No. of women examined	Note
Detected cytologically			
(A) *Non-gravid women*			
REAGAN *et al.* (1955)			(1)
(a) non-white	1.34	2,995	
(b) white	0.53	7,555	
STERN and NEELY (1963)	0.54	19,192	(2)
PATTEN (1966)	0.98	57,469	
CARROW *et al.* (1967)	0.56	1,249	(3)
BUTLER and LANGLEY (1969)	0.29	42,700	(4)
BIBBO *et al.* (1971)			(5)
All women	1.33	140,505	
using oral contraceptives	2.31	18,380	
using intrauterine device	3.12	2,624	
not using oral or intra- uterine contraceptives	1.15	127,731	
(B) *Gravid women*			
SLATE (1959)	0.15	10,044	
DALIAN *et al.* (1959)	0.50	6,652	
REAGAN *et al.* (1961)	3.00	930	
BUTLER (1969)			
antenatal	0.14	2,177	
postnatal	0.08	10,117	
BIBBO *et al.* (1971)	1.23	8,230	
Detected by histological examination			
(A) *Non-gravid women*			
GUSBERG (1951)	2.0	500	(cone biopsy)
LAPID and GOLDBERGER (1951)	2.3	556	(cone biopsy)
GUIN (1953)	3.1	419	(cervical biopsy, necropsy, etc.)
REAGAN *et al.* (1955)	3.2	3,200	
McKAY *et al.* (1959)	1.2	20,029	
FIGGE *et al.* (1962)	3.8	847	(6)
(B) *Gravid women*			
EPPERSON *et al.* (1951)	14.7	286	
NESBITT *et al.* (1952)	1.0	300	

(1) The smears were collected in physicians' offices and in large survey centres, regarded as "more representative of the general population than would be true of hospital sources".
(2) From a cancer detection clinic; biopsies were not performed on all cases.
(3) Detected by irrigation smears and confirmed histologically.
(4) Mostly from hospital patients but includes smears taken from women attending family planning clinics, venereal disease clinics and in prison. Diagnoses confirmed histologically.
(5) From planned parenthood clinics.
(6) From a group of healthy women surveyed by smear and biopsy over a period of seven years.

cytologically, but this difference almost certainly reflects selection of cases for biopsy and this selection is particularly likely to occur in pregnancy. The table also shows that the lesion may occur more commonly in the pregnant than the non-pregnant woman (REAGAN *et al.* 1955, 1961). In our own clinic this again is probably related to the selection of cases for biopsy (BUTLER 1969).

The mean age of detection of dysplasia varies from centre to centre, as seen in Table 4.1., but is usually earlier than the mean age of detection of carcinoma *in situ*. REAGAN *et al.* (1955) found the mean age for women to be 34.2 ± 1.16 years when there was only slight abnormality and 41.4 ± 3.0 years when the dysplasia was classified as severe. McKAY *et al.* (1959) reported a mean age of 28.5 years in women having a reaction which regressed and a mean age of 34.5 years in patients with a persisting lesion. These observations support the concept of dysplasia as an epithelial abnormality which may precede carcinoma *in situ*. PATTEN (1969) has pointed out that in the United States dysplasia occurs approximately 7 years earlier in non-

Table 4.11. Age-specific prevalence of women with cervical dysplasia

Source Age	(1) Cases	(2) Cases	Age	(3) Cases	Rate/ 1,000	(4) Cases	Rate 1,000	Age	(5) Rate/ 1,000
<21	23	3	<20	—	—	18	1.5	<15	9.9
21—30	85	43	20—29	15	10.9	192	3.9	20—24	17.0
31—40	33	53	30—39	31	7.1	163	3.5	25—29	17.5
41—50	15	39	40—49	21	4.3	85	2.6	30—34	16.0
51—60	4	9	50—59	19	4.2	34	1.8	49+	2.9
61—70	3	8	60—69	14	4.8	18	1.6		
71+	0	3	70+	3	3.0	6	1.3		
Total	163	158		103		516			

(1) KRAMER and KAY (1967). Diagnosis was made by cytology, colpomicroscopy and biopsy.

(2) VILLASANTA (1968). Diagnosis was made on a cone biopsy following a smear and, or, biopsy. The mean age of this group was 38.1 years compared with 37.3 years for carcinoma *in situ*.

(3) STERN and NEELY (1963). Cases were discovered by cytological screening and confirmed by biopsy.

(4) DUNN and MARTIN (1967). Cases discovered by cytological screening and confirmed by biopsy.

(5) BIBBO *et al.* (1971). Diagnosis made by cytology.

white than in white patients. This difference is related to socio-economic status, age at initial intercourse, etc., rather than to ethnic factors. Table 4.11 shows the age distribution of cases of dysplasia when first diagnosed, i.e. the age-specific prevalence rate, in five investigations. It is evident that the figures just quoted for the mean age of occurrence of dysplasia generally fail to reveal the relative youth of the population of the dysplastic pool.

d) Progression and Regression of Precancerous Lesions

Following up cases of dysplasia provides some useful, but incomplete, information about the regression of the lesion or its evolution to *in-situ* cancer. RICHART and BARRON (1969) have quoted a large number of such investigations and similar studies are summarized in Table 4.12. Most earlier investigations involved surgical interference with the lesion which may well have modified its course. However, broadly speaking, the progression rate corresponds with the 12% calculated on

Table 4.12. Outcome of dysplasia cases

	Regression to normal	Persisting	Progression to CIS or invasion	No. of cases	Period of follow-up
SIMON and SHEEHAN (1961) 4 quadrant biopsy	54.5%	40.9%	4.6%	44	
SCOTT and BALLARD (1962) Diagnosis: cytological and/or histological					
(a) Cone and follow-up	80.7	15.2	4.1	73	
(b) Positive biopsy and follow-up	48.9	43.9	7.2	223	10 years
(c) No biopsy or negative biopsy and follow-up	60.0	38.3	1.7	120	
STERN and NEELY (1963)	40.0	48.0	12.0	94	3 years
PATTEN (1966) Diagnosis: cytological Progression confirmed by histology					
(a) Slight dysplasia	71.9	—	0		
(b) Moderate dysplasia	44.2	—	0	364	9 months to
(c) Severe dysplasia	16.3	—	11.6		2 years
Pregnancy					
SLATE and MERRITT (1961)	45.0	29.0	25.0	120	
REAGAN (1964)	75.0	—	—	102	Regression within 6 months of delivery

population studies in Los Angeles by STERN and NEELY (1963); but they have pointed out that the eventual outcome of each case may be influenced by a number of complex variables such as the number of visits, the cytological diagnosis on each visit and the biopsy procedure (if any) used. Similarly, KRAMER and KAY (1967) have stressed that biospy strongly influences the natural history of dysplasia. Biopsy alone was followed by cytological regression in 50 of 80 cases of dysplasia whilst, of 28 untreated cases of dysplasia, 3 progressed to *in-situ* carcinoma in 1.5, 7 and 8 years respectively. SCOTT (1966) has estimated that *in-situ* carcinoma was usually demonstrated about 3.2 years after initial cellular detection of dysplasia.

RICHART (1967) has stressed that even a single punch biopsy may eradicate a focus of dysplasia and thus be equivalent to a hysterectomy. Colpomicroscopic studies have shown changes in the distribution of areas of dysplasia following biopsy and that alterations and even regression may occur after considerable delay. In order to follow a group of patients with dysplasia without altering the lesion, it is necessary to use diagnostic sampling techniques which are accurate and do not interfere with the disease process. RICHART considers that exfoliative cytology and colpomicroscopy fulfil these criteria. By these methods he has carried out a long-term study of 518 patients with dysplasia, following them up for varying periods up to 900 days and found that 22 of them progressed to *in-situ* carcinoma. The rate of progression increases with increasing severity of the dysplasia. Spontaneous regressions occurred but only in patients in whom the atypical cells in the smear were confined to the superficial and intermediate cellular layers. In a later study RICHART and BARRON (1969) analysed their results using the statistical technique of the Markov chain. The median transit time to carcinoma *in situ* was calculated to be 86 months for a patient with very mild dysplasia, 58 months for mild dysplasia, 38 months for moderate dysplasia and 12 months for severe dysplasia. The median transit time for all dysplasias was 44 months, which is comparable to SCOTT's figure of 3.2 years, quoted above. However, the curves from which these calculations are made approach an asymptotic limit so that a substantial proportion of patients will remain in the stage in which they were detected and not progress to a more severe lesion over a definite period of time.

STERN and NEELY (1963) and STERN (1969) stress two important observations. First, among women who showed regression to normality there was a recurrence of dysplasia in approximately 33%. Second, although in their studies the incidence of "pre-invasive" cancer and invasive cancer was 0.04 per 1,000 in each condition, in women with previous dysplasia the incidence of "pre-invasive" cancer was 49.0 per 1,000 and of invasive cancer 4.0 per 1,000.

PATTEN (1969) has raised the question as to whether or not the cells comprising the morphological lesions described as carcinoma *in situ* are to be regarded as cancer cells, i.e. are they capable of invasion and metastasis? RICHART and BARRON (1969) regard dysplasia and carcinoma *in situ* as a sequence of changes leading to invasive carcinoma. KASHGARIN and DUNN (1970) when estimating the duration of the intraepithelial phase assumed that all intraepithelial carcinomas progressed to invasive carcinoma. If this is true, then the incidence of intraepithelial carcinoma must equal the incidence of invasive carcinoma. However, BOYES *et al.* (1962) found that, whereas the baseline incidence of invasive carcinoma in British Columbia was 28.4 per 100,000, that of carcinoma *in situ* was 46.0 per 100,000; thus only 60% of the *in-situ* cases became invasive. A more recent estimate using more extensive information (FIDLER *et al.* 1968) indicates that probably only 43% of *in situ* lesions became invasive. It seems probable, provided the demographic factors are comparable, that the two groups of workers (KASHGARIAN and DUNN, BOYES *et al.*) have not used identical histological criteria when distinguishing dysplasia from carcinoma *in situ*. Although the British Columbia workers clearly distinguish dysplasia and carcinoma *in situ* (FIDLER *et al.* 1968b and c), their published photomicrographs suggest that they regard some lesions as carcinoma *in situ* which others might place in the dysplastic category. If these workers distinguish between dysplasia and carcinoma *in situ* in their population studies, it is surprising that they have not published information about the prevalence and incidence of dysplasia in British Columbia. STERN (1969) estimated the incidence of pre-invasive cancer in Los Angeles in a rescreened population as 31 per 100,000 and the incidence of invasive cancer as 15 per 100,000 giving a conversion rate of pre-invasive to invasive cancer of 50%, closely agreeing with the British Columbia finding. PATTEN (1969) has emphasized that in addition to the confusion surrounding the use of histopathological and cytological criteria from one institution to another, differences in the type of sample, the size of the sample and the composition of the population surveyed affect the reported rates of dysplasia.

In contrast to these views, GREEN (1966) has concluded that either the length of the pre-invasive phase is much longer than 20 years or very few *in situ* cancers ever become invasive. He bases this conclusion on an analysis of incidence rates of invasive carcinoma in New Zealand, British Columbia and San Diego and also on mortality rates from cervical cancers in the first two locations. In a later study GREEN and DONOVAN (1970) reported that, of a total of 576 patients with cervical carcinoma *in situ*, 75 have shown evidence of persistent disease after various initial treatments but none of these has developed invasive cervical cancer during follow-up. Using this result they obtained confidence limits for the probability with which carcinoma *in situ* will become invasive and for the latent period prior to invasion. Two models were used to make these calculations. First, a model based on a Poisson process indicated that, if there is a 25% probability of every *in-situ* carcinoma invading, the mean interval before invasion would exceed 25 years, or if the probability of invasion is 10%, then the latent period (at the 95% confidence limit) would exceed 7 years. Second, a model based on a fixed latent period but with the incidence age-related, indicated that if the probability of *in-situ* carcinoma progressing to invasion is 25%, then the latent period would exceed 16 years. It is of interest to recall that Fig. 4.3. indicated the likelihood of a Poisson model.

These various views emphasize the inadequacy of the present state of knowledge of the biological potential of dysplasia and carcinoma *in situ*.

e) Relationship of Dysplasia to Invasive Carcinoma

REAGAN and PATTEN (1962) have described a detailed study of 200 cervical neoplasms in relation to the overlying epithelium. Of these neoplasms, 55 were keratinizing, 104 were large-cell, non-keratinizing tumours and 41 small-cell tumours. The surface overlying 54 of the 55 keratinizing neoplasms was dysplastic and in one specimen the overlying lesion was *in-situ* carcinoma. In 17 of the 104 large-cell, non-keratinizing tumours the surface reaction was dysplastic and in the remaining 87 it was *in-situ* carcinoma, either alone or in combination with dysplasia. Of the 41 small-cell tumours, 40 had the surface changes of *in-situ* carcinoma and one those of dysplasia. These results are summarized in Table 4.13.

Table 4.13. The surface epithelium in relation to 200 cervical neoplasms (REAGAN and PATTEN, 1962)

Type of tumour	No. of cases	Surface epithelium	
		Dysplasia	In-situ carcinoma
Keratinizing	55	54	1
Non-keratinizing			
Large-cell	104	17	87
Small-cell	41	1	40

REAGAN has shown (*vide infra*) that the areas of distribution of dysplasia and carcinoma *in situ* in the cervix are not identical although overlapping. REAGAN and PATTEN (1962) found that all the keratinizing cancers were within the area of distribution described for dysplasia. The distribution of the large-cell non-keratinizing cancers was comparable to that of carcinoma *in situ*. The average age of patients with keratinizing cancer was 40.22 ± 13.45 years and of large-cell, non-keratinizing tumours 46.46 ± 14.81 years, paralleling the differences in the average ages of dysplasia and carcinoma *in situ*.

BANGLE *et al.* (1963) carried out a careful topographic-histological study of 35 selected squamous carcinomas of the cervix. They were all occult invasive tumours not exceeding 0.5 cm in maximum dimension. Of these tumours, 10 were keratinizing, 17 were of large-cell, non-keratinizing type and 8 of small-cell, undifferentiated type. The surface overlying the neoplastic epithelium, at the level of stromal invasion, in the keratinizing tumours presented variations from an almost normal structure to that of dysplasia. The large-cell, non-keratinizing cancers usually originated from a surface epithelium showing varying degrees of dysplasia. However, *in-situ* carcinoma was often, but not always, present in the cervical epithelium adjacent to the invasive site. The small-cell cancers arose from a surface zone of undifferentiated carcinomatous epithelium, usually associated with a variable distribution of carcinoma *in situ* and dysplasia in the surrounding cervical epithelium.

The following case of our own illustrates the relation between dysplasia and invasive carcinoma.

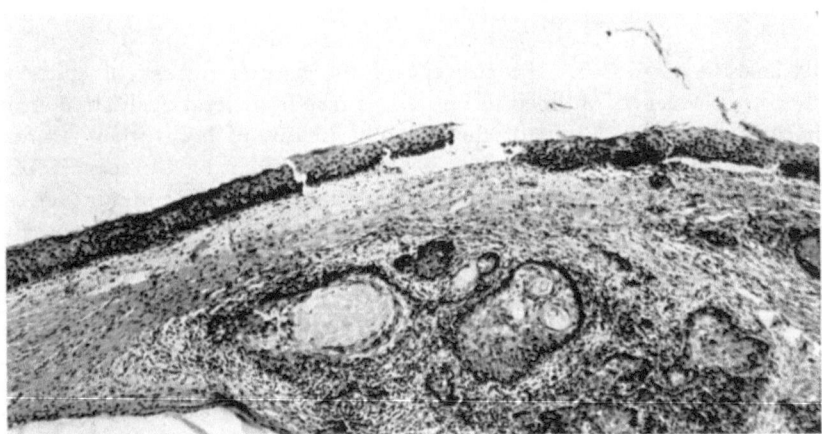

Fig. 4.4. A small invasive carcinoma underlies normal and dysplastic epithelium. Normal squamous epithelium is on the left and dysplastic epithelium on the right (H. & E. × 50)

Mrs. E.V. aged 33. Three consecutive cervical smears taken over a period of 9 months showed increasingly abnormal cells indicative of dysplasia and possible carcinoma *in situ*. A cone biopsy was performed and the specimen cut into ten blocks in sequence. Sections from two adjacent blocks showed chronic cervicitis and squamous metaplasia. Six of the remaining blocks showed severe dysplasia, one showed severe dysplasia bordering on carcinoma *in situ*. In sections from a block taken from the middle of the abnormal area there was a focus of micro-invasive carcinoma. This tumour was of keratinizing type. It lay under dysplastic epithelium adjacent to the junction of the epithelium with normal squamous epithelium (Fig. 4.4.).

KLAVINS (1963) described invasive lesions with well-differentiated or normal cells on the surface. He distinguished intra-epithelial carcinoma with surface differentiation from dysplasia. To separate the two conditions he introduced a new criterion.

This was the retention of the polarity of the basal cell layer at the basement membrane in dysplasia and the loss of this polarity in intra-epithelial carcinoma. GRUBB and JANOTA (1967) compared the morphology of "severe dysplasia" with that of invasive carcinoma. A cellular analysis of the biopsies showed that the two categories have a number of features in common: chiefly the presence of atypical and normal mitoses, nucleoli, horn cells and giant cells. The stratification of the epithelium in "severe dysplasia" is invariably abnormal and the architecture closely resembles that of invasive carcinoma. They suggest that, on the basis of these observations, the term severe dysplasia should be interpreted as differentiated carcinoma *in situ*. If this suggestion were accepted, it would present a number of practical difficulties in interpretation; in particular the borderline between severe and moderate dysplasia which is, on any count, hazy would become the borderline between carcinoma *in situ* and dysplasia. This would increase rather than clarify the difficulties when comparing population studies.

3. Resumé of the Natural History of Epithelial Abnormalities of the Cervix

This analysis shows that the concept of the natural history of epithelial abnormalities of the cervix outlined in Fig. 4.1. is true in general qualitative terms, but quantitatively the relationship of the different phases to each other is uncertain. Squamous-cell carcinoma of the cervix is usually preceded by a precancerous phase but sometimes this may be very short or even non-existent, the tumour then appears to arise directly from normal squamous epithelium. The precancerous phase can be subdivided into one of dysplasia and one of carcinoma *in situ*. Many tumours evolve by transition of dysplasia to carcinoma *in situ* to invasive squamous-cell carcinoma. Sometimes, however, the transition may be directly from dysplasia to squamous carcinoma (Fig. 4.5.).

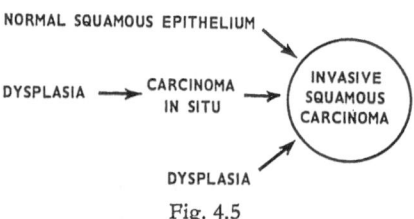

Fig. 4.5

It appears that a high proportion of *in-situ* carcinomas, if undisturbed, progress to invasive squamous carcinoma, but a few regress. A lower proportion of dysplasias progress to carcinoma *in situ* and a higher proportion probably regress, whilst an appreciable number of cases probably remain stationary.

The natural history of microinvasive carcinoma is difficult to investigate because diagnosis must be made on biopsy specimens and the removal of these naturally interferes with the progress of the disease. Thus at the present time GLÜCKSMANN and CHERRY's (1964) division of microcarcinoma into three types (see Chapter 3) must remain a theoretical concept.

It is possible that carcinoma *in situ* may arise directly from normal squamous epithelium without passing through a dysplastic phase but there is no well-documented evidence to support or deny such a contention.

The quantitative assessment of these changes is complicated by a number of factors, the major ones being: (1) There is inconsistency in terminology and diagnostic criteria between different centres. (2) Therapeutic intervention interferes with the course of the disease, which is frustrating to the student of these conditions because interference presupposes that the course is already known. The more widespread use of colposcopy and colpomicroscopy together with exfoliative cytology might reduce the need for surgical interference. (3) The composition of the populations studied varies from centre to centre and, even in one centre, economic factors or social practices may vary from time to time, as suggested by the cohort analysis of HILL and ADELSTEIN (1967).

Chapter 5

The Morphology and Morphogenesis of Epithelial Abnormalities of the Cervix

The object of this chapter is, first, to explore in greater detail the morphological types of dysplasia, carcinoma *in situ* and microinvasive carcinoma, their anatomical distribution and possible morphogenesis. Second, the morphology, fine structure and the genetic constitution of the cells is discussed in order to gain insight into the fundamental cytological changes of the lesions and their relation to the evolution of the abnormalities.

1. Types of Epithelial Abnormality

a) Dysplasia

"Dysplasia" is not a very precise morphological term but is used to describe epithelial abnormalities which are less severe than those seen in carcinoma *in situ* but more severe than those found in squamous metaplasia, basal cell hyperplasia and other bland abnormalities. Corresponding to this rather wide concept, the histological appearances described under this term are very varied. However, the differences in appearance do not necessarily imply differences in aetiology or behaviour because in any one cervix a variety of patterns may be seen.

For descriptive purposes it is convenient and important to describe four features of a dysplastic lesion: its severity, its pattern, its anatomical extent and its relation to adjacent lesions. The first two of these features will be considered here and the last two in the next section of this chapter.

When analysing the cytological changes in dysplastic epithelium it is useful to consider them under two headings—cytoplasmic changes, which are usually changes in differentiation, and nuclear changes, which are usually disorders of maturation. Degenerative changes may be superimposed on these. The lesions may be graded into mild and severe but the borderline between these grades is subjective and a large ill-defined middle group tends to remain. However, prognostically, it may be of value to make the distinction. If nuclear immaturity persists high in the epithelium and differentiation is slight, the changes should be regarded as severe. If nuclear immaturity is confined to the lower layers and differentiation is not greatly disturbed the lesion is considered mild.

Three cytological features occurring in dysplasia are worthy of special note:

(1) the frequency and type of mitosis,
(2) individual cell keratinization, and
(3) koilocytotic atypia.

PATTEN (1969) has stated that mitotic activity was present in 90% of the specimens examined in his laboratory. The average number of mitoses was 2.1 ± 1.3 per high-power field, unfortunately he does not state the size of this field or even the magnification used. These mitoses were usually confined to the lower half of the epithelium and both normal and abnormal forms were present. Mitoses were rare in the upper half of the epithelium. Cells showing individual cell keratinization may be seen scattered through the epithelium; because of their isolated appearance and

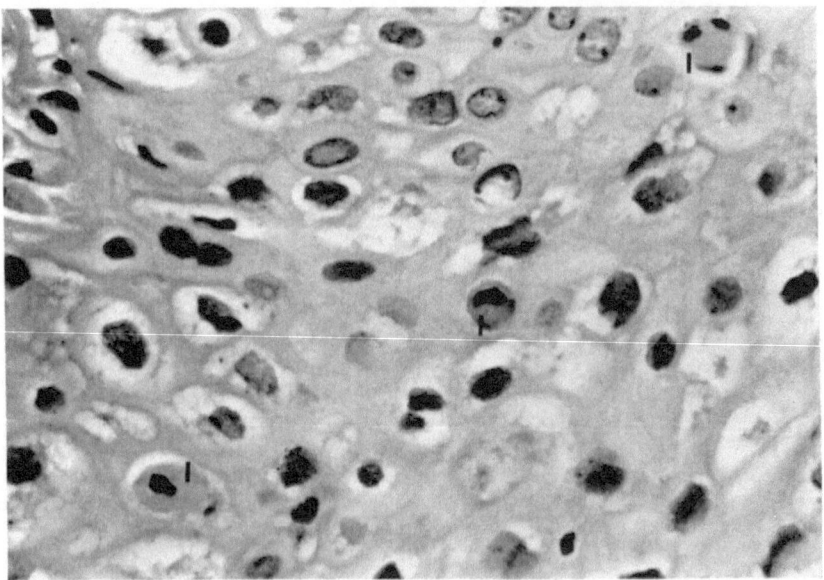

Fig. 5.1. A small area of mildly dysplastic epithelium. The cells marked I show individual cell keratinization; their cytoplasm is homogeneous and the nuclei show pyknosis or karyorrhexis. (H. & E. × 480)

intensely acidophilic and rounded cytoplasm they are readily recognized. The nucleus of such cells usually shows karryorrhexis. The changes should therefore be regarded as degenerative. PATTEN (1969) reports seeing such cells in 45.5% of dysplastic lesions (Fig. 5.1.).

Koilocytotic atypia may be seen both in section of dysplastic lesions and in exfoliated cells. These atypia must be distinguished from the perinuclear haloes described by PAPANICOLAOU in 1933 as "perinuclear or paranuclear vacuoles". In vaginal smears perinuclear haloes are usually associated with trichomoniasis but SAPHIR et al. (1959) have produced perinuclear haloes by applying podophyllin to the uterine cervix. The term "koilocytotic atypia" refers to cells with slightly abnormal nuclei which have large, irregular, clear perinuclear areas often crossed by stands of cytoplasm. This change was first described by AYRE in 1949. DE GIROLAMI (1967) has published a critical study of these two changes, both in smears and histological sections. In sections the simple perinuclear haloes are mostly found in the superficial layers and show a uniform narrow clear rim round a pyknotic nucleus. Intercellular oedema and other changes associated with inflammation may also be present. Cells showing koilocytotic atypia usually occur in the intermediate layer, a few in each low-power field and usually surrounded by small satellite squamous cells lacking maturation and stratification. Occasionally these cells are seen in clusters (Fig. 5.2.).

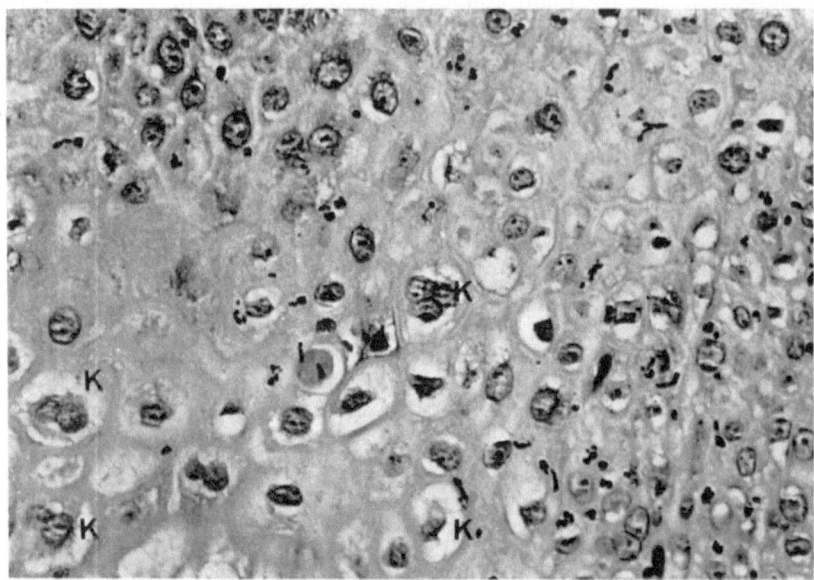

Fig. 5.2. A small area of mildly dyplasic epithelium. The cells marked K show koilocytotic (warty) atypia; their nuclei are degenerate or multiple and they are surrounded by an empty halo crossed by a few strands of cytoplasm. (H. & E. × 300)

Cells similar to these are seen in condyloma acuminatum, thus suggesting a possible relation to virus infection. Indeed Koss (1968) terms these changes "warty atypia". However, PATTEN (1969) states that the perinuclear clear zone has been attributed to shrinkage and SAGIROGLU (1963) considers it an artefact.

    There are a number of different descriptions of the patterns of dysplasia. DE BRUX and DUPRÉ-FROMENT (1961a and b) and DE BRUX and WENNER-MANGEN (1961) introduced a complex classification of the patterns based on a theoretical analysis of the abnormalities of cervical epithelium. They divided dysplasia into two types: (a) regular, distinguished by the persistence of a regular architecture with some anomalies in relation either to slight disturbances of cellular maturation or to the hyperactivity of the basal cells, and (b) irregular, characterized by more or less complete loss of stratification because of delayed cellular differentiation. In the later paper DE BRUX and WENNER-MANGEN (1961) give a useful table correlating their terminology with that of other authors especially that of GLATTHAAR (1955) and BAJARDI (1961b). The classification given by PATTEN (1969) is perhaps the most

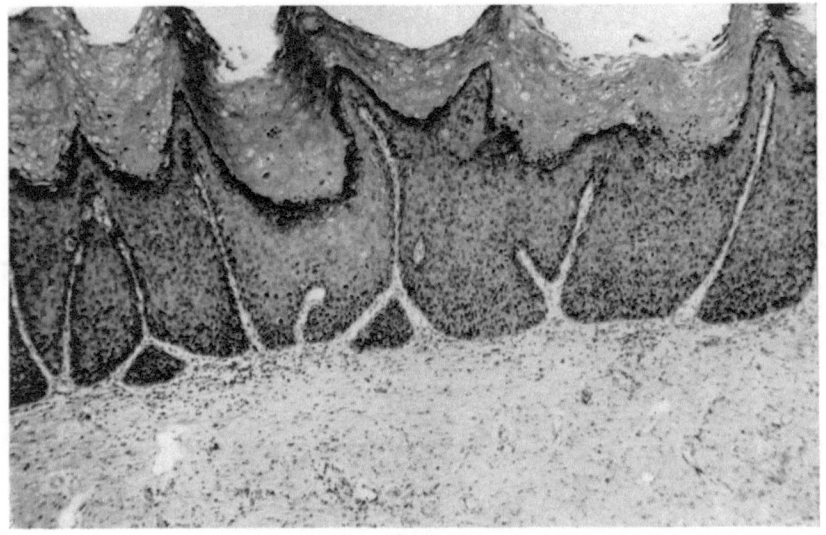

a

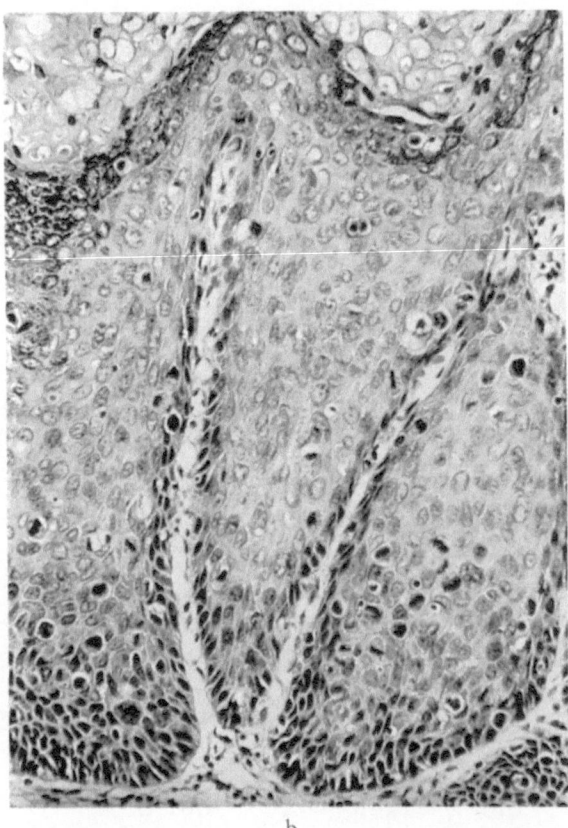

b

Fig. 5.3. a and b. Keratinizing dysplasia. a. The squamous epithelium is covered by a thick layer of keratin and there is a little parakeratosis. The granular layer is very conspicuous. (H. & E. × 60), b. This is a higher magnification of the deeper layers and shows the marked proliferative activity in the lower strata and also a number of cells showing nuclear abnormalities. (H. & E. × 180) useful and carries few theoretical implications. Table 5.1. shows a modification of this classification.

The keratinizing type of dysplasia is especially interesting. Sometimes the hyperkeratosis may be so marked as to make it difficult, if at all possible, to differentiate this condition from leukoplakia cervicis (using the term leukoplakia in the sense employed by pathologists and not by colposcopists). Parakeratosis may sometimes be seen, the lower limits of the change often coinciding with the intraepithelial

Table 5.1. Types of cervical dysplasia

Type	Origin
Keratinizing (ectocervical) Figs. 5.3. (a and b)	(a) normal squamous epithelium (b) basal-cell hyperplasia
Non-keratinizing Figs. 3.8. and 3.9.	(a) normal squamous epithelium (b) basal-cell hyperplasia (c) incomplete squamous metaplasia
Metaplastic, Figs. 5.4. and 5.5.	squamous metaplasia, especially in glands

layer (*Verhornungszone*) of DIERKS. Whether the excess keratin is produced normally, as in reactive hyperplasia, or whether it is abnormal as in psoriasis (BRODY 1964b) remains to be investigated. In psoriasis some of the enzymes linked to fundamental cellular processes such as succinic dehydrogenase, cytochrome oxidase and ribonuclease show greater activity than normal. It may be that the variability in enzyme

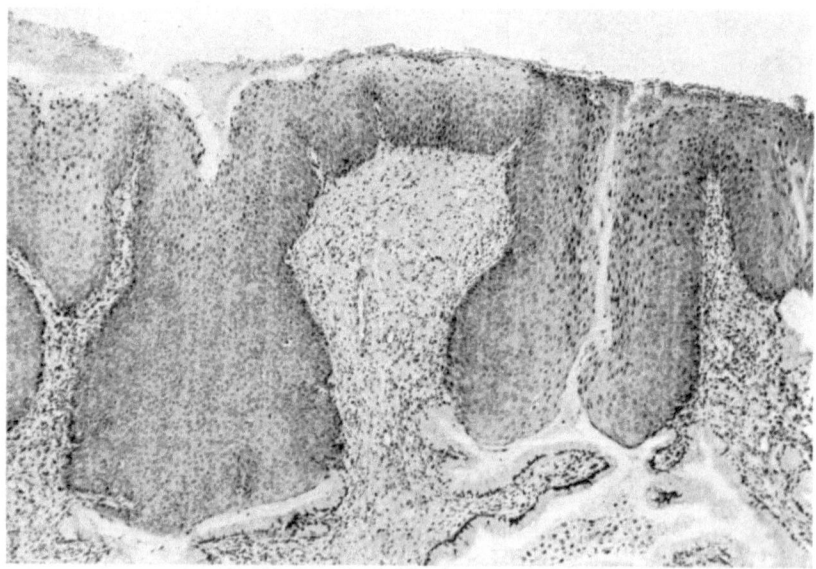

Fig. 5.4. Metaplastic type of dysplasia. The metaplastic squamous epithelium is well formed and involves the necks of endocervical glands. Under higher magnification mild atypia can be seen. (H. & E. × 50)

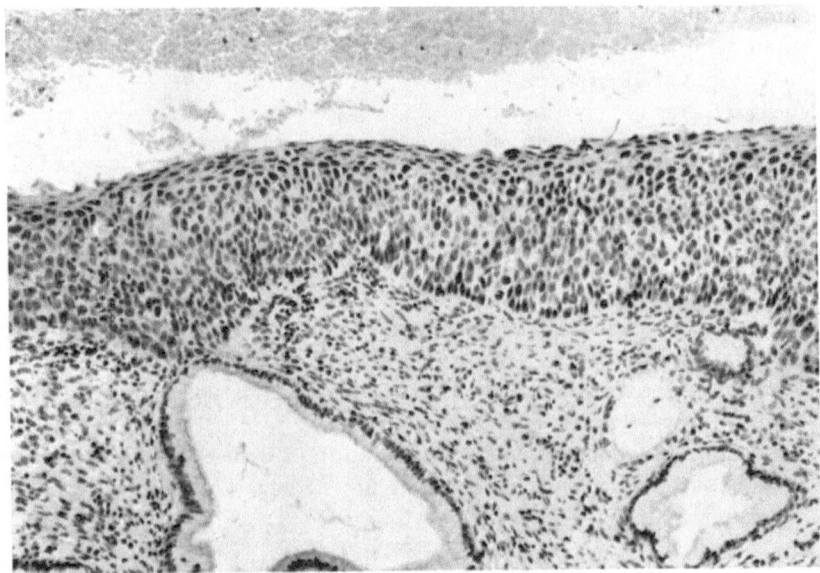

Fig. 5.5. Metaplastic epithelium showing moderately severe dysplasia. The squamous epithelium is immature and poorly organized; some nucelar atypia are also present. (H. & E. × 120)

patterns in dysplasia is related to the degree and type of keratinization or other forms of cytoplasmic differentiation. This needs further study.

A more comprehensive analysis of the morphology of dysplasia has been made by REAGAN (1964) and PATTEN (1969).

It must be remembered that dysplastic lesions are not peculiar to the cervix uteri. There is, for example, an extensive literature on dysplasia of the bronchial mucosa where it may be found unassociated with intraepithelial carcinoma (FORD et al. 1961).

b) Carcinoma *in situ*

A general description of this condition was given in Chapter 3. This followed the criteria laid down in 1961 by the International Committee on Histological Definitions at Vienna, and is illustrated in the papers of GOVAN et al. (1966 and 1969). It must, however, be recognized that there is a variety of histological patterns included under the term of carcinoma *in situ*. FLUHMANN (1961) has suggested three types. His Type I, or undifferentiated pattern, is the "typical lesion" which presents no diagnostic problem. Type II is usually composed of polygonal cells, although there is considerable variation in size and shape and there may be giant nuclei and multiple nuclei. Abnormal mitoses are frequent. Type III contains differentiated and stratified cells and probably does not satisfy the 1961 criteria. BAJARDI (1961a) has described undifferentiated and differentiated carcinoma *in situ*. GORE and HERTIG (1964) included under the designation carcinoma *in situ*, epithelium with surface differentiation and even keratinization. More recently TWEEDALE and RODDICK (1969) have described four histological types:

(1) parabasal-cell type,
(2) keratinizing-cell type,
(3) pleomorphic-cell type and
(4) small-cell type.

They found the keratinizing-cell type more common in older women than in younger women. It is clear from their photomicrographs that this type should be regarded as dysplasia.

Recognizing that a spectrum of histological changes can be seen in carcinoma *in situ*, VON HAAM and OLD (1964) have employed a subclassification of four groups:

(1) Alpha type—questionable carcinoma *in situ* not recognized as such by all observers, possibly regarded by some as dysplasia or a borderline lesion.

(2) Beta type—showing definite evidence of cellular atypism and proliferation.

(3) Gamma type—typical *in-situ* carcinoma.

(4) Delta type—advanced atypical proliferation of epithelial cells without sharp demarcation between epithelium and underlying stroma. This type may show early stromal invasion.

PATTEN (1969) regards the concept of "differentiated" carcinoma *in situ* as incongruous with the definition of this lesion. He has therefore adopted the subclassification of REAGAN and HARMONIC (1956a) which utilizes the terms *small cell carcinoma in situ* and *large cell carcinoma in situ*. This classification is useful in studying morphogenesis. REAGAN *et al.* (1962) have described both histological and cytological patterns characterizing developmental stages of *in-situ* carcinoma. Generally the morphological changes were less than those associated with carcinoma *in situ* and not within the definition of dysplasia. Histologically there were two different patterns. In one, the component reserve cells were predominantly undifferentiated; in another the reserve cells had undergone variable degrees of differentiation towards a squamous-like metaplastic epithelium. These lesions PATTEN (1969) regards as similar to those depicted as "carcinoma *in situ*, beta type", by VON HAAM and OLD (1964). It is undoubtedly true that, from time to time, it is difficult to distinguish reserve cell hyperplasia from carcinoma *in situ* especially if abnormal mitoses are lacking, but it is perhaps open to question whether or not such lesions should be characterized as developmental stages in the evolution of carcinoma *in situ*.

The distinctions so far considered are essentially cytological. HAMPERL (1959), who has a wider concept of carcinoma *in situ* than is now generally employed, has distinguished five types of lesion depending on arrangement of the malign tissue:

(1) simple replacement, including endocervical gland involvement,
(2) bulky downgrowth,
(3) early stromal invasion,
(4) advanced stromal invasion (preclinical carcinoma) and
(5) advanced bulky downgrowth.

Most other workers would probably regard the latter two groups as invasive carcinoma. With this limitation in mind, it is probable that a very adequate morphological classification of carcinoma *in situ* is provided by combining HAMPERL's terminology with REAGAN and HARMONIC's (1956) grouping into large and small cell types.

c) Microinvasive Squamous-cell Carcinoma of the Cervix

In Chapter 3 reference was made to the concept of microinvasive carcinoma as elaborated by GLÜCKSMANN and CHERRY in 1964. More recently (1968) GLÜCKS-MANN has developed the theoretical background more fully. In his view micro-invasive carcinoma is characterized by penetration of the basement membrane by groups of tumour cells which show a "reversal of architecture of the focus: the centre as well as some parts of the periphery are formed by enlarged usually cornify-ing cells which replace the small basal cells of the periphery lining the basement membrane." Lack of xenoplasia, that is lack of capacity to reproduce indefinitely in the stroma, is shown by maturation and death of the cells in their new environment unprotected by a basement membrane. Xenoplasia can be identified positively in the next stage of carcinogenesis by the persistence in the stroma of basal or small tumour cells unprotected by a basement membrane and by their mitotic activity in such sites. If these concepts should prove to be true, then clearly HAMPERL's inclusion of stromal invasion into the category of carcinoma *in situ* would be justified. GLÜCKSMANN has described four stages of xenoplasia, ability:

(1) to grow outside the basement membrane at the primary site,
(2) to grow as embolic metastases at certain sites, such as the regional lymph nodes,
(3) to grow anywhere in the host, and
(4) to proliferate on transplantation into heterogenetic animals.

As GLÜCKSMANN has pointed out, tumour embolism is not synonymous with the establishment of metastases since normal structures may become embolic. He has described the presence of uterine tubules in the pelvic lymph nodes of almost 20% of postmenopausal women as an innocuous occurrence. GRICOUROFF (1962) has described benign deposits of thyroid tissue in the lymph glands of the neck and there is reason to suppose that embolism of trophoblastic cells to the lungs is not an uncommon event in labour. Thus, microinvasive carcinoma can be regarded as a stage in carcinogenesis in which tumour autonomy has not been fully acquired. Autonomy is acquired gradually and can be identified by advancing degrees of xenoplasia shown initially by proliferation of small cells at the primary site and later by capacity to grow at other sites. GLÜCKSMANN has described experimental studies on rats which suggested that X-irradiation and hormones may modify the rate of progress of carcinogenesis. FETTIG (1964) studied 84 microcarcinomas and concluded that growth in size of the tumour is not the only factor determining malignant growth but that changes in the surrounding tissue, especially inflammation, play an important role.

A detailed review of 66 cases of microinvasive carcinoma has recently been reported by NG and REAGAN (1969). Most women were asymptomatic at the time of detection and clinical findings were either normal or non-specific. Thus they were usually detected by exfoliative cytology. The microinvasive neoplasm did not exceed a depth of 5.0 mm and originated predominantly from carcinoma *in situ* and/or dysplasia in the transitional zone of the anterior lip of the cervix. Table 5.2. summarizes some of their observations. Using the classification of WENTZ and REAGAN (1959), 89.4% of the microinvasive cancers were of large-cell type and 10.6% were of keratinizing type and none were of small-cell type. This observed pattern of cell type contrasts with GLÜCKMANN's more speculative views. NG and REAGAN found the pattern of invasion to be variable. A single discrete focus of epithelium was seen in 7.5% of cases, multicentric foci of discrete epithelial cell infiltration in continuity with the parent epithelium were found in 19.7% but in 33.3% the discrete epithelial infiltrations could not be traced to their parent epithelium in the sections examined. Lymphatic involvement by tumour cells was present in 7.6% of cases. The five-years survival rate was 95.8%. This description of microinvasive carcinoma corresponds closely with HAMPERL's early and advanced stromal invasion and advanced bulky downgrowth.

Table 5.2. Microinvasive carcinoma of the cervix uteri (NG and REAGAN 1969)

Depth of penetration	0.1—1.0 mm	1.1—3.0 mm	3.1—5.0 mm	Total
No of cases	13	30	23	66
Unicentric	38.5%	0%	0%	7.5%
Multicentric	61.5%	100%	100%	92.5%
Tissue of origin:				
Carcinoma *in situ*	72.7%	73.1%	85.7%	68.2%
Junction CIS/DYS	18.2%	15.4%	14.3%	13.6%
Dysplasia	9.1%	7.7%	—	4.6%
Normal epithelium	—	3.8%	—	1.5%
Uncertain [a]	—	—	—	12.1%

[a] Surface ulceration at the site of microinvasion was so extensive that it was impossible to identify the nature of the surface alteration.

MUSSEY *et al.* (1969) have reviewed 91 cases of cervical carcinoma with stromal invasion of 5 mm or less. In 69 women there was unequivocal stromal invasion and, in 10 of these, invasion of vascular spaces. In 22 cases there was borderline stromal invasion. Regional lymph node excision was performed in 53 patients and yielded only one cancer-bearing obturator lymph-node metastasis. Metastasis occurred in two patients: one was alive and well five years after a Wertheim hysterectomy and pelvic lymphadenectomy, and the other died during the sixth year after vaginal hysterectomy. They concluded that simple hysterectomy cures many of the so-called early lesions, including those exhibiting borderline stromal invasion, but that this treatment is inadequate for a carcinoma with the metastatic potential implied by the presence of tumour cells in vascular spaces. They regarded lesions with definite but limited (3 mm or less) invasion of the stroma and no discernible invasion of vessels as of less serious import.

The discussion following the paper of MUSSEY *et al.* (1969) indicates that there is no agreement as to the precise meaning to be attached to the term microinvasive carcinoma. FIDLER and BOYES (1959) used the term to mean very small clusters of invasive cells usually found adjacent to *in-situ* carcinoma. When confluence of invasive cells had occurred, forming a measurable tumour mass, FIDLER and BOYD (1960) called the lesion "occult" carcinoma. They found vascular metastases in a lesion 2 mm in diameter.

2. Topography and Morphogenesis of Malign Lesions of the Cervix Uteri

Topographic studies of the distribution of dysplasia and carcinoma *in situ* in the cervix are difficult because there is no well-defined anatomical point of reference. FENNELL (1955, 1956) used the squamo-columnar junction as a fixed reference point indicative of the external os. KAUFMANN and OBER (1959) have shown that this junction moves relative to the anatomical external os and thus is unacceptable as a fixed point of reference. Moreover, whilst the anatomical os is well defined in many cervices, it is less so in others. PRZYBORA and PLUTOWA (1959) carried out a very careful study of 100 cervices. They regarded the external os as the dividing border between the portion visible through the speculum and the portion concealed in the canal. This border does not take the form of a line but forms a ring-like area in the lower canal about 0.2 cm in extent. In their analysis they also made corrections for the effect of contraction of the tissues as a result of fixation. COPPLESON and REID (1967) have more recently pointed out that the speculum actually opens the cervical canal so that the cervix as seen *in vivo* and as seen in the fixed specimen may differ. A similar observation had previously been made by MORICARD and CARTIER (1956).

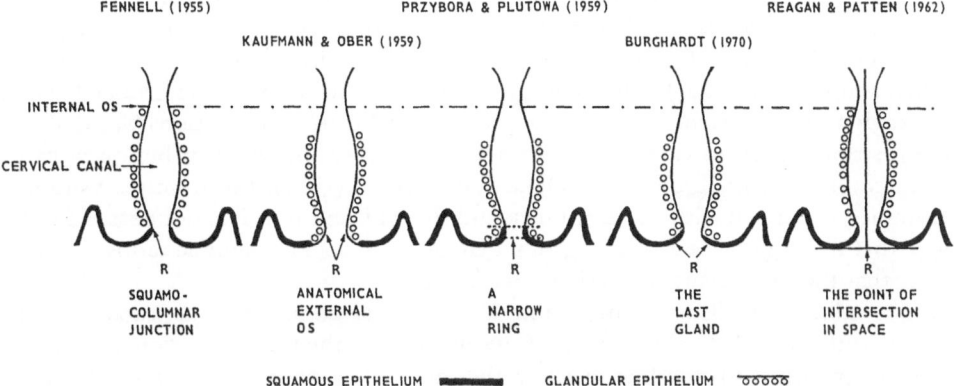

Fig. 5.6. This diagram shows the point of reference used by various authors when describing the topography of the cervix

BURGHARDT (1970) has commented on these difficulties and employs the last endocervical gland as a reference point; this may often lie underneath squamous epithelium. REAGAN and PATTEN (1962) made their measurements in relation to a point where a vertical line passing through the axis of the cervical canal intersects a horizontal line passing through the outermost portion of the portio vaginalis. These various reference points are illustrated in Fig. 5.6. The problem is similar to that of defining where an estuary ends and the open sea begins and there can only be arbitrary answers.

FOOTE and STEWART (1948) were the first to investigate the topography of carcinoma *in situ* of the cervix uteri. Of 27 cases studied, 14 involved both the portio vaginalis and the endocervical canal, 10 involved only the portio and 3 only the endocervical canal. Similarly, HELD (1957) remarked on the rarity of endocervical carcinomas. Thus he found only 2.5% of in-situ carcinomas, 2.4% of microinvasive carcinomas and 4% of clinical carcinomas situated in the endocervical canal. PRZY-BORA and PLUTOWA (1959) studied 100 cases, 79 of which were in situ, 18 showed incipient invasion and 3 an invasive focus (clinical stage IA). Ten of these lesions involved only the region of the external os, 33 the os and portio vaginalis, 10 lesions were in the os and endocervical canal, and 44 involved both the endocervical canal and portio vaginalis. The least extensive cancers were those involving only the os, the two smallest had diameters of scarcely 0.12 cm. In 5 specimens the cancerous epithelium involved the vaginal fornices. Unfortunately, these workers do not refer to the concomitant presence of dysplasia and since this is fairly common, it may be supposed that their histological criteria of carcinoma in situ included at least severe dysplasia.

REAGAN and PATTEN (1962) and PATTEN (1969) have analysed the relation of carcinoma in situ, dysplasia, metaplasia and reserve cell hyperplasia to their reference point. As would be expected, reserve cell hyperplasia and squamous metaplasia had a similar distribution to the columnar epithelium. Surprisingly, perhaps, carcinoma in situ was similar distributed. Dysplasia largely involved squamous epithelium or metaplastic epithelium. When dysplasia and carcinoma in situ co-existed in the uterine cervix, the latter always lay proximally and dysplasia lay distally.

LOHE (1969) described the location of the lesion in 73 cases of cervical dysplasia and found the distribution to be similar to that of carcinoma in situ as described by OBER and BONTKE (1959). Almost 60% of his dysplastic lesions were grouped about the region of the external os. A curious feature of LOHE's observations was that the age distribution of his cases of dysplasia was similar to the age distribution of cases of carcinoma in situ described by OBER and BONTKE (1959). LOHE's cases were not examined in parallel with those of OBER and BONTKE and thus it is not possible to be sure that they represent a similar group of women in socio-economic terms, nor is it clear that the same diagnostic criteria were used.

COPPLESON and REID (1967) found that atypical colposcopic appearances consistent with a histological diagnosis of dysplasia lay in the transformation zone inside (that is, proximal to) the line marking the junction of native squamous epithelium with metaplastic squamous epithelium. This is precisely the site at which Stage 0 carcinoma occurs. They explain the rare occurrence of dysplasia and carcinoma in situ at the vaginal vault on the supposition that such foci represent atypical metaplasia which developed in embryological vestiges of columnar epithelium.

Although there are differences in detail between the findings of various workers it is clear, from the above review, that dysplasia and carcinoma in situ arise in, or about, the metaplastic epithelium lying between the mature squamous epithelium and the columnar epithelium. The evidence suggests that dysplasia tends to arise more distally than carcinoma in situ. When dysplasia is succeeded by carcinoma in situ two possibilities exist. First, either the dysplastic epithelium is proliferating so rapidly that it never matures sufficiently to differentiate and become stratified before the surface layers are shed, or the noxious agent first affects squamous or metaplastic epithelium and then extends to the columnar epithelium. The second possibility is that dysplasia and carcinoma in situ are on a par, the one being a reaction of squamous (or metaplastic) epithelium, the other of glandular epithelium.

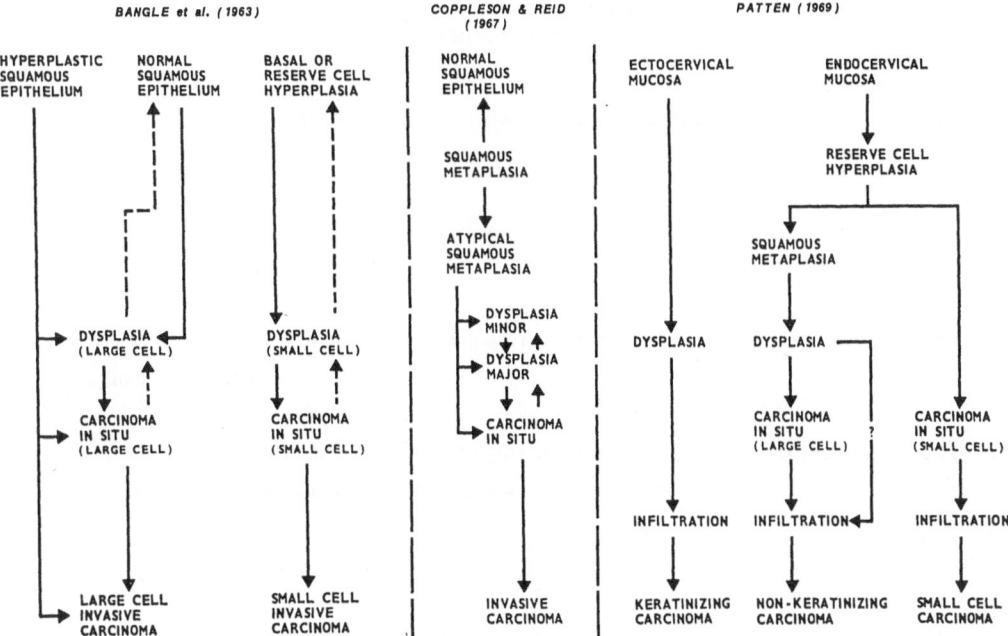

Fig. 5.7. This diagram summarises various views as to the mode of development of epithelial abnormalities of the cervix

Several schemes have been put forward to illustrate the developmental stages in the morphogenesis of squamous cell carcinoma of the cervix. These are illustrated in Fig. 5.7. None is entirely satisfactory but each stresses some aspect of importance. The scheme of BANGLE *et al.* (1963) indicates the occasional development of squamous cell carcinoma from normal, or nearly normal, squamous epithelium but does not sufficiently distinguish between basal and reserve cell hyperplasia. COPPLESON and REID (1967) in their scheme stress the relationship of epithelial abnormalities of the cervix to squamous metaplasia but ignore other possible routes of morphogenesis. PATTEN (1969) gives perhaps the most comprehensive picture but he does not accept the direct route of development from normal squamous epithelium to invasive carcinoma without an intermediate stage. The development of keratinizing carcinoma from the ectocervical mucosa *via* a dysplastic phase parallels the mode of progression in the rodent cervix following carcinogenic stimulation.

PRZYBORA (1966) has shown that the pattern of carcinogenesis in the cervix and at other sites depends on the rate of progress of the condition and the interplay between two factors—proliferative and transformative progression. Proliferative progression, as the term indicates, consists of the proliferation of tissues affected by the carcinogenic process. Transformative progression finds its morphological expression in disorder of tissue differentiation and maturation, chaotic architecture and cellular atypia. He has described four schemes of carcinogenesis as shown in Fig. 5.8. The transformative scheme is the classical pattern of development of cervical carcinoma.

VARIETIES OF CARCINOGENESIS
PRZYBORA (1966)

RAPID   NORMAL EPITHELIUM ➤INVASIVE CARCINOMA

UNIFORM   NORMAL EPITHELIUM ➤HYPERPLASIA + PRECANCER ➤INVASIVE Ca.

PROLIFERATIVE   NORMAL EPITHELIUM ➤HYPERPLASIA ➤ HYPERPLASIA + PRECANCER
                                                          ➤ INVASIVE CARCINOMA

TRANSFORMATIVE   NORMAL EPITHELIUM ➤PRECANCER ➤IN SITU CARCINOMA
                                           ➤INCIPIENT INVASION ➤INVASIVE CARCINOMA

Fig. 5.8. Przybora's scheme

The pattern of development is also modified in the later stages by whether or not the invasion is unicentric or multicentric (PRZYBORA and PLUTOWA 1959; BURGHARDT 1970). BURGHARDT (1970) has stressed the sharp changes in pattern between adjacent areas of dysplastic epithelium, suggesting differences in biological properties of adjacent fields. These differences may be a result of focal changes in chromosomal constitution (see later) and they may ultimately be reflected in the type of invasion—unicentric or multicentric.

3. The Ultramicroscopic Structure of Dysplasia, Carcinoma *in situ* and Invasive Carcinoma

GLATTHAAR and VOGEL (1958) were two of the earliest workers to study carcinoma of the cervix under the electron microscope. They found that the surface area of the cells was greatly increased by the presence of microvillus-like projections, whereas the number of intercellular bridges was greatly reduced. In the same year BERGER et al. (1958) using the electron microscope examined specimens of cervix showing "marked atypical epithelium", so-called carcinoma *in situ* and invasive carcinoma. At the magnification employed they could find no differences in the structure of the cells and nuclei in these conditions. In simple atypical epithelium at a magnification of 6,000 they occasionally found cells with irregular nuclei and notched nuclear membranes but intercellular bridges could still be seen. However in "marked atypical epithelium", carcinoma *in situ* and invasive carcinoma these bridges could no longer be seen.

More recent studies have confirmed and enlarged upon this earlier work. ASHWORTH et al. (1961) stated that in invasive carcinoma and carcinoma *in situ*, in contrast to normal squamous epithelium, there was a condensation of nuclear granules just inside the nuclear membrane and around enlarged nucleoli and that there were marked clefts and infoldings of the nuclear membrane. Within the cytoplasm there was scarcity or absence of glycogen droplets, enlargement and vacuolation of the mitochondria and increased density and clumping of RNA protein granules. The cell membranes showed a decrease in number of the intercellular bridges, many of which were imperfect, but villus-like projections of the cell margin were present. MORICARD and CARTIER (1964) have summarized and illustrated the changes in fine structure of these lesions. In invasive carcinoma they found that the nuclei were often extremely polylobed and the nucleolar modifications were complex. The differentiation of the desmosomes was variable. In invasive cancer of the basal-cell type there was little or no differentiation of the desmosomes; in the spinal-cell type differentiation of the desmosomes appeared almost normal but sometimes the middle stratum was missing. In carcinoma *in situ* it was possible to observe an absence, or only partial differentiation, of the desmosomes. The attachment plaques were incompletely formed and a widening could be seen in the clear middle zone between them. Sometimes there was complete lack of differentiation of desmosomes as was found in the basal-cell type of squamous-cell carcinoma. These lesions are beautifully illustrated by MORICARD and CARTIER in their account.

SHINGLETON *et al.* (1968) have reported a carefully controlled study of dysplasia and carcinoma *in situ* using somewhat higher magnifications. The nuclei of dysplastic cells were much enlarged and often multilobed. The nuclear membranes exhibited numerous invaginations and the nuclear chromatin was coarsely clumped while the nucleoli were often multiple and irregularly shaped. In the cytoplasm glycogen was scanty or absent. There was no consistent change in the mitochondria. The Golgi apparatus and lysosomes appeared normal but there was a striking increase in non-membrane associated ribosomes which were often arranged in aggregates. There was a smaller increase in rough-surfaced endoplasmic reticulum. The cell surface was altered in all cases. Desmosomes were decreased in number in the advanced lesions but retained their usual structure and there was a parallel decrease in the number of tonofibrils. Microvilli were increased in numbers and they were frequently elongated and branched. The half desmosomes attached to the basement membrane appeared normal. In carcinoma *in situ* the nuclei were intermediate in size between those in dysplastic and normal epithelia. The nuclei were more regular in shape than in dysplasia but the nucleoli were frequently multiple and irregular. No glycogen was found in the cytoplasm. Mitochondria were found throughout all levels of the epithelium and the numbers of non-membrane associated ribosomes and cisternae of the granular endoplasmic reticulum were similar to those seen in the cells of dysplastic lesions. There were fewer desmosomes than in dysplasia and tonofibrils were correspondingly diminished in numbers. The half-desmosomes attached to the basement membrane were relatively normal. Microvilli were very numerous and similar to those seen in dysplasia.

HANSHKE and SCHULZ (1960) studied smears obtained from the portio vaginalis of 15 women, 5 of whom had cervical carcinoma. They concluded that the electron microscope revealed no changes pathognomonic of malignancy but that, as under the light microscope, tumour cells are recognised by the sum of their individual characteristics. GREIDER and SCARPELLI (1964) examined scrapings from the surface of a stage II carcinoma of the cervix. The outer rim of nuclear chromatin was dense and the nucleoli were composed of thicker strands, less densely packed than the chromatin. Most of the cytoplasm contained tonofilaments. Few mitochondria or elements of endoplasmic reticulum were seen but in some areas membrane-bound vesicles occurred. The cell membrane contained many microvilli but desmosomes were not as highly developed as those in normal epithelial cells of the cervix.

The diagnosis of the invasive status of cervical carcinoma depends on whether or not the tumour cells are confined by the underlying stroma and basement membrane. ASHWORTH et al. (1961) carried out a correlated study of the basement membrane identified both histochemically and by electron microscopy. In carcinoma in situ electron microscopy showed a continuous intact basement membrane, the structure and thickness of which appeared normal. However, there was a notable straightness of the membrane reflecting an absence of foot-like projections. SHINGLETON et al. (1968) agree that the basement membrane in carcinoma in situ is less undulating than in dysplasia, where it is normal.

In invasive carcinoma ASHWORTH et al. (1961) found several distinctive alterations in the basement membrane. Electron microscopy showed that most of the infiltrating groups of cells lacked a basement membrane. This was confirmed by PAS-alcian blue and by colloidal iron stains in histological sections. There were, however, exceptions to this rule. Occasionally electron microscopy and histochemical preparations revealed varying amounts of basement membrane investing the groups of cells. Around invading carcinoma nests they frequently found that the PAS stain revealed a thick, condensed zone, somewhat resembling a basement membrane. Careful study of this PAS-positive layer and evaluation of the alcian blue and colloidal iron stains indicated that this was usually a compressed layer of stromal elements rather than a true basement membrane. MASSON (1956) has shown that a continuous reticular basal membrane (the basement membrane of light microscopy, see Chapter 1) may be present in carcinomas in which there is a pronounced stromal reaction. MORICARD and CARTIER (1964) have found that in such cases polynuclear cells may pass through the electron-dense basement membrane. However, when there was a dispersion of isolated tumour cells in the connective tissue, there was no electron-dense basement membrane separating the cells from the ground substance of the connective tissue.

The most striking features revealed by electron microscopy, but not necessarily the most fundamental, are the changes in the cell surface and in the basement membrane. The decrease in the number of desmosomes accords with the finding that neoplastic cells are more loosely attached to one another than are normal cells. Ability to form desmosomes may explain the close apposition of normal cervical epithelial cells grown in tissue culture (WILBANKS and SHINGLETON 1970) whilst inability to form desmosomes would account for the lack of such apposition in cells cultured from dysplasia and carcinoma in situ (WILBANKS and RICHART 1966). SHINGLETON et al. (1968) point out that the increase in ribosomes in all layers of the epithelia in dysplasia and carcinoma in situ and their occurrence in aggregates is consistent with a high level of RNA and protein synthesis, whereas the disaggregation or disappearance of ribosomes, as seen in the upper layers of normal cervical squamous epithelium, denotes a decrease or cessation of cellular synthesis of these substances.

4. The Biochemistry of Malignant and Pre-malignant Lesions of the Cervix

Studies of cervical epithelium by conventional biochemical methods are relatively few but nevertheless illuminating. PEDERSEN (1968) has remarked that among the numerous biochemical abnormalities which have been demonstrated in malignant tissue the high rate of glycolysis, first described by OTTO WARBURG, is the only one which, so far, has been found characteristic of malignant tumours. PEDERSEN studied the oxygen consumption and the aerobic and anaerobic glycolysis in cervical biopsies taken from patients with malignant and non-malignant diesease. The oxygen uptake was measured by the conventional Warburg technique and glucose and lactate by specific enzymatic methods. The metabolic balance expressed as the Warburg ratio of lactate accumulation to oxygen uptake was found to be elevated in both the non-malignant and malignant tissue, but the absolute values of oxygen consumption, glucose consumption and lactate production were much higher in the malignant than the non-malignant tissue. He states, however, that there was no correlation between these parameters and the clinical stage of the disease. Moreover, no differences were found between the parameters in tissues with cellular atypia, the non-malignant portion of the cervix adjacent to the tumour and non-malignant tissue from normal cervices. This does not agree with the observations of BRIAND (1967) (quoted by PEDERSEN) who found a "malignant Warburg quotient of 2.0 to 3.1 in biopsies of the human ectocervix showing various degrees of atypia." In non-malignant tissue the Warburg quotient is usually below 1.5.

Studies of the isoenzymes of lactate dehydrogenase (LDH) support the contention disputed by PEDERSEN, that at an early stage in the development of cervical cancer there is a metabolic change in the tissue. TURNER (1964) and SUTCLIFFE and EMERY (1968) have shown that in invasive carcinoma of the cervix there is a considerable increase in the isoenzyme LDH-5 compared with normal cervical tissue. LATNER et al. (1966) found an increase in the proportion of LDH-5 in epithelium exhibiting carcinoma in situ, and SUTCLIFFE and EMERY (1968) found an increase in LDH-5 in the stroma beneath an in-situ carcinoma; this had probably diffused from the epithelium. LANGVAD and PEDERSEN (1969) studied the LDH-isoenzyme pattern in the cervix of 64 patients without malignancy and in 54 patients with different stages of cervical malignancy. The ratio of the isoenzyme LDH-4 to LDH-2, which in other malignancies has proved a sensitive parameter, showed no significant increase in malignancy of the uterine cervix. This ratio, however, in the non-malignant cervix, showed a significant variation with the phase of the menstrual cycle. In patients with suspected or manifest carcinomas of the uterine cervix no significant isoenzyme variations were noted. This finding was independent of the presence, or absence, of tumour tissue in the fragment of epithelium examined biochemically. This may indicate a "dedifferentiation" of tissue which normally is highly responsive to the inductive effect of progesterone on LDH synthesis. LANGVAD and PEDERSEN point out that the starch-gel electrophoretic technique used by LATNER et al. (1966) in determining the LDH-isoenzyme pattern of cervical carcinoma did not allow quantitative separation of LDH-5 from LDH-4. However, in the hands of SUTCLIFFE and EMERY these two isoenzymes were estimated separately and show a fall in LDH-4 in malignancy and a rise in LDH-5. Clearly more studies of the LDH-isoenzyme pattern are needed both in cervical malignancy itself and in comparison with malignancies elsewhere in the body.

a) Glucose-6-phosphate dehydrogenase

PARK and JONES (1968) have examined the blood and cancerous and non-cancerous epithelium of the cervix of 18 patients of African origin who were heterozygous for the A and B variants of glucose-6-phosphate dehydrogenase. Among 10 patients without cancer of the cervix, the cervical epithelium contained both variants in 9 cases and one variant in the other. Of 8 patients with cervical cancer, 5 contained a single variant in the cervical tissue (one was A, the other four B) and 3 contained both variants, but it is probable that in these 3 cases normal adjacent tissue was included. Polymorphism for the gene for glucose-6-phosphate dehydrogenase is found in about a third of individuals of African origin but seldom in Caucasians, and the gene is located on the X-chromosomes. Because of the Lyon phenomenon, Africans with a gene polymorphic for glucose-6-phosphate dehydrogenase have individual cells which have only the A or the B or one of the other infrequent forms of the enzyme. If in a patient, polymorphic for the gene in question, a tumour arose from a single cell the tissue of the tumour would yield only one variant of the enzyme although adjacent tissues might yield both. From this study PARK and JONES concluded that squamous-cell carcinoma of the cervix arises in one of the following ways: (1) from a single cell; (2) from one clone of cells with the same X-inactivation; (3) from multiple single cells with the same X-inactivation; (4) from multiple clones of cells with the same X-inactivation; or (5) from tissue which is a mixture of cells with both Xs active but with selective elimination during proliferation of one cell line with the same X-inactivation.

SMITH et al. (1971) investigated the electrophoretic variants of glucose-6-phosphate dehydrogenase in cervical biopsies of 5 negro patients with dysplasia, one with carcinoma in situ and 7 with invasive carcinoma. In each of the preinvasive lesions they found only one variant, which is consistent with a unicellular origin. Findings in 5 patients with invasive carcinoma are compatible with a unicellular origin of the neoplasm. In two invasive carcinomas both variants of the enzyme were found. They think the most likely explanation of this is that these tumours arose from more than one cell. Other possible, but less likely, explanations are: (1) that normal tissue or blood was mixed with the tissue that was assayed, or (2) that the Lyon hypothesis does not always apply to malignant tissue.

b) Vaginal Enzymology

A number of different enzymes have been studied in vaginal fluid in an attempt to develop a diagnostic screening test for cervical carcinoma and its precursors. Notable among the enzymes are β-glucuronidase (FISHMAN et al. 1954; LAWSON 1959a and b; and RAURAMO 1959), 6-phosphogluconate dehydrogenase (BONHAM and GIBBS 1962; BONHAM 1964; NERDRUM 1964; MUIR et al. 1964; BELL and EGERTON 1965; HOFFMAN and MERRIT 1965; JÜTTING et al. 1965; LAWSON and WATKINS 1965; MOUKHTAR and HIGGINS 1965; LONGNECKER and WHITE 1967, and GOLDBERG et al. 1968), ribonuclease (GOLDBERG et al. 1968), α-mannosidase, β-galactosidase and β-N-acetylglucosamidase (LAWSON 1964).

Unfortunately these studies have added little to our understanding of the development of cervical neoplasia, nor have they as yet provided a satisfactory diagnostic test (MUIR and VALTERIS 1969).

5. The Histochemistry of Epithelial Abnormalities of the Cervix

The histochemical changes will be considered under three heads: (1) the cytoplasmic enzymes, (2) the non-enzymic cytoplasmic components and (3) the nuclear components, especially DNA.

a) The Cytoplasmic Enzymes

Extensive histochemical investigations of the cytoplasmic enzymes have been made by a number of workers: FISHMAN and MITCHELL (1959); LOUIS (1960); HOPMAN (1960); FORAKER and MARINO (1961); FISHMAN et al. (1963); MORI et al. (1963); THIERY and WILLIGHAGEN (1964); WARONSKI (1964); ISHIHARA et al. (1964); MOUKHTAR and HIGGINS (1965); COHEN and WAY (1966); JONEK et al. (1966a and b); THIERY and WILLIGHAGEN (1966); DAWSON and FILIPE (1967); WIDY and KIERSKI (1967); FILIPE and DAWSON (1968); ISHIHARA et al. (1968); BLONK (1969) and WATTS and GOLDBERG (1969).

Although in many of these studies there is broad agreement between the workers, there are also noticeable differences. These may well arise from differences in technique, including differences in fixation, but they may also be a result of differences in the severity of the changes in the tissue examined. DAWSON and FILIPE (1967) write, "We know that in inflammatory conditions such as chronic cervicitis mitotic activity also increases, yet it is precisely from such conditions that we wish reliably to separate carcinoma *in situ*. We have not found any qualitative differences in enzyme distribution between these two conditions; and a quantitative one is improbable if both types of cell are hyperactive." Although enzyme studies of invasive carcinoma are fairly numerous, studies of dysplasia and carcinoma *in situ* are scanty. To date it is not possible to discern a pattern of enzyme change in invasive or pre-invasive carcinoma. Hence at present these studies contribute little to our understanding of the development of cervical neoplasia and they will not be discussed further.

b) The Non-enzymic Cytoplasmic Components

Glycogen, keratin, prekeratin and allied substances, and RNA are the most easily studied non-enzymic cytoplasmic components. Very few recent studies have been made of these in abnormal cervical epithelium and these have been confined to glycogen. MORICARD and CARTIER (1964) have summarized much of our knowledge of the distribution of glycogen in atypical epithelia. They use the presence or absence of glycogen to distinguish two types of basal-cell hyperactivity: (a) If glycogen is present in the squamous epithelium, the basal-cell hyperactivity may correspond to an oestrogenic hormonal hypersecretion. (b) If there is an absence or reduction of glycogen the basal-cell hyperactivity may be associated with cervicitis in a transformation zone. Glycogen is lacking in dysplasia and in carcinoma *in situ*. These findings are consistent with the reduced activity of the glycogen-metabolizing enzymes amylo-1, 6-glucosidase and amylophophorylase in dysplasia (FORAKER and MARINO 1961; FIENBERG and COHEN 1968). Indeed, it seems likely that the loss of enzyme activity is the prior metabolic lesion in these atypical epithelia. Although glycogen may be present in the more differentiated part of an invasive squamous-cell carcinoma, it is usually absent. These changes in glycogen content of cervical epithelia form the basis of SCHILLER's test.

c) The Nuclear Components

When assessing malignancy the diagnostic cytologist lays stress primarily on the nuclear changes and only secondarily on the cytoplasmic changes. It is indeed probable that, for the most part, the cytoplasmic changes are consequent on the nuclear abnormalities. Studies of the DNA content of cell nuclei are of importance because of their theoretical implications as to the nature of the cell changes and their practical value for devising automated screening techniques.

ATKIN (1964a and b, 1966a) has shown that the DNA content of the interphase nucleus of tumour cells is closely related both to the size and the ploidy of the nucleus. He compared (1966a) the modal DNA content and the modal chromosome number of 50 human malignant tumours and found that the two were in close agreement although the DNA content exceeded that expected on the basis of the chromosome number by an average of about 4%. It appears that in tumours the average chromosome size is very slightly greater than for normal cells. ATKIN et al. (1959) and ATKIN (1964a) have shown that, according to their modal DNA content, uterine

Table 5.3. Proportion of squamous lesions of the cervix uteri with small or large nuclei (ATKIN 1964a)

	Small nuclei	Large nuclei	Total cases
Basal-cell hyperplasia	17	1	18
Carcinoma in situ			
— squamous	23	54	77
— basocolumnar	6	4	10
Microcarcinoma			
— squamous	10	9	19
— basocolumnar	0	5	5

and other tumour groups may fall into two fairly distinct ploidy classes. From a study of the size of the nuclei in histological sections of cervical carcinoma, it was possible to make a correct estimate of the ploidy group in the majority of cases. About half the tumours were found to have a predominantly small nucleus, corresponding to a near-diploid DNA content, and about half the tumours had large nuclei, corresponding to near-tetraploid DNA content. ATKIN (1964a) studied 77 in situ squamous lesions of the cervix and found large nuclei in 54 cases; this proportion (70%) differed significantly from that of invasive carcinoma. His findings are shown in more detail in Table 5.3. The histological terminology used is that of GLÜCKS-MANN and no photomicrographs are provided to assist the reader. ATKIN suggested that these results indicated three possibilities: (1) Perhaps carcinoma in situ with large nuclei progresses less often and more slowly to invasive carcinoma than lesions with small nuclei. (2) Alternatively, a change from large to small cell type occurs when invasion begins. (3) Possibly in carcinoma *in situ* the majority of cells are near-tetraploid but a few are near-diploid and these become predominant when invasion occurs. These suggestions are highly speculative but are not inconsistent with ASHLEY's suggestion (1966) quoted above (Chapter 4) that there are two types of carcinoma of the cervix.

WILBANKS *et al.* (1967) and RICHART (1967) have studied the DNA content of cervical intraepithelial neoplasia by two-wavelength Feulgen cytophotometry. They found that the nuclei of normal cervical squamous epithelium had the expected distribution of DNA content round a modal diploid value. Histograms prepared from lesions of mild dysplasia and carcinoma *in situ* showed cells outside the normal diploid-tetraploid range including some with an extremely high DNA content (from 8N to nearly 16N). No distinct difference could be found between dysplasia and carcinoma *in situ*. A continuous spectrum of changes was found with a broader range of DNA values in the more severe lesions than in mild dysplasias. In addition to the heteroploid values, a significant proportion were in the diploid range, suggesting that the lesions included a diploid population of cells.

SANDRITTER *et al.* (1966) studied the DNA content of cells from a variety of human tumours including 5 cases of cervical carcinoma (2 described as epidermoid and 3 as squamous-cell). Many of these tumours were characterised by the presence of DNA-stem lines but in other there were multiple DNA peaks indicative of chromosomal mosaicism. In tumours with a DNA-stem line most of the nuclei were probably in the S-phase of the mitotic cycle and, presumably, rapidly growing. Of the cervical carcinomas, one had a hypotetraploid stem line, three had hyperdiploid stem lines and one had no well-defined stem line and was probably a mosaic. Earlier work (SANDRITTER 1964) had shown that *in-situ* and invasive carcinoma of the cervix had the same stem line, like primary and metastatic deposits of certain neoplasms.

VALERI *et al.* (1967) have investigated the relationship between the nuclear volume of cells and their DNA content. Sixteen cases of carcinoma *in situ* and 8 cases of invasive carcinoma were examined. In agreement with other workers, they found that the DNA values of carcinomatous cells were higher than those of control cells (lymphocytes and endocervical cells). In 11 cases of carcinoma *in situ* and all those of invasive carcinoma, the ratio of nuclear volume to DNA content was less than in control epithelium. In one case the ratio was the same as in the control tissue, and in two it was greater. In one of these latter cases the DNA content of the cells varied from two to almost eight times and in the other the DNA content was sixteen times the normal value. VALERI *et al.* point out that the increase in DNA per nucleus might result from polyploidy, from a polytenic chromosome, an increase in preprophase DNA, or aneuploidy. They suggest that the variations from normal in the ratio of nuclear volume to nuclear DNA content could be because other components of the nucleus (proteins, for example) have not been synthesized in the same proportions as DNA. Such a dissociation may be normally seen in actively growing tissues (BLOCH and GODMAN 1955; ALFERT 1958).

In summary, it appears that the nuclei of malign and malignant lesions of the cervix uteri usually have an increased DNA content. Often the increase indicates an aneuploid state of the nuclei and the presence of DNA-stem lines, but sometimes there is no well-defined stem line and the epithelium shows DNA nuclear mosaicism. Parallel with these changes in nuclear DNA there may be a dissociation of nuclear synthesis. The studies just reviewed were made on the epithelium in histological sections or on scrapings from the surface of the tissue. The following studies, which are broadly in accord with these, were made on exfoliated cells.

CASPERSSON (1964) measured the total content of DNA, RNA and protein in individual cells by cytochemical methods. The cells were obtained as scrapings from the cervix of patients with cervical carcinoma, premalignant cervical changes and atypical cervical epithelium, as well as from women with normal cervices. The DNA findings were similar to those described above. The dry mass (protein) values were extremely low in the tumour cell populations. This is probably because the rapidly growing tumour cell does not synthesize such large amounts of cytoplasm as a normal cell. The absolute amounts of RNA appeared to be lower in tumour cells than in normal cells but there was a higher average total nucleic acid content per unit mass of the cell. CASPERSSON found similar deviations from the normal in cells derived from premalignant epithelium although, in some cases, the deviations were less pronounced than in cell populations from invasive tumours.

WIED et al. (1966) used quantitative DNA measurements on Feulgen-stained cells exfoliated from the cervix. They compared the DNA content of these cells with that of thymus lymphocytes and related their results to the phases of the mitotic cycle (Fig. 5.9.). In non-specific infections they found that 13.3% of the cell population has

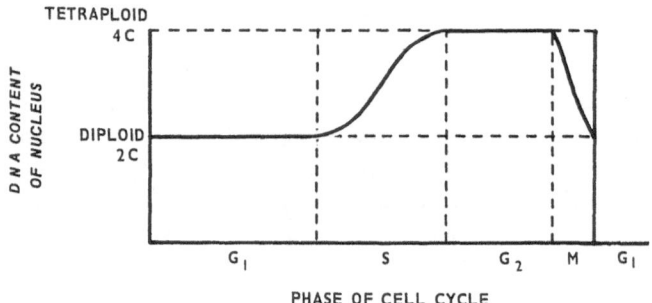

Fig. 5.9. The cell cycle

a 2cDNA content, 86% of cells are in the process of DNA synthesis and 0.6% are already at the 4cDNA level, i. e. the G_2 phase. Similar results were obtained from cells showing inflammatory changes due to trichomonad infection. Analysis of both these groups indicates a proliferating population of diploid cells. Of the cells originating from dysplasia, 82% had a higher than tetraploid DNA content, indicating that they had not followed the normal cycle but had by-passed or delayed the process of mitosis. All the tumour cells derived from carcinoma *in situ* had three to five times the normal diploid amount of DNA, whilst the cell population from invasive carcinoma had a slightly lower DNA content.

It is evident from these studies that the DNA content of cells derived from malign cervical epithelium may be raised by two processes — first, increased cell proliferation, and second, aneuploidy or changes in nuclear ploidy.

6. Cell Morphometry of Epithelial Abnormalities of the Cervix Uteri

Morphometric studies of cells in sections have been made by a number of workers, notably HILLEMANNS and co-workers and CASTAÑO-ALMENDRAL and BEATO.

With the Zeiss integrating ocular (HILLEMANNS et al. 1968 b) and the Zeiss particle-size analyser (HILLEMANNS and PRESTEL 1968) it has been shown that the mean nuclear volume increases from normal epithelium to dysplasia and to carcinoma in situ, where it reaches a maximum. The mean nuclear volume in invasive carcinoma is less than in carcinoma in situ. As the nuclear volume increases the nuclear/cytoplasmic ratio rises and is a maximum in carcinoma in situ. The decrease in nuclear/cytoplasmic ratio in invasive carcinoma represents an increase in the amount of cytoplasm. CASTAÑO-ALMENDRAL and BEATO (1968) used somewhat similar methods and analysed the results statistically. They found that the atypical changes in squamous epithelium are characterized by a change in nuclear/cytoplasmic ratio and an increase in the number of cells per unit area. These parameters reach a peak in carcinoma in situ and level off in invasive carcinoma without reaching normal values. The changes in nuclear size in atypical epithelium indicate a loss of "biological unity" compared with normal squamous epithelium. This is shown by the occurrence of more than one class of cell, as judged by nuclear size. They suggest that this may be explained by aneuploidy. These results parallel those for DNA content of cells described above. CASTAÑO-ALMENDRAL and BEATO (1968) caution that the development of a general concept, based on observations such as these, to explain the evolution of squamous-cell carcinoma of the cervix, is limited by the fact that these results are obtained from stationary states which do not reflect the dynamics of the pathological process. Similar reservations apply to ATKIN's speculations (1966 a) based on the DNA content of the cells.

HILLEMANNS et al. (1968 a) have investigated the development of carcinoma of the cervix in relation to cell count per unit area and the frequency of mitoses. They examined 354 cases of pre-cancer and 61 of microcarcinoma. The cell count per unit area increases with the severity of dysplasia and reaches a maximum in carcinoma in situ, with 278 % of the normal count. This count represents the "critical cell number" necessary for infiltration. When invasion occurs the cell count per unit area falls to 128 % in microcarcinoma and 95 % in invasive carcinoma, but rises again in advanced carcinoma to 140 %. In carcinoma in situ the frequency of mitoses is sixteen times normal but in invasive carcinoma it is only ten times normal. They regard the pressure produced by the increased number of cells and the change in the mode of growth of the cells as one of the decisive factors determining invasion.

7. Structural Abnormalities of the Nucleus

a) Mitotic Abnormalities

Disorders of mitosis in pre-invasive cancer of the cervix have been described by MORICARD and PAPATHEODOROU (1953), MORICARD and CARTIER (1959, 1964) and more recently by KIRKLAND et al. (1967). The mitotic abnormalities can be seen both in histological sections and in squash preparations. They may be classified as follows:

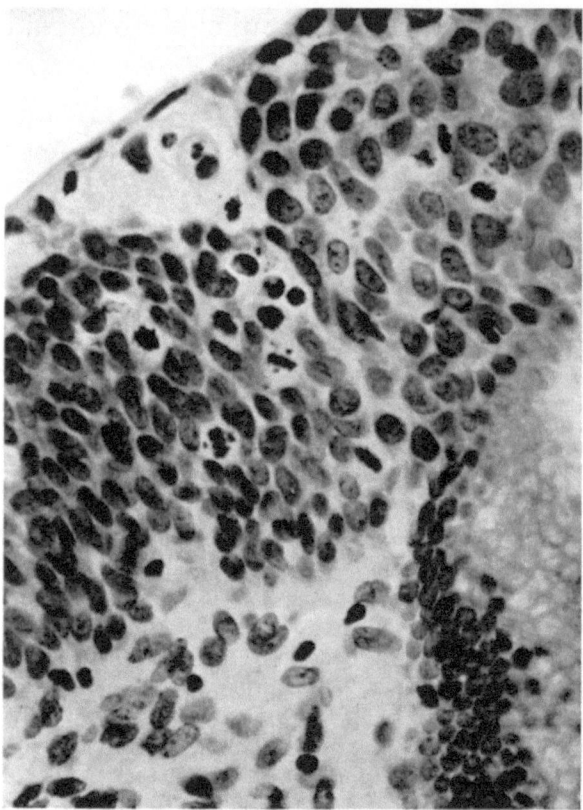

Fig. 5.10. a

Fig. 5.10. a Atypical epithelium showing numerous mitoses some arranged in the form of "three-group metaphase". b. Epithelium in an adjacent field showing "two-group metaphase". (H. & E. × 480)

(1) Disorders of metaphase; two-group metaphase which has a small collection of chromosomes detached and to one side of the metaphase plate (Fig. 5.10. b), and three-group metaphase in which there is a collection of detached chromosomes on both sides of the metaphase plate (Fig. 5.10. a) These abnormalities are easily recognized when the metaphase plate is in profile. Disorders of metaphase are the most easily seen abnormality, a phenomenon related to the longer duration of this phase in mitosis. (2) Abnormal anaphase; the relative positions of the chromosomes are abnormal or the size of the chromosome masses is unequal. These anaphase abnormalities are uncommon and difficult to observe. (3) Multipolar mitoses, such as triaster and quadraster. (4) Polyploidy, shown by the occurence of giant mitoses which have at least double the normal chromosome content. Less common variants are: (5) ring mitoses, in which there is a clearly defined circular structure; (6) V-mitoses, in which there is a partially split metaphase plate; and (7) leader mitoses, in which at least one elongated chromosome protrudes from the metaphase plate.

MORICARD and PAPATHEODOROU (1953) counted the number of mitoses in histological sections of 27 cases of carcinoma *in situ* in non-pregnant women and in 3 cases

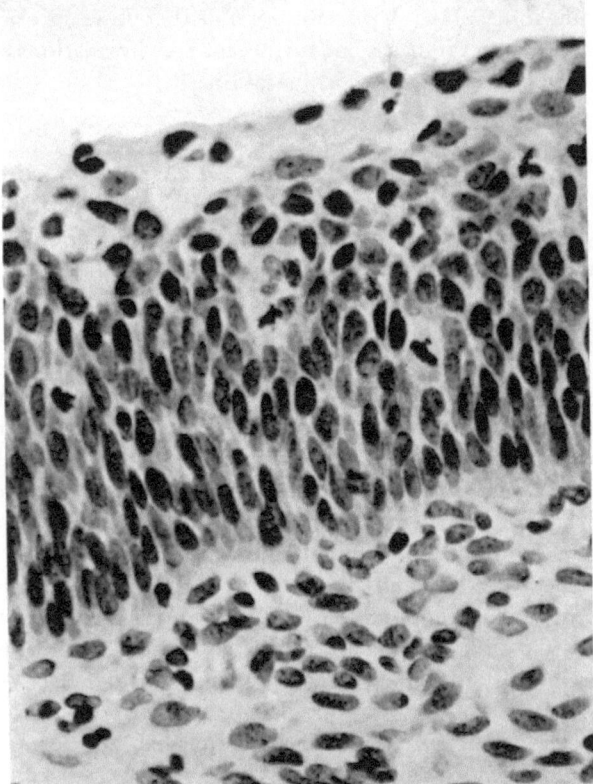

Fig. 5.10.b

in pregnant women. The abnormal mitoses constituted 50% or more of the total. They did not think that abnormal mitoses occured with such frequency in banal inflammations and in benign dystrophies e. g. metaplasia of the cervix. KIRKLAND et. al. (1967) did not find such a high proportion of abnormal mitoses. In dysplasia 84.2% were normal; in carcinoma in situ normal mitoses ranged on the average from 67.2 to 70.4% depending on whether the lesion was of small, mixed- or large-cell type; and in invasive carcinoma from 73.6 to 85.6%. The proportion of normal cells in dysplasia was in close agreement with the proportion of chromosome counts in the diploid range (81.5%). Such close agreement was not present in other situations although the "small-cell" tumours showed better agreement between the proportion of normal mitoses and the proportion of cells with diploid counts than did the "large-cell" tumours or those of mixed-cell type.

Although bizarre mitotic figures are well recognized in malignant tumours, PAYLING WRIGHT (1950) considered that the great majority of mitoses in tumour cells pursue a normal course. He indicated that multipolar and asymmetrical mitoses are not diagnostic of malignancy since they can be seen in normal and regenerating epithelium. Moreover PARMENTIER and DUSTIN (1954) have shown that the mitotic poison hydroquinone can produce mitoses with "three-group metaphase" and mitoses with polar chromosomes. Hence, it seems possible that these mitotic abnormalities are the product, rather than the cause, of malignant transformation and may be the precursors of cell death rather than of proliferation.

b) Variations in Chromosome Numbers

Aneuploidy is a common accompaniment of malignancy but it is not yet known whether the chromosomal changes are the essence of malignancy, or primarily responsible for malignant change, or only secondary to it. Nor, indeed, can it be stated that finding chromosomal changes of the types described below is to be regarded as a criterion of malignancy.

A number of different techniques have been used in studying the chromosomes of the cervix. RICHART and CORFMAN (1964) and RICHART and WILBANKS (1966) studied monolayer cultures of tissue obtained by using the colpomicroscope. Their technique ensured that only cells from cervical intraepithelial neoplasia (dysplasia and carcinoma *in situ*) were explanted. RICHART and coworkers found that the vast majority of cells derived from these epithelia were diploid with a karyotype indistinguishable from that of normal cervical epithelium. These results contrast with those of most other workers who have usually used some form of squash preparation. In these studies chromosomal aneuploidy is the usual finding. KIRKLAND *et al.* (1967) have suggested that this difference may be explained by the selective effects of culture but added that possibly a specific *in vivo* environment exists which is essential for the maintenance of abnormal cell populations. RICHART (1967) has discussed possible reasons for this discrepancy. First, it has been shown in experimental systems that cells containing highly abnormal chromosome numbers are less likely to complete mitosis than those with normal chromosomes, or if mitosis does proceed to completion, it is often prolonged. Second, the mitotic abnormalities presumably occur because of difficulties in chromosome arrangement on the mitotic spindle which probably causes delay in the mitotic cycle. Now, the number of cells in the tissue in each phase of the mitotic cycle is proportional to the duration of that phase. Hence the increased proportion of cells in abnormal metaphase is due to prolongation of this phase of the cycle. Since the squash technique selects only those cells which are in metaphase, chromosome numbers might be skewed in favour of the delayed heteroploid mitoses.

SPRIGGS *et al.* (1962) originally investigated cytogenetic abnormalities in direct squashes. Because of technical difficulties it was not possible to present satisfactory karyotype assays. Hence, they modified their method (BODDINGTON *et al.* 1965). Before preparing the squashes they cultured the tissue for 1 hour in medium 199 containing colchicine. A similar method has been used by ATKIN and BAKER (1966) and KIRKLAND *et al.* (1967) and also by WAKONIG-VAARTAJA and HUGHES (1965), who omitted the colchicine treatment

Tables 5.4., 5.5. and 5.6., are based on the paper of JONES *et al.* (1968) and summarize chromosome counts in dysplasia, carcinoma *in situ* and invasive carcinoma. It must be emphasised that there is some variation in histological criteria between the workers quoted. Although in each type of lesion a high proportion of the cells examined were near-diploid, there was a range of modal values. Thus in dysplasia 73% were near-diploid, 10% were near-triploid and 17% near-tetraploid. A similar high pro-

Table 5.4. Chromosomes in dysplasia (squash technique)

Reference	Patients	Chromosome mode		
		Diploid	Triploid	Tetraploid
Spriggs *et al.* (1962)	1	0	0	1
Boddington *et al.* (1965)	4	2	1	1
Auersberg *et al.* (1967)	9	9	2	1
Jones *et al.* (1967)	4	2	0	0
Kirkland *et al.* (1967)	8	8	0	0
Jones *et al.* (1968)	8	5	0	3
Total	34	26	3	6

Table 5.5. Chromosomes in carcinoma in situ (squash technique)

References	Patients	Chromosome mode			No mode
		Diploid	Triploid	Tetraploid	
Spriggs *et al.* (1962)	5	1	1	3	
Boddington *et al.* (1965)	6	4	2	0	
Auersberg *et al.* (1967)	7	4	5	2	
Jones *et al.* (1967)	2	1	0	1	
Kirkland *et al.* (1967)	47	8	4	15	20
Jones *et al.* (1968)	5	2	0	3	
Total	72	20	12	24	20

Table 5.6. Chromosomes in invasive squamous-cell carcinoma (squash technique)

References	Patients	Chromosome mode			No mode
		Diploid	Triploid	Tetraploid	
Spriggs *et al.* (1962)	1	0	1	0	
Atkin and Baker (1966)	5	4	1	0	
Atkin *et al.* (1966)	20	11	8	1	
Auersberg and Worth (1966)	14	9	3	2	
Atkin *et al.* (1967)	4	3	1	0	
Jones *et al.* (1967)	5	1	3	1	
Kirkland *et al.* (1967)	54	25	10	5	14
Total	103	53	27	9	14

portion of cells was diploid in invasive carcinoma but in *in situ* carcinoma triploid and tetraploid cells tend to predominate. The terms diploid, triploid and tetraploid in this context do not mean that there were precisely 46, 69 or 92 chromosomes per cell, but a range about these values. Kirkland *et al.* (1967) used a range of 35—56 chromosomes for the diploid state, 57—78 for the triploid state and 78—103 for the tetraploid state. Even using such wide ranges, they found that an appreciable number of lesions had no modal value, there being a wide scatter of chromosome values. Other workers have found that, when there is a clearly defined mode, a few cells have a very different chromosome complement. Thus, JONES et al. (1968) describe an example of atypical cervical epithelium with a well-defined mode of 93 chromosomes per cell, but one cell contained 362 chromosomes and another 504. WAKONIG-VAARTAJA and HUGHES (1965) expressed their results rather differently from other workers. They examined 4 cases of dysplasia. The range of chromosome numbers was 40—80 but there was a clear diploid mode at 46 in 37.3% of the cell population. In 22 cases of carcinoma in situ the chromosome numbers varied from less than 40 to more than 100, the numbers between 75 and 90 being the most frequent, apart from the diploid number which formed 10% of the cell population. In 35 cases of invasive carcinoma there was a similar wide chromosomal range and diploid cells formed 12% of the population. The in-situ and invasive cell populations were very similar.

It is important to compare these results with a control population of cells derived from normal epithelium or an epithelium with only bland lesions. This is difficult because of the low frequency of mitoses in cervical epithelium. TJIO and PUCK (1958) found that cultured cervical cell populations were almost entirely diploid, with less than 3% of tetraploid cells. JONES et al. (1968) using a squash technique examined the cervical epithelium of 25 women with normal cervices, or with cervicitis or mild atypia, and also 15 pregnant women. Efforts to secure adequate spreads were difficult and better results were obtained in regenerating epithelium after destruction of a small area by freezing. All the countable cells were diploid and had normal karyotypes.

When assessing the significance of these changes, the following considerations adduced by JONES et al. (1968) must be borne in mind. (1) Except for abortuses and some congenital abnormalities, malignant tumours are the only known source of chromosomal aneuploidy. (2) Except for aneuploidy, there is no consistent chromosomal abnormality characteristic of malignancy. They consider that early cervical epidermoid tumours tend to have a specific modal number of chromosomes as part of a characteristic and unique karyotype, so that each early cervical tumour may be thought of as having a chromosomal fingerprint. Later tumours appear to have a shifting karyotype. (3) With rare exceptions, chromosomal fingerprints are similar when cervical tumours are sampled at multiple sites or at intervals. (4) In a few instances when it has been possible to sample cervical atypia (dysplasia) at intervals the chromosomal fingerprints has been found to be essentially the same. (5) Samples of atypical epithelium associated with carcinoma in situ show aneuploid chromosomes. Such considerations support the stem-cell theory that a malign lesion arises from a single cell or clone of cells of identical karyotype. Against these observations it must be remembered that KIRKLAND et al. (1967) found, in a significant number of cases, no characteristic mode or stem line. All 8 of their dysplasias contained a mode but 20 of 47 carcinomas in situ and 14 of 54 invasive carcinomas did not have a demonstrable mode. KIRKLAND et al. (1967) found that in invasive carcinomas there was no difference in distribution of chromosomal count between two biopsies. In a few cases of in-situ carcinoma differences were observed between biopsies, and this was accompanied by a difference in the cell size of the lesion. This parallels the observations of SANDRITTER et al. (1966) previously mentioned (page 121). Using the DNA content of the nucleus as an index, they found that 4 of 5 cervical carcinomas, were composed of a single stem line of cells, but the fifth was not. Thus it appears that, while a majority of malign and malignant lesions of the cervix exhibit a stem line of cells, a significant proportion do not.

c) Karyotypes

Studies of the disorders of karyotype lend some support to the stem line hypothesis.

Detailed analysis of karyotypes of cervical lesions have been included in a number of reports (carcinoma *in situ*, WAKONIG-VAARTAJA 1963; dysplasia and carcinoma *in situ*, BODDINGTON *et al.* 1965; invasive carcinoma, ATKIN and BAKER 1966; ATKIN *et al.* 1967, and all three types of lesion by JONES *et al.* 1968). Perhaps the most significant findings in these investigations are: (1) the differences in karyotype from tumour to tumour, and (2) the occurrence of marker chromosomes in a number of tumours. Marker chromosomes are abnormal chromosomes which do not fall into the normal categories by length and arm ratio. ATKIN *et al.* (1967) carried out chromosome studies on 4 cervical carcinomas. Most of the cell metaphases had a karyotype characteristic of the tumour of origin. Although random loss of chromosomes from the characteristic karyotype might occur, these losses were probably artefactual. Three of the tumours were near-diploid, with characteristic ("stem-line") karyotypes having 47, 48 and 44 chromosomes, respectively; out of 37 metaphases from these tumours, 22 had the karyotype characteristic of the tumour, 14 had a random loss from this karyotype and only one had a single additional chromosome. Material was obtained from the fourth tumour on two occasions; both specimens were characterized by having 77 chromosomes. Three of the 4 tumours had marker chromosomes characterizing the karyotype. BODDINGTON *et al.* (1965) had previously described a long marker chromosome in several metaphases from a case of carcinoma *in situ*. ATKIN *et al.* (1967) concluded that their results suggest that it may be relatively easy, with recently devised techniques, to determine the stem-line karyotype of cervical carcinomas and that usually only one such line (but occasionally a small number of stemlines) will be found for each tumour.

GRANBERG (1971) found that the normal diploid karyotype was common in carcinoma *in situ* but absent in microinvasive and invasive carcinomas. Gains and losses in the modal population were associated with the same chromosome types in the different stages of malignancy. Chromosomes were usually in excess in group C while deficits were found in group B and, more often, in groups D and G. Structural aberrations appeared occasionally in preinvasive and microinvasive lesions and more often in invasive tumours, usually as an integral part of the modal karyotype. There was a statistically significant increase in the severity of the chromosome changes with the degree of malignancy.

d) Sex Chromatin Anomalies and Related Changes

In the preceding section the relationship between chromosomal abnormalities and malign and malignant lesions of the cervix uteri was discussed. Abnormalities of one particular chromosome, the X-chromosome, may reveal themselves in changes in the Barr body of the cell nucleus. These changes are relatively easy to see and will be considered in this section.

Sexual dimorphism of nuclei was first described by BARR and BERTRAM (1949) in nerve cells of cats. The sex chromatin (or Barr body) is a small, fairly distinctive mass of chromatin visible in the nuclei of somatic cells of females of most mammalian species studied. With the exception of the opossum, the sex chromatin is rarely visible in the nuclei of males. BARR and CARR (1962) and GRUMBACH and MORISHIMA (1962) have summarized the evidence that the sex-chromatin body is a chromosomal derivative arising from a single X-chromosome with heteropyknotic properties. Further, it is a general rule that an X-chromosome does not display positive heteropyknosis in the interphase nucleus unless there is more than one X-chromosome in the sex-chromosome complex.

TAVARES (1962) has reviewed the occurrence of sex chromatin in tumour cells. Generally, with the exception of teratomas, benign and malignant neoplasms reveal a nuclear sex identical with that of the bearer. However, some undifferentiated tumours show anomalous sex-chromatin behaviour. Using a squash technique, ATKIN (1958) showed the presence of two chromocentres in 7 malignant tumours out of a group of 65. In the same series 8 cases had low sex-chromatin frequencies. AMARAL FERREIRA (1962) has doubted whether we can speak of the presence or absence of sex chromatin in cancer cells, the disturbance of chromatin pattern producing clumps which mask the sex-chromatin in most cells. DE WITT (1962) found that in studying sex-chromatin bodies in tissue culture it was necessary to use very rigid criteria, otherwise many small paranuclear chromatin particles might be erroneously identified as sex chromocentres. Her criteria were, "(1) the sex chromocentre must be Feulgen positive; (2) it must be at least 1 μ in length; (3) it should be located against the inner surface of the nuclear membrane and (4) the flat surface should be against the nuclear membrane." Presumably similar criteria should be employed when studying the sex-chromatin body in tumour cells.

HANSCHE (1960) was the first to describe the morphology of the Barr body in cervical carcinoma. In tumours from 50 patients the chromatin body was found in 55 to 76% of nuclei and he regarded the chromosomal sex of these tumours as invariably female. ATKIN (1966b, 1967c), using squash preparations, found that of 363 cervical carcinomas half were characterized by single sex chromatin, about 10% by double sex chromatin and 0.6% (four tumours) by triple sex chromatin; the sex chromatin body appeared to be absent in 40% of tumours. THIELE (1967) examined 100 cases of cervical carcinoma; 69 were of intermediate type, 7 showed a tendency to keratinize and 24 were anaplastic. Seven of the tumours were regarded as sex chromatin-negative (0 to 4% of cells with Barr bodies), in 15 the chromosomal sex was questionable (7 to 13% of cells with Barr bodies) and 78 tumours were sex chromosome-positive (18 to 52% of cells with Barr bodies).

FORNI and MILES (1966) examined 23 cervical smears from 20 patients. The smears from 11 patients contained no malignant cells. The remaining 9 patients had cervical "epidermal" carcinoma, 4 being *in situ*. When the sex-chromatin body was present in malignant cells it was often double or abnormally large. They considered the most likely cause of this phenomenon to be an increased number of tetraploid or near-tetraploid nuclei in cancer cells. Another possible explanation is that in malignant tissue there will be more cells synthesizing DNA and hence probably more cells in the S and G₂ phases. They considered this second explanation to be inadequate. NAUJOKS (1969) has also investigated the occurrence of sex chromatin in cervical smears from 61 cases of carcinoma *in situ*. He discussed the problem of assessing the presence of the Barr body, especially in cells with coarsely granular nuclei. The average frequency of the sex-chromatin body was 13% (range 0 to 40%). A single cell with two sex-chromatin bodies was found in 6 cases, and one cell with a triple sex-chromatin body in another case.

The sex-chromatin body has been studied in histological sections of carcinoma *in situ* by LISKA (1961) and by TREBBIN (1968). LISKA found 9 to 44% of chromatin-positive nuclei (average 27%) in sections from 25 cases of precancerous cervical lesions. The average proportion of sex chromatin-positive nuclei in normal cervical epithelium was 35% and in cancerous epithelium 12%. TREBBIN found 7 to 36% of sex chromatin-positive nuclei in 11 cases of carcinoma *in situ*. However, the sections exhibited such dense cellular patterns that examination was difficult.

ATKIN (1966b) has commented, "Taken as a whole, the data supports the view that the varying sex-chromatin content of tumour cells in females is directly related to chromosomal changes, and depends on whether the late replicating X-chromosome that forms sex chromatin is unaffected by these changes, or is lost, duplicated, etc. Apparently, the changes involving this chromosome occur more or less at random. The greater the number of chromosomes that are replicated, the more likely is the sex chromatin-forming X to be included among these but it is not clear, however, why near-tetraploid tumours frequently lack sex chromatin". He went on to point out that cells with double or enlarged sex chromatin can only be regarded as malignant if it can be assumed that none of the non-malignant cells in the preparation are polyploid or have completed DNA synthesis.

e) Nuclear Protrusions

In one case of *in-situ* carcinoma NAUJOKS (1969) found that many nuclei had a protrusion similar to that described by UYEDA *et al.* (1966). UYEDA *et al.* described a nuclear protrusion in about 5% of cells collected by a sponge from the surface of an *in-situ* carcinoma showing microinvasion. The protrusion was seen in well-preserved malignant cells and in cells which they regarded as only mildly dyskaryotic. Tissue sections from the same patient disclosed similar nuclear protruberances and also an identifiable giant chromosome in several metaphase plates. Similar nuclear protrusions have been described by ATKIN and BAKER (1964) in tumour cells from malignant ascites of ovarian origin. This protrusion was formed by the long arm of a large abnormal subacrocentric chromosome present in the tumour karyotype.

Whether or not this protruberance is similar to that sometimes seen in normal endocervical cells at the time of ovulation probably merits further investigation.

f) Telophase Chromatin Pattern in Cervical Carcinoma Cells

Most observers have seen a condensed chromatin pattern in cervical carcinoma cells. As described by ATKIN (1967a) the chromatin consists of thick discrete threads or blocks of varying size, each probably constituting an individual chromosome. This pattern is best seen in squash preparations. This telophase pattern has been seen in about 10% of invasive carcinomas of the cervix and also in carcinoma *in situ*. In histological sections the phenomenon is seen in actively growing regions. Measurements on cells from a squamous-cell carcinoma of the cervix showed that the majority of the nuclei had a diploid amount of DNA. Thus in structure and DNA content such nuclei are probably in the telophase part of the mitotic cycle. ATKIN concluded that this phenomenon represents a prolongation of telophase or a retention of a telophase pattern during the first part of interphase.

If ATKIN's argument is correct, this change is probably similar to the prolongation of metaphase which is indicated by the high frequency of the metaphase pattern in malign cervical epithelia.

g) Changes in the Late-replicating X-chromosome in Leucocytes Associated with Cervical Lesions

BAMFORD et al. (1969) have made studies of the late-replicating chromosome of lymphocytes which raise questions as to the aetiological significance of chromosomal changes in adenocarcinoma of the endometrium, squamous cell carcinoma of the cervix and carcinoma in situ.

The late replicating X-chromosome has been described as heteropyknotic and its size has been shown to correlate directly with the size of the sex-chromatin body i.e. the Barr body of epithelial cells and the neutrophil drumstick appendage of peripheral blood. It appears from the work of BAMFORD et al. (1969) that a statistically demonstrable relationship exists between the size of the late-replicating X-chromosome in circulating leucocytes and the occurence of pre-malignant and malignant changes in the female reproductive tract. If the larger size in such conditions is caused by added genetic material, the question arises as to whether this alteration occurs concomitantly with the development of the lesion, or before or after carcinogenesis. It is possible that these changes are the result of viral transformation or that they are genetically determined. Their studies suggest that the changes are more readily attributed to environmental influences than to early embryonic changes.

8. The Kinetics of Cell Proliferation in Cervical Epithelial Abnormalities

Analysis of the kinetics of cellular proliferation in abnormal cervical epithelium presents many difficulties, both theoretical and technical. RICHART (1967) has pointed out that cells containing highly abnormal chromosome numbers are less likely to complete mitosis than are those with normal chromosomes or, if mitosis does proceed to completion, it is often prolonged. These abnormalities probably result from disorder in chromosome arrangement on the mitotic spindle. Many foci of carcinoma in situ contain large numbers of mitotic figures, usually in metaphase. Since the number of cells in each phase of the cycle is proportional to the time spent in that phase, it seems likely that mitosis in general and metaphase in particular are markedly prolonged. RICHART also pointed out that, even though mitotic activity is increased in the more severe grades of carcinoma in situ, mitotic activity alone does not account for the large number of mitoses seen in histological sections. If it is assumed that prolongation of mitosis is a consequence of abnormal chromosome numbers, then it might be expected that the majority of cells in visible mitosis would be heteroploid. Since the neoplastic diploid cell might be expected to pass through mitosis more rapidly than a heteroploid cell, a relatively small proportion of metaphases at any given time would be present in diploid cells and a relatively large number in hetero-ploid cells. TIMONEN's studies (1955) of the prophase index (the ratio of the frequencies of metaphases to prophases) suggest that there is an increased duration of metaphase in precancerous and invasive lesion of the cervix. Correspondingly, the cycle time of the cells, and thus the generation of the tissue, would tend to differ from that of normal epithelium and would show greater scatter in values.

A number of workers have studied the uptake of tritiated thymidine by explants of cervical tissue, using the autoradiographic technique. There are technical problems in the use of this method, particularly the relationship of the size of the tissue fragment explanted to the diffusion of the culture medium into the fragment. JOHNSON et al. (1960a and b) have compared radioactive labelling of mouse tumours in vivo and in vitro and found good agreement in the uptake of tritiated thymidine. This has been confirmed by the studies of BASERGA et al. (1962).

RICHART (1963) placed fragments of cervical tissue in PUCK's solution containing 1 μ Ci/ml of tritiated thymidine and incubated them for 1 hour at 37 °C. The labelling index (labelled cells/total number of cells) was determined in the most heavily labelled portion of each biopsy and the information grouped according to a 6-point scale of severity ranging from normal cervical tissue (1 +) to carcinoma in situ (6 +). The results are summarized in Table 5.7.

Table 5.7. Labelling indices of tissue cultured with tritiated thymidine in relation to the severity of the lesion (after RICHART 1963)

Severity	Mean labelling index (%)
1+ Normal	4.6
2+ Minimal dysplasia	5.6
3+ Mild dysplasia	10.3
4+ Moderate dysplasia	15.2
5+ Severe dysplasia	20.3
6+ Carcinoma in situ	46.5

The labelling index increases logarithmically with the severity of the lesion. RICHART used the relationship:

$$T_g = T_s \times 100/T_L$$

(where T_g is the generation time, T_s the time required for DNA synthesis, and T_L the labelling index) to calculate the generation time. He assumed the average period of DNA synthesis to be 6 hours (JOHNSON and BOND 1961). Whence the generation time for normal epithelium is approximately 138 hours and for carcinoma in situ 12 hours; that is, in carcinoma in situ the full thickness of the neoplastic epithelium is replaced twice a day.

REID and COPPLESON (1964) carried out a similar investigation on biopsies from women aged 30—50 years. They cultured the tissue in medium 199 enriched by foetal calf serum in an atmosphere of 95% air and 5% carbon dioxide for 4 hours at 37°C. The final concentration of radioactive thymidine in the medium was 10 μ Ci/ml. In normal squamous epithelium more parabasal than basal cells were marked and there was much variation in labelling from one site to another. This variation was also found in atypical epithelium. Although the labelling of carcinoma *in situ*, restless and abnormal epithelium was usually greater than that of normal epithelium it was sometimes less. They did not find any correlation such as that found by RICHART (1963) and other workers (*vide infra*).

FETTIG and OEHLERT (1964) and FETTIG and SIEVERS (1966) incubated tissue at 37°C for 30 minutes in a medium containing tritiated thymidine at a concentration

Table 5.8. Labelling indices of tissue cultured with tritiated thymidine in relation to the type of lesion

Lesion	FETTIG and SIEVERS (1966)		FEIT and STANÍČEK (1967)	
	Mean labelling index (%)	Generation time	Mean labelling index (%)	Generation time
Normal epithelium	6.25	96 hours	6.4	93 hours
Abnormal epithelium	11.90	50 hours	11.2	53 hours
Restless epithelium	14.97	46 hours	—	—
Atypical epithelium	15.69	38 hours	15.9	37 hours
Carcinoma (pre-invasive)	22.90	26 hours	23.2	25 hours

of 4 μ Ci/ml. They state that in normal squamous epithelium the parabasal cells are labelled but not the basal cells, although their illustrations seem to show labelled basal cells. Like RICHART, they found a relationship between the severity of the lesion and the labelling index and using a value of 6 hours for the sythetic phase as suggested by JOHNSON *et al*. (1960a and b) they calculated the generation time. Their results are summarized in Table 5.8. and are very similar to those of RICHART (1963) and FEIT and STANIČEK (1967).

In restless epithelium (unruhiges Plattenepithel der Portio), FETTIG and OEHLERT (1964) found labelling of the nuclei in the lower strata but the upper strata were free from labelled cells. However, in atypical epithelium (atypisches-carcinomatöses Epithel der Portio) there was labelling of nuclei in all layers. This distribution corresponds to that of mitotic activity in these conditions. ILIYA and AZAR (1967) incubated tissue for 30 minutes with tritiated thymidine. They found that, whilst only 5% of the basal and parabasal cells were labelled in normal epithelium, the labelling index was as high as 75% in severe dysplasia and carcinoma *in situ*. However, this high index of labelling did not occur in invasive carcinoma. In mild dysplasia there was an uptake of radioactive thymidine in the lower third of the epithelium, in moderately severe dysplasia nuclei in the lower half were labelled, and in carcinoma *in situ* nuclei throughout the whole thickness.

Except for REID and COPPLESON (1964), investigators are in general agreement that the number of labelled nuclei increases with the severity of the lesion until invasion occurs. Moreover, the labelled cells in abnormal epithelia are not confined to the basal and parabasal cells but occur at a level in the tissue which is higher the more severe the lesion. This, of course, corresponds to the distribution of mitoses as seen in conventional histological preparations. It follows that the dividing compartment of the cell population increases in size with a corresponding diminution in the size of the non-dividing, functional compartment.

There are probably two sources of error in the calculation of generation times by the workers just cited: (1) According to CLEAVER (1967) and BRESCIANI (1968), the expression $T_g = T_s \times 100/T_L$, used to calculate the generation time relates to an asynchronously replicating cell population with uniform age distribution in the p-compartment (Fig. 1.16); a correction factor must be introduced for a growing population of cells as in a solid tumour (JOHNSON *et al.* 1960a). Whether or not an *in-vitro* culture of squamous epithelium is to be regarded as in a steady state or as an expanding population remains to be determined. (2) In the calculation of the generation time it has been tacitly supposed that T_s is about 6 hours, as in normal human squamous epithelium. The evidence is against this assumption. MEYER and DONALD-SON (1969) have measured the duration of DNA synthesis *in vivo* in two squamous-cell carcinomas in the oral cavity, in one it was 39.0 hours and in the other 4.6 hours. BRESCIANI (1968) has tabulated *in-vivo* estimates for other human tumours; these show considerable variation and are all considerably longer than six hours. A much more carefully planned study of the cell kinetics of abnormal cervical epithelium is necessary before any useful conclusions can be drawn.

9. Resumé

It is important at this stage to draw together some of the themes outlined in this chapter.

The evidence from investigations of the X-linked glucose-6-phosphate dehydrogenase, nuclear DNA studies and the direct investigations of chromosomes indicates that in many cases of dysplasia, carcinoma *in situ* and invasive carcinoma single, well-defined aneuploid or heteroploid cell lines are established. However, in a minority of cases there may be more than one cell line, or no well-defined stem line. The presence of a well-defined cell line with a specific karyotype suggests that the atypical epithelium started as an individual cell and, as the normal epithelium exfoliated, it was replaced by cells derived from the abnormal cell. This concept of the focal origin of malignant epithelium implies that once the initial transformation has taken place, the subsequent development and growth proceed exclusively by division of abnormal cells, as opposed to the idea of the continous conversion of surrounding normal cells. In his general discussion of the nature of a tumour growth BERENBLUM (1970) contrasts this focal origin of tumours with the field theory of WILLIS (1960). However, a number of workers have shown that in certain cases carcinoma *in situ* and microinvasive carcinoma of the cervix are multicentric in origin (FOOTE and STEWART 1948; PRZYBORA and PLUTOWA 1959; NG and PATTEN 1969), whilst a number of studies have shown a fairly frequent association between cervical carcinoma *in situ* or invasive carcinoma with similar lesions in the vagina, vulva or perianal skin. The spatial and temporal multicentricity of female genital cancers has been reviewed by JIMERSON and MERRILL

(1969). In their own series of 41 primary carcinomas of the vulva there were 15 patients with a simultaneous, or previously diagnosed, primary squamous carcinoma (*in situ* or invasive) of the cervix, and we have seen cervical dysplasia associated with a separate focus of vaginal dysplasia and Bowen's disease of the vulva.

It would appear then that occurrence of cancer or precancer in the cervix is associated with a field change, probably of varying extent, in the epithelium of the adjacent part of the lower genital tract, i. e. the part derived from the urogenital sinus (see chapter 1). Chemical carcinogenesis affords a useful comparison. Some substances, such as 3,4-benzpyrene, when applied to the skin of animals initiate malignant transformation of cells which is only revealed after the application of a promoting agent such as croton oil (BERENBLUM 1970). The initiating substance need not be applied locally, for RITCHIE and SAFFOITI (1955) have shown that orally administered 2-acetamidofluorene renders the skin responsive to the application of croton oil. Taking such animal experiments as a model, it may be supposed that when cancer or precancer occurs in the cervix the adjacent part of the lower genital tract has been subjected to an initiating process which is revealed when the promoting stimulus is applied. If the promoting stimulus is effective at one point, then a single cell may be transformed and give rise to atypical epithelium composed of one stem line, but if the promoting stimulus is effective at more than one point, then the malignant change will be multicentric and the stem lines may be different (GRANBERG 1971). If the two foci are close together, the abnormal epithelia may mix and there may be more than one stem line at that site.

The field affected by the initiating agent may be small and confined to the transformation zone, or wide and extend to the vulva. This concept is of considerable clinical importance since it implies that, once cervical neoplasia has occurred, the rest of the lower genital tract may be at risk, and the patient needs constant surveillance. This field theory also has important epidemiological implications since some of the aetiological factors may be associated with initiating agents and others with promoting agents.

RICHART (1969) has developed a theory of cervical carcinogenesis based on the failure of the malignly transformed cells to produce epidermal chalone (chapter 1) or, alternatively, their failure to respond to chalone produced by the adjacent squamous epithelium. The following discussion is based on Richart's hypothesis. He has drawn attention to the following observations: (1) malign lesions of the cervix usually begin at the squamo-columnar junction with one edge of the lesion bordering the columnar epithelium; (2) a malign lesion extends by direct replacement into the transformation zone on the portio and into the endocervix; (3) the exposed portion of the lesion is usually well differentiated, of dysplastic type, whilst the endocervical portion is less well differentiated and of carcinoma *in situ* type. Thus there is usually a gradient from a well differentiated lesion on the vaginal side to a poorly differentiated lesion in the endocervix. When a single cell receives a "carcinogenic hit", it develops a resistance to the ordinary control mechanisms, especially those of the microenvironment, and its progeny possesses a similar resistance or relative non-reactivity. When a clone of malign cells has developed, the cells nearest the normal squamous epithelium will be under the influence of epidermal chalone and may be constrained to differentiate, at least partially, giving rise to a dysplastic lesion. The cells of the clone growing nearest the endocervix will be more remote from the squamous epithelium and hence less under the influence of epidermal chalone and thus will remain undifferentiated as carcinoma *in situ*. This hypothesis would account for the fact that 80% of patients with carcinoma *in situ* have a coexisting dysplasia, but would appear to leave unexplained the temporal relationship of these two lesions, namely that dysplasia generally occurs at an earlier age than carcinoma *in situ*. However, the evidence discussed in chapter 3 seems to suggest that only a fairly low proportion of cases of dysplasia progress to *in-situ* carcinoma, and we do not know the age distribution of the two moieties. It may be that the women with dysplasias that progress to *in-situ* carcinoma are older than those whose lesions regress. Indeed the age-specific incidences of such progressive dysplasias may be the same as the *in-situ* lesions but because of the larger proportion of regressing, or stationary, dysplastic lesions this would not be evident in population studies.

The central point in the immunological theory of cancer, advanced by GREEN (1954) and developed in greater detail by GREEN *et al.* (1967), is that malignant cells are malignant because they have lost tissue-specific antigens — the "identity proteins" or "recognition factors" — and are no longer subject to tissue homeostatic control mechanisms. Antigenic deletion has been demonstrated in a number of experimentally induced tumours and in some spontaneous human tumours, including those of the cervix uteri. HILLEMANNS (1962) found that fluorescein-labelled antiserum against cervical squamous epithelium labelled carcinoma of the cervix only weakly. DAVIDSOHN and KOVARIK (1969) have also shown that, whereas squamous epithelium of the normal cervix contains the AB0 blood-group antigen proper to the patient, this antigen is lost in carcinoma *in situ*.

If a mutation in a cell causes deletion of some portion or the whole of the identity proteins postulated by GREEN, the specific labels by which cells can be recognized outside their normal boundaries will have disappeared. Because of this loss of identity, there is no mechanism to dispose of them outside their normal confines and they can infiltrate other organs with impunity. Thus deletion of "identity proteins", whilst not accounting for the mechanism of invasion of tumour cells, is the physical basis of xenoplasia described by GLÜCKSMANN.

HAMPERL (1966) as a result of his studies of the reticulum network adjacent to early invasive cervical carcinoma regards the internal pressure of the tumour tissue as the active force in invasion. Moreover, the superficial layers of the squamous epithelium of the cervix are said to show much greater cohesion than the epithelial cells of the more basal layers. "This fact", he says, "may provide an explanation as to why, when the internal pressure increases precisely in these layers, the epithelium with its back to a cohesive surface 'escapes' towards the stroma." He contends that there is no evidence of lytic enzyme action of the tumour cells directed against any component of normal tissue nor is there any indication of amoeboid motility of the tumour cells which would carry single tumour cells far into the normal tissue. HILLEMANNS *et al.* (1968a) on the basis of cell counts per unit area reached a similar conclusion (*vide supra*). This pressure hypothesis is not entirely convincing, for it might have been supposed that a tumour would burst outwards to the surface rather than inwards, but lack of knowledge of the pressures involved renders speculation unprofitable.

Chapter 6

The Aetiology of Epithelial Abnormalities of the Cervix Uteri

In this chapter an examination is made of the factors which may be of aetiological importance in the development of invasive carcinoma, carcinoma *in situ* and dysplasia of the uterine cervix. Since invasive carcinoma has been much more extensively investigated than *in situ* carcinoma or dysplasia, and since invasive carcinoma may be the final outcome of the other abnormalities, it is appropriate to consider first the factors associated with the invasive lesion.

1. The Epidemiology and Geographic Distribution of Invasive Carcinoma of the Cervix

The epidemiological factors affecting invasive carcinoma of the cervix have been reviewed by BOYD and DOLL (1964), CLEMMESEN (1965), and COPPLESON and REID (1967). It is relevant here to summarize the findings only briefly.

a) Socio-economic Status

CLEMMESEN and NIELSON (1951) have shown that in Copenhagen, during the years 1943—47, the average prevalence of carcinoma of the cervix was higher among the poorer members of the population than among the more wealthy. LOGAN (1954), using a 1 % sample of deaths, was able to show that the mortality from cervical cancer in England and Wales was higher the poorer the economic status of the women. This gradient did not apply to corpus carcinoma. DORN and CUTLER (1959) found a similar relation between social class and cervical carcinoma in the Ten City Survey in the U.S.A. In Buffalo, N.Y., GRAHAM *et al.* (1960) also found a lower incidence of carcinoma of the cervix in the more economically favoured population than in the less favoured. However, COHART (1955) failed to show any such relation in New Haven, Connecticut. Similarly, BOYD and DOLL (1964) using groups of carefully matched hospital patients found no relation between cervical carcinoma and social status.

b) Heredity

In assessing the role of heredity, systematic statistical studies encounter difficulty in distinguishing between cervical and endometrial cancer. A number of comparisons have been made of probands with controls, but there is difficulty in matching the two groups, especially with regard to socio-economic factors. However, the studies of

NIELSON and CLEMMESEN (1957) and HARVALD and HAUGE (1963) failed to show coincidence of uterine cancer in pairs of twins. STERN et al. (1967) using correlation analysis have shown that family history is of some importance in discriminating between women with preinvasive and invasive cancer of the cervix, suggesting the possible role of a genetic factor in this disease.

c) Marital Factors

GAGNON (1950) examined the medical records of Canadian nuns, covering an annual average of 13,000 women during a 20-year period. He found 14 cases of carcinoma of the uterine corpus but none of cervical carcinoma. In a separate study of the pathology records in Montreal and the eastern part of Quebec he found 19 cases of corpus carcinoma in nuns but only 3 of cervical carcinoma. Further, in a population of 3,280 nuns from four different religious orders he found only 130 malignant neoplasms during a period of twenty years. Two of these were in the corpus uteri and none in the cervix. The extreme rarity of cervical carcinoma in nuns was confirmed by Towne's study (1955). Unfortunately neither GAGNON nor TOWNE give any information about the number of nuns married before their entrance into the religious life. However, outside this special class of women, BOYD and DOLL (1964) and TERRIS et al. (1967) have shown that cervical carcinoma is much less frequent in unmarried than in married women.

Age at marriage. TERRIS et al. (1967) found that early marriage was more frequent among patients with cervical carcinoma than among controls; 28% of patients were married before the age seventeen compared with 16% of controls. This is in agreement with the observations of BOYD and DOLL (1964) who found that the average age at marriage of 280 married women with cervical carcinoma was 22.7 years compared with 23.9 years for 553 married women in a gynaecological control group; this difference is statistically significant. ROTKIN (1967) found the mean age at marriage of cervical cancer patients to be 19.9 years and of controls 22.5 years. The age at marriage has been put forward as a possible explanation for much of the difference between various national and socio-economic groups (WYNDER et al. 1954, and HAENSZEL and HILLHOUSE 1959) but how this operates is unknown. BOYD and DOLL (1964) suggest it may be partly because early marriage results in more frequent coitus but it may also be that young tissue is more susceptible. STERN and DIXON (1961) investigated a population of women attending a cancer detection clinic and identified the type of lesion by cervical cytology. They found a correlation coefficient between age at marriage and dysplasia of −0.04 and of carcinoma *in situ* of −0.06, but between the age at marriage and invasive carcinoma there was a positive correlation coefficient of 0.20.

Parity. Although a relationship has sometimes been demonstrated between parity and the occurrence of cervical carcinoma (MALIPHANT 1949; SHE et al. 1962; BARRON and RICHART 1971), according to BOYD and DOLL (1964) this has only been found when no account was taken of the interrelationship between multiparity and early marriage.

Age at first pregnancy. This has been investigated by BOYD and DOLL (1964) who showed that a higher proportion of patients with cervical cancer gave a history of pregnancy at an early age than did women in the control group. The mean age of first pregnancy was 23.1 years in the cancer patient compared with 25.1 years in the control group; the difference is statistically significant. Similarly, CHRISTOPHERSON and PARKER (1965) found that 25.7% of their sample who became pregnant before the age of twenty accounted for 47.6% of cases of invasive carcinoma of the cervix and 41.5% of *in situ* carcinoma. Likewise, BARRON and RICHART (1971) found an association, in Barbados, between a positive smear and an early first pregnancy.

Age at first coitus. Strangely enough, although the age at first pregnancy can be determined easily and accurately, the age at first coitus which can be ascertained with much less reliability has attracted more attention. WYNDER *et al.* (1954) showed that within a group of non-Jewish white women only 14% of women with cervical cancer had their first coital experience after the age of 25, against 25% of control patients without cervical cancer. MARTIN (1967) and TERRIS *et al.* (1967) have also produced evidence of earlier commencement of coitus in women with cervical cancer. On the basis of cytological diagnosis, BARRON and RICHART (1971) have shown that in Barbados there is an excess of women with dysplasia and carcinoma *in situ* who reported having coitus before the age of seventeen compared with women with a negative smear.

Frequency of sexual intercourse. This may be regarded as an index of sexual activity. The observations of BOYD and DOLL (1964) suggest that cervical cancer patients experience more frequent intercourse than women in the control group. Thus the average frequency was 6.2 per month in the cancer group and 5.2 in the control group and the difference is statistically significant. When the results are standardized for the age at marriage the trend persists but is no longer statistically significant. TERRIS *et al.* (1967) and MARTIN (1967) found no significant difference between patients and controls in the reported frequency of coitus.

Marital instability. This has been reviewed by MARTIN (1967). In nine studies cited from the literature, it is evident either that there has been a more frequent dissolution of the first marriage in cervical cancer cases than in controls or that the cancer patients have been more frequently married more than once. These general statements need some qualification. BOYD and DOLL (1964) considered the frequency of broken first marriages, whether caused by the death of the husband or by separation or divorce. For women married under twenty years of age the frequency was high but there was no striking difference between cases and controls. With later marriage the proportion broken was significantly greater in the cervical cancer patients than in the controls. However, the frequency of remarriage after the first marriage had broken was practically the same in both cases and controls. Slightly different results were reported by TERRIS *et al.* (1967). A history of more than one marriage was given by 35% of women with cervical cancer but by only 22% of controls. This difference could be explained in part by the earlier marriage of the patients. The incidence of multiple marriages was higher for those marrying before the age of seventeen and there was no difference between patients and controls in this group. However, for those marrying at the age of seventeen and over the incidence of multiple marriages was significantly greater in the patients than in the controls.

TERRIS *et al.* (1967) in their study, based on four hospitals in New York City, found no difference in the numbers of sexual partners in cervical cancer cases compared with controls. On the contrary, ROTKIN (1967) working in the San Francisco Bay area and the Los Angeles metropolitan regions of California found that patients with cervical carcinoma had an excess of sexual mates compared with controls.

d) Syphilis

The relation between syphilis and cervical carcinoma has been extensively reviewed by CLEMMESEN (1965). Perhaps the most extensive study of this relationship has been made by RØJEL (1953). He used carefully defined diagnostic criteria for syphilis and found that this disease occurred about three times as frequently among cervical cancer patients as among controls. Further, the proportion of loose women was 6.1 % among cervical cancer patients as compared with 1.2 % among controls.

e) Circumcision

The relation of circumcision to cervical cancer has been extensively studied by a number of workers. However, the assessment of whether or not the male partner has been circumcised is extremely difficult. The interpretation and significance of the observations is therefore uncertain. BOYD and DOLL (1964) found that the evidence was essentially negative; closely similar proportions of women both in the cervical carcinoma group and in the controls said that at one time they had been married to an uncircumcised man. CLEMMESEN (1965) questioned whether a demonstration of an association between cervical carcinoma and lack of circumcision can be demonstrated in a mixed population. Earlier, HANDLEY (1936) had investigated the occurrence of cervical cancer in the Fiji Islands where 90,000 Fijians lived side by side with 70,000 Indians; the Fijians practised circumcision but the Indians did not.

Table 6.1. Average annual incidence per 100,000 population (from DOLL et al., 1966)

	Penile carcinoma	Cervical carcinoma
Mozambique	1.9	18.6
Nigeria	0.1	8.2
Canada	0.9	24.4
Colombia	2.3	62.0
Puerto Rico	5.1	36.6
Connecticut	0.9	16.0
New York State	0.8	17.4
Israel	0.1	5.5
Singapore (Chinese)	0.8	14.6
Denmark	1.3	34.0
Birmingham	1.1	16.8
Liverpool	1.2	18.6
England (S. W. Metropolitan)	1.2	16.1
Finland	0.7	18.3
Iceland	1.0	15.7
Netherlands	1.1	23.3
Norway	1.0	19.3
Sweden	1.3	22.1
Yugoslavia	0.7	29.3
New Zealand	0.8	15.0

HANDLEY found in reports of the Colonial War Memorial Hospital at Suva that from 1925 to 1932 three cases of cervical cancer occured in Fijian women and twenty-six in Indian women. He attributed the difference to the hygienic effect of circumcision.

If circumcision has any effect in this way it seems likely that smegma or infected material retained by the prepuce has some carcinogenic action. This should reveal its effect both in the cervix and, more particularly in the penis. Table 6.1. is based on the report by DOLL *et al.* (1966) on cancer incidence in five continents. It can be seen that, broadly, there is a correlation between the incidence of penile cancer and cervical cancer. Thus Nigeria and Israel with the lowest incidence of cervical carcinoma also have the lowest incidence of penile carcinoma, and Colombia and Puerto Rico with the highest incidence of cervical carcinoma have the highest of penile carcinoma. Although there is a marked parallelism the correlation is not complete, suggesting that other factors also operate in the two conditions.

f) Contraceptives

The relationship between epithelial abnormalities of the cervix and the use of contraceptives will be considered in more detail later in this chapter. BOYD and DOLL (1964) found that obstructive contraceptives were less frequently used in the group of women with cervix cancer than in the gynaecological control group. ROTKIN (1967) found that his controls showed a significantly greater use of diaphragm, jelly or rhythm methods of contraception, whilst cancer patients showed a significant excess using a douche. It could be suggested that the lower frequently of cervical malignancy when obstructive methods are used is because smegma, or similar material, is prevented from coming into contact with the cervix.

g) Race, Religion and Culture

These three factors are inextricably mixed and make comparison difficult. OETTLÉ (1961) gave a picture of the various races in South Africa. He showed that when the Bantu population was standardized directly to the United States population, the age-specific incidence rates for carcinoma of the cervix of the Bantu approximated closely to that of the United States Negro.

Using cervical smears and biopsies, JORDAN *et al.* (1969) have investigated the frequency of cervical carcinoma in South Western America Indians and Caucasian residents of New Mexico. The two groups were matched as closely as possible for age and socio-economic level. Despite conditions of poverty, multiple pregnancies, early coitus and uncircumcised consorts, South Western Indian women apparently have a lower rate of cervical carcinoma than age-matched Caucasian controls. This lower frequency in Indian women was interpreted to be at least in part the result of delay in first births relative to Caucasian women. The delay in first pregnancies is probably a result of transient adolescent sterility. JORDAN *et al.* concluded that in this population the age at first childbirth seemed to be a more significant determinant of subsequent cervical carcinoma than the age at first coitus.

WAHI *et al.* (1969) have analysed 693 cases of cervical carcinoma from a population of 39,587 women attending hospitals in the Agra district of India. These women were screened by a vaginal smear examination. A biopsy was obtained from 342 women, the remaining cases were diagnosed either on the basis of clinical or cytological findings. The study included seventeen cases of carcinoma *in situ*. The average age at marriage of women in the group with cancer was 13.6 years compared with 15.6 years for the control groups. The prevalence of cancer of the cervix was higher in those Hindu women who gave birth to the first child at or before the age of seventeen, whereas in Muslim women it was highest in those who had their first childbirth between eighteen and twentyone years of age. This difference in age between Hindu and Muslim women was considered to be of little significance because Muslim women marry somewhat later than Hindu women. They found a direct correlation between the number of pregnancies and the incidence of cervical carcinoma. The majority of patients with cervical carcinoma belonged to a low socio-economic group but, since no information about the size of the various economic groups was given no estimate of the importance of this factor can be made. In childless married women the rate was twice as high as in unmarried women, and in nulliparous women in general the rate was far less than in women with one child. The prevalence of cervical carcinoma was lower in Muslim women than in Hindus; WAHI *et al.* regard this as probably the result of the lack of smegma in the circumcised Muslim males. This study shows the same cluster of factors operating in India as elsewhere.

In contrast, the study of Amish women by CROSS *et al.* (1968) shows that when these factors are absent the prevalence of malignant disease of the cervix is low. The records of 10,314 Papanicolaou smears were analysed to determine the prevalence of cervical cancer among the rural inhabitants of Holmes County, Ohio. The smears were from two populations of women; 3,606 were considered typical of rural American populations whilst 2,068 were members of a highly chaste religious group known as the Old Amish. The Amish are small groups of people who are descended from the extreme left of the Protestant Reformation in Europe. They emigrated to America where they still live a life little changed from European conditions of the seventeenth and early eighteenth centuries (PAYNE 1965). This sect is highly religious and enforces isolation from the "world". Marriages with non-Amish partners are forbidden and no attempt is made to proselytize. Movies, dances and commercial entertainment are regarded askance. The prevalence of cancer of the cervix was considerably lower among Amish women in spite of a higher birth rate and the absence of contraceptives (Table 6.2.). CROSS *et al.* concluded that certain culturally determined practices among the Amish may have limited the spread of some factor which is responsible for the disease.

Table 6.2. Prevalence of cervical cancer (per 1,000 women) found on first examination among Amish and non-Amish women compared with other studies (modified, after CROSS *et al.* 1968). All ages

Amish	2.0	
Non-Amish	12.4	
San Diego	10.1	DUNN *et al.* (1954)
Floyd County	4.2	NIEBURGS *et al.* (1957)
Memphis (Caucasian)	4.58	KAISER *et al.* (1960)

CLEMMESEN (1965) has reviewed the literature pertaining to the morbidity of cervical carcinoma in Jewesses. The rates for New York in 1952 showed 4.7 cases of cervical carcinoma per 100,000 Jewish women with 17.1 for other white women. He comments "the rarity of cervical carcinoma among Jewish women has been reported and commented on more frequently than subjected to relevant statistical analysis. Judged from the few detailed statistics on the difference between Jewish and other women within the same city, it does not seem more pronounced than differences between various parts of the city, e. g., København". He suggests that the Jewish rite of Niddah, which is frequently offered as an explanation of the low prevalence of cervical carcinoma among Jewesses, may not have its main influences through the circumcision of the male but through the regulation of sexual life and its concept of cleanliness and hygiene.

h) Various Hypotheses

After reviewing the various aetiological factors discussed above, MARTIN (1967) concluded that squamous-cell carcinoma of the cervix shares many characteristics of communicable disease which follows a venereal mode of transmission. He suggested the existence of an infectious agent which is a necessary but not the sole condition needed for the development of cancer. The agent must be (a) asymptomatic for the carrier, (b) carried by both sexes, (c) primarily, or solely, transmitted by coitus and (d) such that many years may intervene between initial infection and its malignant manifestation. Support for such an hypothesis follows from the observations that virgin women are rarely affected, women once married are less frequently affected than women twice married or leading an irregular sexual life. Moreover, Muslim, Amish, Jewish, Seventh-Day Adventist and other religiously oriented groups are at low risk for cervical cancer. These groups are not only circumspect in marital and sexual conduct for doctrinal reasons but also practice religious endogamy — that is, most members marry within the faith. Martin considers that these groups are exceptionally free of the disease because of three mechanisms: (a) their high rate of endogamous marriage presents a barrier to the introduction of a venereally infectious agent into the community, (b) their maintenance of monogamous sexual patterns restricts the propagation of infection within the membership and (c) in the case of an agent dependent upon venereal transmission, the passing of each generation helps to deplete any existing infection.

CLEMMESEN (1965) has suggested that the association of cervical carcinoma with the early beginning of sexual activity might be conditioned by a high oestrogen level as the background of both. It could be assumed that some feedback mechanism may influence the hormonal pattern, and that early and intensive sexual activity may have a tendency to continue, leading to less regular sexual habits than a strongly traditional monogamous pattern of life.

ROTKIN (1962) has suggested that the adolescent cervix is more susceptible to the action of a carcinogenic agent, introduced by the male during coitus, than is the cervix of older women. This agent produces carcinoma after a latent period of several years. This hypothesis does not require a relationship of risk to total dose of carcinogen, hence the frequency of exposure is not a factor. However, the number of partners may be relevant unless it is supposed that every male carries the carcinogenic agent.

LUNDIN *et al.* (1964) suggested that some change which occurs after the first pregnancy may be significant in the genesis of cancer. They have pointed out that the squamo-columnar junction, which is the site of predilection of squamous cell carcinoma of the cervix, is proximal to the external os in the nulliparous cervix but is situated on the vaginal surface following delivery. Thus the first pregnancy may be important in exposing the squamo-columnar junction to a noxious agent whereas subsequent pregnancies have no further effect (but see page 56 above and COPPLESON and REID, 1967).

One of the most common hypotheses is that the male carries a carcinogen, presumably in smegma, which causes cervical cancer. This hypothesis suggests that the disease may be associated with frequent coitus since the risk of disease would be expected to increase with the degree of exposure to the agent. This view is strongly supported by the studies on Jewish women, Muslims and Fijians.

There is thus a multiplicity of hypotheses each of which explains many of the epidemiological observations. It will be the task of the remainder of this chapter to explore some of these in greater detail.

2. Viral and Allied Infections of the Cervix

One of the emerging lines of investigation of cervical pathology is an assessment of the role played by viruses both as simple infecting agents and as carcinogens. There is a parallelism between the epidemiology of viral infections of the vagina and cervix, venereal infections and cervical cancer, but at present there is no indisputable evidence that viruses are inculpated in cervical carcinogenesis. Nevertheless, it is quite probable that some of the epithelial abnormalities of the cervix which masquerade under the term dysplasia are, in reality, viral in origin. Unfortunately, no criteria equivalent to Koch's postulates as yet exist to enable us to determine whether or not any tumour is of viral origin, nor has an experimental model been devised to support any such contention in the cervix.

Viral oncogenesis represents the mutual adaptation of virus and host cell, each undergoing genotypic transformations so that the new state can flourish (FRAENKEL-CONRAT 1969). The key to such development is the integration of some genetic material, and thus information, from both partners. Viruses may be divided into two broad groups, DNA viruses and RNA viruses. There are tumour viruses among most of the major groups of DNA viruses, the most frequently studied being the polyoma, papilloma and adenoviruses. Almost all the oncogenic RNA viruses belong to one or two closely related groups — the leukoviruses.

a) Viruses and Cell Growth

Most of the well known viruses, such as that of poliomyelitis, kill the cells in which they multiply. Such infections are termed "lytic" or "cytocidal" and, since they cause the death of cells they invade, they cannot give rise to a tumour. Tumour viruses infect cells without killing them and changes in the function of the surviving cells then follow. Any non-cytocidal infection by a tumour virus may lead to the appearance among the survivors of cells with permanently altered behaviour, in particular altered growth potential (STOKER 1970). These are called transformed cells and they form clones which can be recognized easily in cultures. Transformed cells have many, but not necessarily all, the characteristics of cells obtained from tumours induced *in vivo*. It is thought that viral transformants represent the initial change to malignancy which occurs before progression takes place by the successive emergence of cell variants during the course of tumour growth. Transformed cells continue to carry the virus which initiated the transformation; thus cells transformed by RNA viruses continue to release new virus particles. In cells transformed by DNA viruses, complete virus synthesis cannot be detected and, if it occurred, would be cytocidal. The viral DNA (genome) can, however, be detected by chemical or genetic procedures and it seems probable that one or more copies of the viral genome are attached to chromosomes of the cell. This is supported by hybridization experiments between mouse cells and SV-40 transformed human cells (WEISS *et al.* 1968). Using Rous sarcoma virus, MACPHERSON (1965) has shown that loss of virus is accompanied by loss of transformed cell characters. Hence, it seems that not only does the virus initiate the change, but its presence is necessary to maintain it. The Rous sarcoma virus is an RNA virus and the transformed cells carry the virus specific antigens.

Virus-induced tumours may carry transplantation-like antigens (HABEL 1961, 1962; SJORGREN *et al.* 1961). These antigens are unrelated to the viral antigen itself. Resistance to polyoma tumours can be transferred to isogenic recipients with lymphoid cells and, less effectively, with serum from virus-infected donors but, as yet, direct *in vitro* methods for demonstrating polyoma-specific transplantation antigens are not available (GREEN *et al.* 1967). BRYAN (1964) suggests that in this group of tumours initiation would occur only if: (a) the virus infected its host at a time prior to the development of immunological competence; or (b) the immunological competence of animals infected later in life, and harbouring subclinical infections of the virus, were destroyed by some other disease, irradiation or treatment with some substance such as cortisone. In addition to the transplantation antigens, HABEL (1965) has also shown the presence of specific complement-fixing antigens in polyoma tumours and transformed cells.

When cells or tissues are invaded by a virus, such as the polyoma virus, only a small proportion of cells show a transformational response; in the others the response is cytocidal (see FRAENKEL-CONRAT 1969). Similar results have been reported in intact animals by STANTON *et al.* (1959). In foetal mice infected with polyoma virus, inclusion bodies were seen in damaged and dying cells, in which the virus was obviously multiplying, but not in the viable neighbouring cells which had undergone transformation. They also saw a range of transformation in the same host from nodules having a fairly benign appearance to small clusters of cells which might be compared with carcinoma *in situ*, and finally to frankly malignant tumours.

From this brief review of viral oncogenesis it will be evident that there are considerable difficulties in establishing the viral nature of human tumours; particularly in the case of DNA viruses, since the process of initiation involves the incorporation of the viral genome into nuclear DNA with a loss of viral antigen. Possibly morphological studies similar to those of STANTON *et al.* (1959) may offer a pointer. If virus-induced changes can be seen in tissue adjacent to the tumour, and particularly if inclusion bodies can be found in this tissue but not in the neoplastic tissue, then there would seem to be a possibility that a virus has initiated the neoplastic transformation.

Clearly, such a possibility would need to be followed by *in vitro* and especially by immunological studies.

There are two near-neoplastic conditions in the human probably caused by viruses. Verrucae can be transmitted by experimental inoculation. STRAUSS *et al.* (1951) regard eosinophilic bodies present in the nuclei of epidermal cells as viral inclusion bodies, but BLANK *et al.* (1931) regard these bodies as nucleoli. However, electron microscopic studies of BUNTING *et al.* (1952), CHARLES (1960) and HOWATSON (1962) indicate that virus particles are present in these warts. Condylomata acuminata are infective and probably also caused by a virus.

b) The Co-carcinogenic Action of Viruses

The co-carcinogenic effect of viruses has been reviewed by BRYAN (1964). Some non-oncogenic viruses of various infectious diseases have been found to be capable of enhancing the activity of chemical carcinogens. These viruses include: (1) pox viruses (fowl pox and vaccinia), (2) a medium-sized DNA virus (herpes) which replicates in the nucleus but has an outer membranous envelope, (3) RNA viruses of the myxovirus group which bud from cell membranes (three strains of influenza), and (4) small RNA strains which replicate in the cytoplasm such as West Nile, polio, Coxsackie B 4 and Echo 9. In most instances the virus merely speeded up the process and produced a higher incidence of lesion at a given dose level than was obtained with the chemical alone. Precancerous and benign precursors of malignant tumours induced in skin were similarly enhanced by virus.

It may well be that the main effect of viral infection of the cervix is co-carcinogenic rather than primarily oncogenic.

c) Infection with Herpes Simplex Virus

The herpes simplex group of viruses has been extensively reviewed in a monograph by KAPLAN (1969) and herpesvirus infection of the genital tract by JOSEY *et al.* (1968). Two different types of herpes virus are usually recognised — herpes simplex virus, type I, and herpes genitalis virus, type II. TEPLITZ *et al.* (1971) have described methods of distinguishing these viruses when cultured cells are infected.

The herpes simplex virus was first isolated from the female genital tract in 1946 by SLAVIN and GAVETT. The disease can present itself both in an acute and in an asymptomatic form. The acute form may occur as a diffuse inflammatory reaction of varying intensity nearly always characterized by hyperaemia. Sometimes it may appear as multiple tiny superficial lesions of the cervix, vagina or vulva. Occasionally larger and deeper ulcers may form and constitutional symptoms and inguinal lymphadenopathy may occur (YEN *et al.* 1965). The asymptomatic lesion is usually detected by cytological changes in the vaginal smear. JOSEY *et al.* (1968) found the asymptomatic form in 0.5% of women screened at the Granly Memorial Hospital, Atlanta. In a family planning clinic WOLINSKA and MELAMED (1970) found cytological evidence of infection in 0.09% of women. Cytological diagnosis may be confirmed by isolation of the virus and identification by tissue culture or by serological methods such as the presence of neutralizing antibodies in a primary infection or complement-fixing antibodies in asymptomatic infection.

The characteristic cytological changes have been described by a number of authors. STERN and LONGO (1963) recorded the typical multinucleated cells and nuclear inclusions in vaginal smears from a young woman with vaginal ulceration from whom they successfully cultured herpes simplex virus. AN (1969) reported eighteen cases of herpes simplex virus cervicitis in which the initial diagnosis was made by routine vaginal smear. Three phases can be recognized in exfoliated cells. In stage I, there is an increased granularity of the nuclear chromatin with clumping which is followed by fine intranuclear vacuolation. In stage II, the nucleus assumes a ground-glass appearance caused by swelling of viral inclusion material and the chromatin is marginated to the nuclear membrane. Stage III is characterized by a typical type A acidophilic nuclear inclusion surrounded by a clear zone of nucleoplasm. NG et al. (1970) described a similar sequence of changes but commented that in the primary infection acidophilic intranuclear inclusions are uncommon and that the majority of infected cells have a "ground-glass" nuclear appearance. In contrast to the initial lesion, cells with a "ground-glass" appearance and those with acidophilic nuclear inclusions occur in about equal numbers in recurrent disease. Electron microscopy shows that the "ground-glass" appearance is produced by viral particles (FRIEDRICH et al. 1969; ROY and WOLMAN 1969). Both columnar and squamous epithelium may be affected. These changes are illustrated in Figs. 6.1. and 6.2..

Correlated cytological, virological and histological studies in cervical herpes simplex infection have been described by NAIB et al. (1966) and by JOSEY et al. (1968). In their first study they described their findings in 62 women whose vaginal smears showed changes compatible with herpes simplex infection; 32 of these women were also examined virologically and by cervical biopsy. In 12 patients it was possible to culture the herpesvirus. The negative virological cases were most likely the result of the lapse of time (averaging 3 weeks) between the original vaginal smear and the return of the patient to the gynaecology virus clinic. Forty-one of the 62 patients had a repeat vaginal, cervical and endocervical smear taken 2—6 weeks after the original diagnosis but only 5 of them had persistent diagnostic inclusion-containing cells. This indicates that the majority of lesions are short-lived and exfoliative cytology is probably unable to detect the real incidence of herpetic infection in the female genital tract. For the same reason histological changes probably do not represent a true picture of the changes in the cervix. One to six weeks ofter the initial cytological diagnosis of herpes infection, cervical biopsies were taken from any grossly visible "Schiller" positive erosions or ulceration. They found carcinoma in situ in 4 cases; squamous atypia in 6 cases, ranging from atypical basal cell hyperplasia to severe dysplasia; acute cervicitis with vascular granulation tissue in 11; chronic cervicitis in 6 and cervical herpes simplex in 5 cases.

In the 5 cases of herpes simplex lesion NAIB et al. (1966) found vesiculation of the epithelium in one case and deep ulceration in the other 4 .Most of the viral changes were localized in the proliferating basal cells. The majority of these cells were swollen with transparent vacuolated cytoplasm. Occasionally, multinucleated giant cells with intranuclear eosinophilic inclusions were seen. The corium was infiltrated with lymphocytes and monocytes. The other lesions showed no features diagnostic of herpes infection. The main feature of the six cases with squamous atypia was the marked basal cell hyperplasia NAIB et al. comment that the possibility of a relation between cervical atypia and herpetic genital infection should be considered.

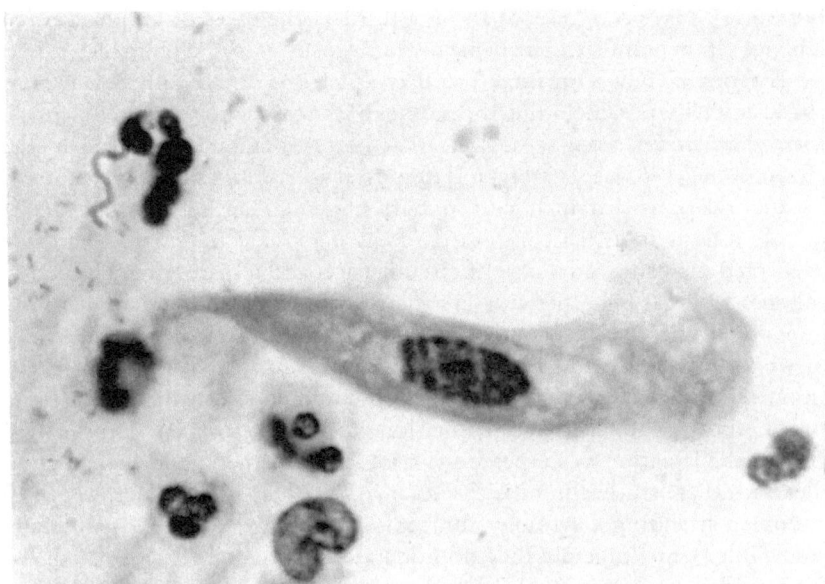

Fig. 6.1. A columnar cell showing increased granularity and clumping of the nuclear chromatin. Described by An (1969) as Stage I. (Papanicolaou's stain × 1,200)

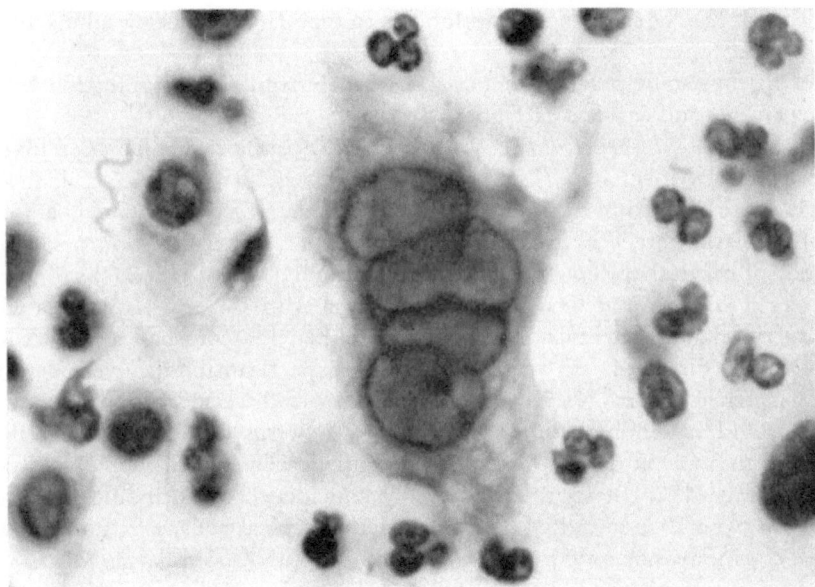

Fig. 6.2. Stage II viral change, showing a multinucleated cell with a ground-glass texture of the nuclei. (Papanicolaou's stain × 1,200)

In the series of NAIB *et al.* (1966) about a third of the cases of herpes were pregnant. Such women may infect their babies. Thus, JOSEY *et al.* (1968) isolated herpesvirus type II from 12 newborn infants and type I from one infant. Seven of these mothers had genital herpes, including the mother of the case with type I virus infection.

Epidemiological studies seem to suggest that herpes genitalis is spread by sexual contact. JOSEY *et al.* (1968) isolated type II herpesvirus from a number of women who had had sexual relations with men with concurrent genital herpes. BARILE *et al.* (1962) studied penile lesions in American armed forces personnel in Japan. Characteristically, the affected men showed a lack of circumcision and a history of repeated venereal infections. In 7 cases herpes was associated with condyloma acuminatum. No herpes infection was found in a control group, two thirds of whom were circumcised and all of whom had refrained from sexual intercourse for 30 days prior to examination. PARKER and BANATVALA (1967) have also commented on the association between penile herpes and the lack of circumcision whilst NAHMIAS and DOWDLE (1968) have recorded the isolation of herpes virus type II from smegma in the male.

Parallel with these studies in men, KLEGER *et al.* (1968) isolated herpesvirus from 0.1% of women attending a cytology clinic and from 1.6% of women from a venereal disease clinic. Unfortunately they do not state the type of virus isolated. RAWLS *et al.* (1969) carried out a seroepidemiological survey using an assay method based on antibody neutralization kinetics. They found that whereas antibodies to type I herpesvirus tended to appear early in life, the antibodies to type II did not appear until adolescence and they occurred more frequently among prostitutes (54%) than among the control population (22%). In a low socio-economic group, 90% of whom were negroes, NAHMIAS *et al.* (1970) found that antibodies to herpesvirus type II began to be detected in young females of about fifteen years of age. After 45 years of age the incidence of types I and II was 100%. ROYSTON and AURELIAN (1970) found that the incidence of antibodies to type II virus decreased up the social scale.

There is thus some parallelism between the epidemiology of infection with herpesvirus type II and cervical carcinoma.

The association of herpes virus type II with carcinoma of the cervix has been investigated more directly. JOSEY *et al.* (1968) found epithelial anaplasia of the cervix in 21.7% (46 of 212 cases) of women with evidence of herpetic infection. Included among the cases of anaplasia were 9 of carcinoma *in situ* and 4 of invasive carcinoma. The overall frequency of cervical epithelial anaplasia in the same hospital was 2.6%.

RAWLS *et al.* (1969) detected herpesvirus type II in 78% of 41 patients with invasive carcinoma of the cervix and in 64% of 24 patients who had been successfully treated for the disease 4—20 years previously. Type II antibodies were detected in 22% of matched control women, 24% of patients with cervical dysplasia and 35% of patients with carcinoma *in situ*. Antibodies to the virus were not found to be associated with tumours at other sites except, possibly, carcinoma of the vulva. ROYSTON and AURELIAN (1970) have reported a 98% incidence of antibodies neutralizing herpesvirus type II *in vitro* in 110 patients with atypical cells, carcinoma *in situ* or invasive carcinoma but only a 55 % incidence in controls. Similarly, NAHMIAS *et al.* (1970) in a group of low socio-economic status, mainly negro, found that patients with invasive carcinoma, carcinoma *in situ* and dysplasia had antibodies to type II herpesvirus.

Skinner et al. (1971) investigated the sera of 335 women with normal and abnormal cervical cytology for neutralizing antibodies to type I and type II herpesvirus. There were no significant differences between the mean k-values of antibodies in the sera of any of the groups of patients against type I herpesvirus. With type II virus, patients with histological evidence of cervical disease had significantly higher mean k-values than both the control gynaecological group and the control group of patients with genital carcinoma of other sites. This difference was independent of age and social class. For patients with carcinoma *in situ* some preliminary evidence suggested that surgical conization of the cervix results in a decline in type II herpesvirus neutralizing antibody activity. Although they accept the association between sexual promiscuity and cervical carcinoma, they suggest that this venereally transmitted virus is more important in the development of cervical carcinoma than the sole factor of promiscuity. First, all their patients with abnormal cytology had higher mean type II k-values than woman attending a venereal disease clinic. Second, the mean type II k-value increased with the degree of severity of the neoplastic process from dysplasia to invasive carcinoma.

The results of Royston and Aurelian (1970) indicate that the peak age for active genital herpes infection in women precedes the peak age for preinvasive disease by at least ten years and the invasive disease by at least twenty years. This is consistent with an aetiological role for this virus. However, in the study of Nahmias et al. (1970) the peak ages of incidence were too low for active infection to precede *in situ* by carncioma ten years.

Rawls et al. (1969) have pointed out that the association between invasive carcinoma of the cervix and herpesvirus type II may not be causal. There are three possible hypotheses: (1) both the virus infection and malignancy are co-variables with sexual promiscuity; (2) the virus infection follows neoplastic change; and (3) the virus infection precedes the neoplastic change and contributes to the formation of the lesion as a carcinogen or co-carcinogen. Further work is needed to decide which possibility is correct. Fleissner (1970) has suggested certain approaches to the general problem of the relation of viruses to human cancer. These may be relevant in the present context. (1) The tissue-culture transformation of human cells has been described for the Rous, adeno- and papova viruses. Up to the present this transformation has not been recorded for herpesvirus. (2) The possibility of the occurence of tumour antigens, such as the transplantation antigen in transformed cells, needs exploring. (3) The rescue of the tumour virus genome in transformed cells by fusion of these cells with sensitized cells might be investigated.

d) Other Viral and Viral-like Infections

Several other viral and viral-like infections of the female genital tract are of importance because they may be transmitted to the foetus and newborn infant causing perinatal infection. Some of these have a rather similar epidemiology to that of herpesvirus type II and must be considered as possible aetiological agents in epithelial abnormalities of the cervix. However, to date, no study of the relation of these viruses to such abnormalities has been reported.

Cytomegaloviruses belong to the same group of viruses as herpes simplex. In a recent survey in the North West of England (1970) cytomegalovirus was isolated from the cervices of 3 to 4% of women attending hospital clinics. When the virus was found in the cervix this was either the only site in which it was present or, if detected elsewhere, it was probably present in the cervix in larger amounts. In Taiwan, ALEXANDER (1967) found cervical excretion of this virus in 18% of Chinese women. In the North West of England survey antibodies were found in 18% of girls by the time they left their primary school (aged about 11 years). The percentage of girls with antibodies then rose steadily to the age of 35 years after which it remained stationary. Antibodies were found more frequently in girls "on remand" then in any other group of the population; however, this might reflect as much their socio-economic background as a higher rate of infection among such girls. Their epidemiological studies indicate that cytomegalovirus infection needs close contact for its spread and should be included among the "kissing diseases". DIOSI et al. (1967) were able to identify cytomegalic inclusions in the columnar cells of the cervix of a woman in pregnancy.

The TRIC agent is responsible for trachoma. It belongs to the PLT (psittacosis, lymphogranuloma venereum, trachoma) group of atypical viruses which are midway between true viruses and bacteria. They are filtrable yet divide by binary fission, have both DNA and RNA, a cell wall like bacteria, and a level of complexity approaching that of bacteria. This agent can cause inclusion blenorrhoea in the newborn (FREEDMAN et al. 1966; WATSON and GAIRDNER 1968). In both these studies the disease was found to be more common when the mothers were promiscuous. The usual source of infection of the infant's eyes is the mother's birth canal and evidence of TRIC infection can frequently be demonstrated in the cervix (JONES et al. 1964). KOTCHER et al. (1962) found large basophilic and minute acidophilic cytoplasmic inclusions in Giemsa-stained smears in 2.8% of nearly 8,000 women examined in a cancer cytology clinic. These were similar to those described in the literature in association with inclusion conjunctivitis. Material from those women positive for inclusion bodies was inoculated into embryonic chicken eggs and acidophilic elementary bodies were grown from two women.

CHIANG et al. (1968) have investigated genital infection by the TRIC agent in Taiwan. They were able to isolate the virus from the genital tract of 5 women. No inclusions could be seen in the smears, in contrast to eye infections. Indeed, the agent was isolated from the cervix of one pregnant patient, no inclusions being seen, but her infant developed blenorrhoea with intracellular inclusions. They were able to examine the cervices of these 5 women histologically; 2 pregnant women had necrotic papillary erosions, two non-pregnant women had simple erosions and one had no significant lesion.

Condyloma acuminatum is often regarded as viral although to date no evidence in support of this view is available (GARDNER and KAUFMAN 1965; MORGAN and BALDUZZI 1967). Adenovirus has been isolated from the female genital tract (MELCZER and HAMAR 1965; NAIB 1966). This virus is of particular interest in that some strains are oncogenic in animals.

From the above brief survey it is clear that, although herpesvirus has been the most studied and best documented virus in relation to malign lesions of the cervix, other viruses may possibly be implicated and should be investigated from this point of view.

The simultaneous presence of antibodies to several viruses (herpes simplex virus, cytomegalovirus and psittacosis, a member of the PLT group of viruses) has been recorded by CROMPTON (1971) in women attending a colposcopy clinic. In a group of 23 women, antibodies were found in all but 3. Of these 3, the cervix of one showed incomplete squamous metaplasia, another basal-cell hyperplasia and a third invasive squamous-cell carcinoma. In one other patient with squamous-cell carcinoma antibodies to all three viruses were present. Significant antibody titres were found in some women with bland cervical abnormalities and were commonly found in patients with dysplasia or carcinoma *in situ*. Apart from these lesions, atypical epithelium was also frequently present. This is illustrated in the following two cases:

Case K 1014. A colposcopic biopsy and the whole cervix were available for histological examination. Fig. 6.3. is from a section of epithelium taken from the

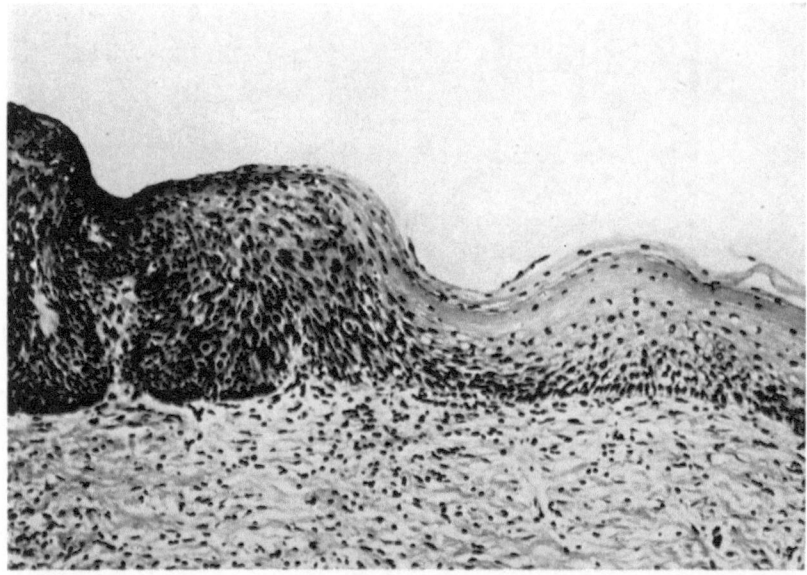

Fig. 6.3. Case K 1014. Normal squamous epithelium is present on the right and dysplastic epithelium on the left. Antibodies to cytomegalovirus were present at a titre of 1 in 32. (H. & E. × 120)

portio vaginalis; it shows the junction of the normal and dysplastic epithelium. Nearer the external cervical os there is a sudden change of pattern from dysplasia to an unusual type of squamous metaplasia, which involves much of the endocervical canal and is very thick. In it there are a number of cysts, or vesicles, and many of the adjacent cells show cytoplasmic swelling and eosinophilia (Fig. 6.4.). The patient's serum contained antibodies to cytomegalovirus at a titre of 1 in 32.

Case 971. Two colposcopic biopsies were available for histological examination. A notable feature is the papillary structure of the surface (Fig. 6.5.). The general architecture is somewhat disordered but stratification is present. A few cells show individual keratinization and koilocytotic atypia are conspicuous. Subsequently other colposcopically similar lesions, which had not been biopsied, disappeared. The pa-

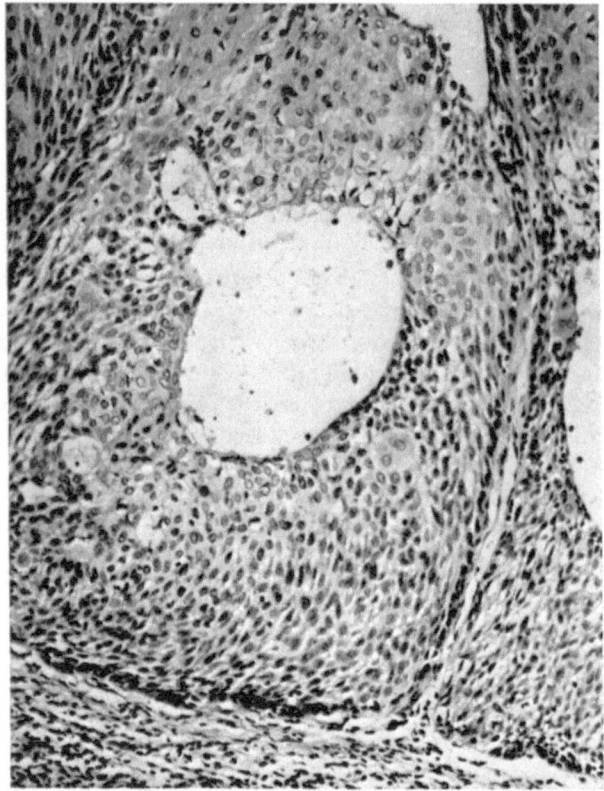

Fig. 6.4. Case K 1014. An intraepithelial cyst in an area of metaplasia. Note the groups of cells with abundant cytoplasm which readily takes up eosin. (H. & E. × 120)

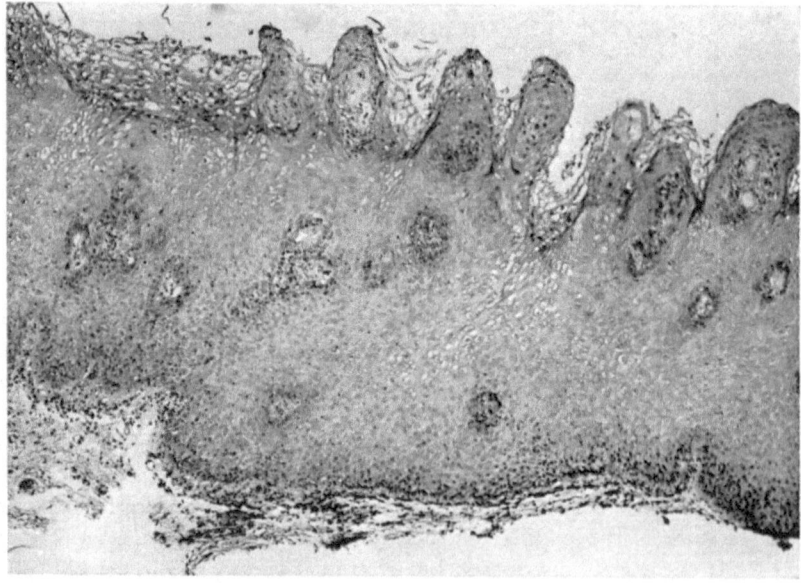

Fig. 6.5. Case 971. A colposcopic biopsy showing the full thickness of the squamous epithelium which has a curious papillary surface. The patient's serum contained antibodies to psittacosis virus, cytomegalovirus and herpes simplex virus. (H. & E. × 50)

tient had raised serum antibody titres, to psittacosis virus 1 in 128, and to herpes simplex and cytomegalovirus each 1 in 32.

e) Trichomoniasis

PATTEN et al. (1963) have shown that epithelial atypia may be produced by repeatedly inoculating mice per vaginam with T. vaginalis. In women a significant association of trichomonad infestation with cervical atypia has been described by a number of workers (BECHTOLD and REICHER 1952; SIMECKOVA et al. 1962; FROST 1962; JORDAN et al. 1964; CHRISTOPHERSON and PARKER 1964). CHRISTOPHERSON and PARKER (1964) do not think the atypias produced by trichomoniasis are sufficiently severe to be confused with the changes of carcinoma in situ. KOSS (1964) takes a similar view.

BERTINI and HORNSTEIN (1970) have recently carried out a survey of trichomoniasis in Israel. They found a significantly higher frequency of Trichomonas infestation among western and young Israeli-born women compared with those originating from eastern countries. This observation is of interest because of the higher standard of living, higher educational backgrounds and better sanitary conditions prevailing among the western and young Israeli-born women. These differences in the incidence of trichomoniasis could be related to the particularly strict observance by the eastern communities of religious laws and principles forbidding extra-marital sexual relations. The cytological findings in the smears showed a higher frequency of dysplasia and endocervical hyperplasia in the presence of trichomoniasis as well as a close association of the infection with benign lesions of the cervix. These cellular abnormalities regressed after treatment, indicating a causal relation between the cytological abnormality and the trichomonad infestation. There was no evidence of a higher incidence of cervical malignancy in these women.

3. Chemical Carcinogenesis of the Cervix Uteri

a) Animal Experiments

The use of rodents as a model for the study of cervical carcinogenesis was catalysed by MURPHY's classical studies (1953). Some workers have used the rat as an experimental animal (VELLIOS and GRIFFIN 1957) but for the most part mice have been employed. The time required to produce lesions depends on the strain of mice used, the carcinogen employed and the mode of application. The type of lesion (dysplasia, invasive carcinoma and so on) depends on the duration of treatment.

VON HAAM and SCARPELLI (1955) produced cervical dysplasia in C3H mice within 12 to 28 weeks by painting the cervix with 3,4-benzpyrene. CHRISTOPHERSON and BROGHAMER (1961) induced dysplasia in the same strain of mice by painting with 1% methylcholanthrene. REAGAN and WENTZ (1959) produced dysplasia in some C3H mice as early as one week after the application to the cervix of a thread impregnated with methylcholanthrene, and invasive carcinoma occurred in 3 out of 10 mice treated for 5 weeks. ALAUDDIN and ZAMAN (1967) produced cervical dysplasia in Swiss-Webster mice within 3—5 weeks of exposure to methylcholanthrene applied by a thread impregnated with the carcinogen. Continued application of the carcinogen led to progressively more abnormal epithelium and invasive squamous-cell carcinoma. WENTZ (1962) recognized four progressive stages: dysplasia, pleomorphic dysplasia, early infiltrative stage and invasive carcinoma. He found that following the cessation of carcinogen treatment all lesions up to the early infiltrative stage reverted to normal. VON HAAM (1961) had earlier observed that some of the dysplastic lesions in mice reverted to normal. However, the studies of CHRISTOPHERSON and BROGHAMER (1961) produced no evidence of regression but indicated that once the stage of dysplasia was reached no further application of carcinogen was needed to ensure progression to invasive carcinoma. Similarly, ALAUDDIN and ZAMAN (1967) found that, following removal of the thread impregnated with methylcholanthrene when there was cytological evidence of dysplasia, within a period of 26 weeks 8% of lesions progressed to invasive carcinoma and 50% to carcinoma *in situ*, 42% remained as dysplasia and none reverted to normal.

These experimentally induced lesions thus behave very similarly to the naturally occurring lesions in women, although they seem to regress less frequently. However, the similarity must not be pushed too far. The epithelium of the mouse cervix and vagina is structurally rather different from that of women and behaves differently in the ovarian cycle (MEYER and ALLEN 1932). Moreover, the studies of cell kinetics (LADINSKY and PECKHAM 1965; EDWARDS and LANGLEY 1971) indicate differences between the proliferating compartments of human and murine cervical and vaginal epithelium. Nevertheless, the mouse cervix affords the most convenient experimental model we have at present.

PARK and KOPROWSKA (1968) have carried out an interesting and illuminating investigation of lesions induced in the mouse cervix by 3,4-benzpyrene. In tissue culture, epithelial cells from these lesions were able to establish "transformed" cell lines. However, none of these cell lines manifested tumorigenic properties when injected subcutaneously into isologous mice. The ability of epithelial cells to establish "transformed" cell lines appeared early in neoplastic progression and was an independent character to be distinguished from tumour-forming abilities. The tumour-forming abilities of induced cervical lesions appeared later and were demonstrable by direct transplantation. They suggest that, since benzpyrene acts on the nucleus, nuclear transformation of epithelial cells occurs first by means of an exchange of the altered genetic material between fibroblasts and epithelial cells of the benzpyrene-painted mice before the cytoplasm has switched to the neoplastic pattern. This switch entails the second stage of transformation with the evolution of another hybrid population of cells endowed with the characteristics of invasiveness. Once both nuclear and cytoplasmic transformations have occurred, the cells manifest their invasiveness *in vivo*. However, in the absence of their own fibroblasts, under *in-vitro* conditions, tumorigenicity of even completely transformed cells may be difficult to demonstrate by bioassays.

The relationship of steroid hormones to the induction of cervical cancer in mice is somewhat complex and confusing. PINCUS (1967) induced cancer of the cervix by Murphy's method, using a methylcholanthrene-impregnated thread passed through the cervix of a mouse. He found that progesterone and at least one other synthetic progestin promoted the rate of cancer formation in the cervix of these mice, whereas oestrogen inhibited the rate of formation. This is the reverse of the effect on breast cancer. The results of Zaman and co-workers on the effects of endogenous hormones on tumorigenesis are consistent with these effects of exogenous steroids

(MUEENUDDIN and ZAMAN 1967; ALAUDDIN and ZAMAN 1967; MANNAN and ZAMAN 1968). They have shown: (1) that ovariectomy did not protect Swiss-Webster mice from developing carcinogen-induced cancer of the cervix uteri; (2) that ovariectomy in these mice gave rise to a relatively large number of methylcholanthrene-induced invasive carcinomas as opposed to *in-situ* carcinomas, and (3) that ovariectomy hastened induced cervical carcinogenesis. In a later study ASHRAF and ZAMAN (1969) investigated the effect of concurrent adrenalectomy and ovariectomy on the induction of cervical cancer in mice. Adrenalectomy not only removes an extraovarian source of oestrogen but produces a state of hormonal imbalance. There was no difference in the incidence of carcinoma in the adrenalectomized-ovariectomized animals as compared with intact mice or ovariectomized mice. However, the average latent period for carcinogenesis was significantly shortened in the adrenalectomized as compared with the intact animal. In contrast to these results, KAMINETZKY (1966) found that in methylcholanthrene-induced cervical atypia in C3H mice, castration reduced the abnormalities, oestrogen promoted stromal penetration by dysplastic epithelium and progesterone counteracted the effect of oestrogen. However, the photomicrographs in this report are unconvincing, the number of mice employed was small and there was no statistical analysis.

EBNER *et al.* (1968), using a chemical carcinogen in the cervical canal of mice, treated half of the animals with a synthetic progesterone compound and used the remainder as untreated controls. Carcinoma of the cervix developed in 50% of the untreated mice while no carcinoma developed in hormone-treated mice. If the hormone was administered at a later stage, after anaplastic changes had occurred, no inhibiting influence was manifested. They concluded that potential and actual cancer cells are no longer responsive to the hormone and that the progestin acted by protecting the cell from carcinogen.

Chromosomal studies have been made of methylcholanthrene- and podophyllin-induced lesions in the mouse cervix (KAMINETZKY and JAGIELLO 1967). Podophyllin is a potent mitotic poison but not a carcinogen. A single application of podophyllin to the mouse cervix produced numerous mitotic figures but all the nuclei contained the species number of chromosomes (40). After repeated application of podophyllin a large number of nuclei contained twice the species number of chromosomes (80); chromosome coalescence occurred and probably accounted for the malignant appearance of podophyllin-treated cells. Among animals receiving repeated methylcholanthrene applications, most chromosomes in the cervical epithelium appeared normal but in some metaphases the chromosomes were grossly distorted.

Some experimental studies have been made using the monkey cervix, which may be supposed to be more comparable to the human cervix than is that of the mouse. OVERHOLZER and ALLEN (1935), in four monkeys, produced squamous metaplasia involving endocervical glands by prolonged injection of oestrogen combined with local trauma to the cervix. In an earlier paper they had regarded the changes in the cervical epithelium as those of early carcinoma. KAMINETZKY and SWERDLOW (1968) applied a 1% suspension of methylcholanthrene in mineral oil to the cervix of 16 mature rhesus monkeys. Eight were allowed to menstruate physiologically and eight were given 20 mg. of oestradiol benzoate three times a week. Only mild abnormalities of the cervix occurred in the monkeys not treated with oestrogen, whereas four of the oestrogen-treated monkeys showed advanced epithelial dysplasia.

b) Changes Induced in the Human Cervix by Steroids
and Other Chemical Agents

α) *Therapeutic and Chemical Agents*

Koss (1961) has observed cytological abnormalities similar to dyskaryosis in the superficial cells of patients treated with alkylating agents. In one such case an abnormality of cervical epithelium was seen in material removed at necropsy from a 12-year-old girl who died of leukaemia. Patients affected in this way may present diagnostic difficulties in the evaluation of the cervical smear or the biopsy. The histological appearance of the lesion may resemble that of spontaneously occurring dysplasia or koilocytotic atypia. Although there is no evidence at present that alkylating agents have a carcinogenic effect on the cervix, Koss (1968) has recorded the development of invasive carcinoma of the cervix after 5 years of busulphan therapy but this may have been a fortuitous occurrence. Other alkylating agents, such as thiotepa, may occasionally induce abnormalities in the squamous epithelium of the cervix.

GURELI et al. (1963) have also described the changes in the cervix of patients treated with busulphan (myleran) for chronic myeloid leukaemia. The squamous epithelium showed atypical hyperplasia with dyskaryosis and many giant cells. The cervical smears showed cellular enlargement of small numbers of isolated cells and also some nuclei of gigantic size, but the nucleo-cytoplasmic ratio was not significantly disturbed. Similar changes may be seen in other organs of patients under busulphan therapy (KIRSCHNER and ESTERLY 1971).

Rather similar changes have been produced in the mouse cervix by the topical application of podophyllin (Koss 1961). SAPHIR et al. (1959) have produced dysplasia-like lesions in women by painting the cervix with the drug for a few days prior to hysterectomy. KAMINETZKY and McGREW (1961) treated the cervices of 50 women with podophyllin prior to hysterectomy: in 25 they found atypical changes in metaplastic squamous epithelium and atypical columnar epithelium in 31 cervices. Topical tetracycline can cause sloughing of atypical epithelium and sometimes apparent cure of carcinoma *in situ* (Koss 1961; Koss et al. 1963).

KAY et al. (1970) found cellular abnormalities in the Papanicolaou smears of 3 of 28 female patients receiving immunosuppressive therapy following renal transplantation. One of the 3 patients showed persistent atypicalities and was found on conization to have carcinoma *in situ*. They point out that whilst there is no definite proof that the cervical changes were caused by the treatment it is important to screen such patients for cervical lesions.

β) *Smegma*

The infrequency of carcinoma of the cervix in Jewesses suggests a possible relation between the uncircumcised state of the male consort and the occurrence of cervical carcinoma in the female partner. The equivocal nature of this relationship has been discussed above, but some support may be lent to this view by BLEICH's observation (1950) that carcinoma of the penis is associated with lack of circumcision. It is thus suggested that smegma, retained by the prepuce, may be a carcinogenic agent. Experiments have been directed to implicating smegma as a chemical carcinogen but it is equally possible that viruses, or other similar agents, present in the smegma might be inculpated.

PLAUT and KOHN-SPEYER (1947) constructed artificial tunnels on the backs of mice into which they injected horse smegma. Four malignant neoplasms developed in the tunnels, 2 in a series of 190 mice treated with whole smegma and 2 in a group of 8 mice treated with the non-saponifiable fraction of smegma. PRATT-THOMAS *et al.* (1956) and HEINS *et al.* (1958) have studied the action of human smegma on mice of the DBA-1 strain. It has been suggested that the bacteria in smegma, particularly the *Myobacterium smegmatis*, might convert cholesterol into a carcinogen. They introduced smegma, the contents of ovarian dermoid cysts and cultures of *M. smegmatis* into the vaginae of these mice using various procedures. Of 160 mice so treated, eighty-eight were available for evaluation. Of these, 8 developed an epidermoid carcinoma, 2 a sarcoma, 1 a malignant papilloma and 22 marked epithelial hyperplasia. To obtain these changes, it was necessary to continue treatment for 14 months. The changes were produced both by smegma and the contents of dermoid cysts. The DBA-1 strain of mice were used because (a) they do not develop cervical carcinoma spontaneously but (b) they are not cancer-resistant, since there is a known incidence of hereditary breast cancer. Further, PRATT-THOMAS *et al.* (1956) showed they were not refractory to the carcinogenic action of methylcholanthrene. In contrast to these results, HEINS *et al.* (1958) were able to show that the bi-weekly application of smegma to the vaginae of a Wistar strain of mice failed to produce any tumours.

In contrast to these observations, FISHMAN *et al.* (1942) found no evidence of a neoplasm after the subcutaneous injection of smegma into twelve mice and the intravaginal injection in twenty. More recently REDDY and BARUAH (1963) have shown that human smegma would produce epithelial hyperplasia but not squamous-cell carcinoma when applied to the vagina of Swiss mice. It took sixteen months to produce the changes and the number of mice surviving so long was small. It is difficult to be sure, from their histological illustrations, that some workers might not regard their "epithelial hyperplasia" as invasive carcinoma.

It is thus not possible at present to state whether or not human smegma is carcinogenic to mice. The results may depend on the strain of mice employed. By the same token, and because the epithelium of the human cervix and vagina is different from that of mice, it cannot be concluded that human smegma is carcinogenic to the cervix or vagina of woman.

c) Oral Progestins, Contraceptives and Related Substances

From the discussion of animal experiments it is clear that the role of steroid hormones in potentiating epithelial abnormalities of the cervix in animals is uncertain. This is also true of women, in whom the effects of these substances have been studied both morphologically and statistically. There is, however, such a wide variety of substances and combinations of substances used both as oral contraceptives and in the treatment of endometriosis that some of the effects may be unrecognized.

RYAN *et al.* (1964) reported increased secretion by the cervical glands as a result of long-term cyclical therapy with norethynodrel. MAQUEO *et al.* (1966) also found increased secretion and also stromal oedema. Squamous metaplasia occurred with continuous progestin dosage, but they found no increase in epithelial abnormalities in the cervices of women receiving contraceptive therapy as compared with control groups of women. DITO and BATSAKIS (1961) recorded slightly more changes in the cervices of women treated by norethynodrel for endometriosis. After 2 months there was increased vascularity and oedema of the cervix, and after 3 months hyperplasia, hypertrophy and hypersecretion of cervical glands. In some women there was thickening of the squamous epithelium of the portio vaginalis and occasionally a submucosal decidual reaction or decidual polyp. Forty per cent of the cervices showed squamous metaplasia; but it is doubtful if this is in excess of normal. The changes described by these various groups of workers are very similar to those seen in pregnancy and cannot be regarded as pathological. PINCUS (1967) has pointed out that in Puerto Rico, where there is possibly the highest prevalence of cervical carcinoma in the world, the occurrence of suspicious PAPANICOLAOU smears was extremely low in the group of women using oestrogen-progestin pills who were originally studied. This was in contrast to his studies of the effect of progesterone and one synthetic progestin on the rate of formation of experimentally induced cervical cancer in mice. Of course, the group of women originally treated by Pincus may have been of a different socio-economic class from the bulk of the population.

In contrast to these observations, GUHR (1964) claimed to observe a marked increase in pathological changes in the cervix with contraceptive levels of oestrogen-progestin combinations. He studied a group of 79 women and found pathological cervical lesions in 67 including intraepithelial carcinoma in 5. More recently, TAYLOR et al. (1967) reported atypical endocervical hyperplasia in 13 patients taking oral contraceptives. The histological appearance of the lesions was so bizarre that the possibility of adenocarcinoma had to be considered. Similar lesions have been found by GOVAN et al. (1969) in 10 women taking contraceptive pills for a considerable time and in 5 pregnant women. Numerous polypoid structures were present on the cervix and these were covered by a single layer of cuboidal cells or a thin layer of stratified epithelium. Beneath this there was a honeycomb or cribriform syncytial mass of cells. There was great variety in size and shape of the glands and in the type of epithelium lining them; a few glands were of large adult type, lined by a single layer of mucus-secreting cells. However, many were lined by a single layer of cells which were mostly flattened and elongated but occasionally cuboidal. The essential changes were cytoplasmic and not nuclear, although in areas of degeneration dark pyknotic nuclei could be seen. The type of change described by these workers is shown in Fig. 6.6. GOVAN et al. suggest that the lesion is formed under the influence of steroids on a cervix which is already pathological. They suggest that two changes are necessary before steroids can have this effect: polypoidal lesions must be present and these must show reserve cell hyperplasia.

In New York MELAMED et al. (1969) have carried out a long-range study of cervical carcinoma among women using contraceptives. Overt cervical carcinoma was not found in the population studied. Occult carcinoma was detected by cytology and confirmed by cervical biopsy or conization. Oral contraceptives were chosen by 27,508 women and the diaphragm by 6,809. A small but statistically significant difference in the prevalence rate of cervical carcinoma *in situ* was found between these two groups of women. It can be attributed either to a decreased prevalence rate for women using the diaphragm or to an increased rate for women using oral contraceptives. The difference was consistently present in subsets for each of the five factors known to influence the prevalence rate of cervical carcinoma: age, ethnic origin, age at first pregnancy, number of live births and family income. When corrections for all five factors were carried out simultaneously, there was still a significantly higher prevalence rate for carcinoma *in situ* within the population choosing and using steroid contraceptives. They point out that before this difference

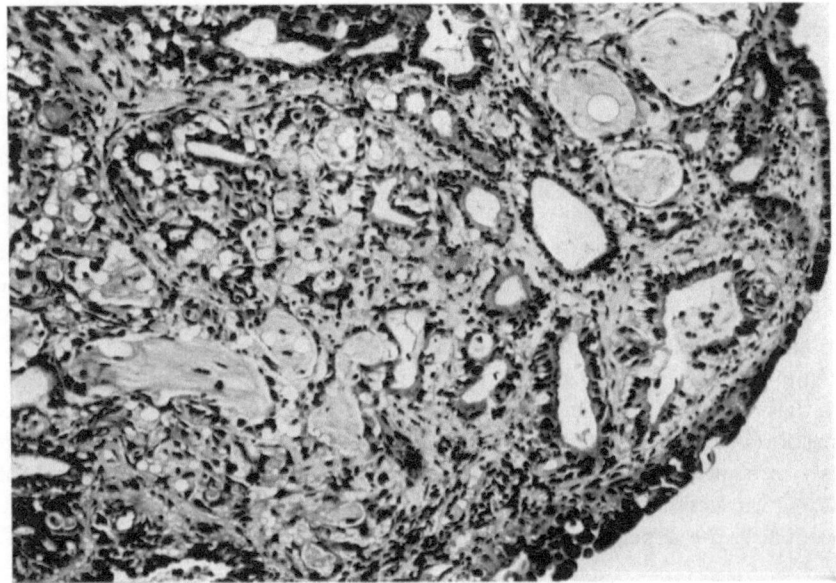

Fig. 6.6. The complex pattern of an endocervical polyp in a patient on oral contraceptives.
(H. & E. × 120)

in effect of oral contraceptives and the diaphragm can be established it will be necessary to confirm the difference by incidence rates of carcinoma *in situ* in the two groups. If the difference is confirmed, it could be suggested that the diaphragm exerts a barrier effect, for example excluding contact of smegma with the cervix or transmission of viruses to the cervix from the penis; alternatively the contraceptive steroids may potentiate carcinogenesis. Comparative studies of women using an intrauterine device would be useful since there is neither a barrier nor a hormonal effect with this contraceptive.

RICHART and BARRON (1967) have carried out some studies which have an indirect bearing on this problem. Two groups of patients with cervical dysplasia were investigated. The first group of 221 women wore no intrauterine contraceptive device and a second group of 114 wore varying types of intrauterine device. They were each followed by cytology and colpomicroscopy but no biopsies were performed. They found no evidence that the intrauterine device increased the rate of progression from dysplasia to carcinoma *in situ*.

The observations of AYRE *et al.* (1969) are pertinent in this context although surprising. They found 27 cases of dysplasia or carcinoma *in situ* among 1,020 women attending a planned parenthood clinic. Following Enavid (combined norethynodrel and mestranol) a third of the lesions showed regression.

4. The Role of Spermatozoa in Cervical Carcinogenesis

a) The Dynamic Phases of Activity of Cervical Epithelium

COPPLESON and REID (1967) have advanced the concept that the dynamic transition from columnar to metaplastic epithelium occupies only a relatively short time, of hours, days or weeks. They have suggested that during this dynamic phase conditions may exist which permit environmental factors which have a neoplastic potential to exert a mutagenic influence on the metaplastic epithelium. They followed the changes in the cervix of some women by serial colposcopic examination and found that the first pregnancy played a major part in producing the greatest area of metaplasia. In some primiparae there was a physiological eversion of the columnar cell lining of the endocervical canal which reached its height in the second or third trimester. The eversion was usually followed immediately by transformation to metaplastic squamous epithelium (COPPLESON and REID 1966). Sometimes mature metaplastic epithelium may be present at the time of the first pregnancy. PIXLEY (1967) has shown that this arises in earlier dynamic phases which may occur at birth or puberty. COPPLESON (1969) has compared the cervices of 300 girls between the ages of 12 and 17 years, remanded on a charge of "exposure to moral danger" with those of 300 virgins. Colposcopic studies of these girls show that an "atypical form of metaplasia is common in the promiscuous adolescent (over 40%) and rare in the virgin".

b) The Role of Spermatozoa

These morphological observations parallel the epidemiological evidence quoted earlier in this chapter indicating the significance of early sexual experience and the importance of the first pregnancy in the aetiology of cervical carcinoma. These findings are consistent with a viral hypothesis and also with the suggestion of REID (1964b, 1965a and b and 1966) and COPPLESON and REID (1967) that spermatozoa may be incriminated. Their evidence may be summarized as follows:

(1) When semen was cultured *in vitro* with biopsy material of mature metaplastic squamous epithelium or with cervical columnar epithelium (i.e. not during the dynamic phase of metaplasia) the spermatozoa were always seen on the surface of the tissue and never gained entry into the cells.

(2) However, when semen was cultured with biopsy material removed during the dynamic phase of metaplasia immediately following the first pregnancy, the immature cells ingested the spermatozoa.

(3) This process was shown to occur *in vivo* as well as *in vitro*. Biopsies of early or immature metaplastic epithelium were taken under colposcopic control seven to nine hours after coitus and occasionally a sperm head was seen ingested by an immature cell.

(4) When tritiated thymidine-labelled sperm were injected among the regenerating cells of a mouse uterus previously damaged by 5% trichloracetic acid, the label from the mouse sperm could be demonstrated within the nucleus of the dividing cells.

(5) Similarly, when tritiated thymidine-labelled mouse sperm was incorporated *in vitro* with human cervical tissue undergoing active metaplasia, there was a rapid uptake of the label first by the cytoplasm and then by the nucleus.

(6) Chemical analysis of sheep macrophages which had been exposed to sperm showed that there had been some change in the chemistry of the nuclear DNA, probably by incorporation of DNA from the spermatozoa.

COPPLESON and REID concluded that this evidence suggested that a mutation is caused by admixture of nucleic acids of the two genomes. It should be emphasized that the experiments in support of the observations just listed were not numerous and often the supporting photomicrographs are not very convincing. In part this is an optical problem; for example, the nuclei of the cells in the sections are by the nature of the technique not in the same plane as the autoradiographic image.

This work needs further confirmation although there is no doubt that spermatozoa can react with the female organism since specific antibodies against spermatozoa can be found in infertile women (FRANKLIN and DUKES 1964; BELL and WOOD 1968). It would be of value to investigate the occurrence of sperm antibodies in women with dysplasia, carcinoma *in situ* and invasive carcinoma.

5. Resumé

Earlier in this chapter it was pointed out that epidemiological evidence indicated that invasive squamous-cell carcinoma of the cervix had many of the characteristics of a communicable disease which follows a venereal mode of transmission. Infections of the female genital tract by cytomegalovirus, the TRIC agent and, particularly, herpesvirus type II have a similar epidemiology and may play a role in cervical oncogenesis. The nature of this role is still unknown. COPPLESON and REID have also adduced evidence that spermatozoa may have a part to play in cervical oncogenesis. Whatever part these agents play in the development of invasive carcinoma of the cervix they must also play a similar role in the preceding stages. However, it is much more difficult to make epidemiological studies of dysplasia and carcinoma *in situ* than of invasive carcinoma and thus extensive information is lacking for these conditions. Moreover, since some cases of dysplasia and of carcinoma *in situ* may regress it is probable that analysis of epidemiological information might be equivocal.

What is termed dysplasia or carcinoma *in situ* on morphological criteria may be a heterogeneous collection of conditions with different biological potentials. Some may be precursors of invasive carcinoma but others may be benign conditions which regress when the causal stimulus is removed, in a similar manner to the podophyllin-treated cervix. Alternatively, dysplasia, carcinoma *in situ* and invasive squamous-cell carcinoma may be one disease entity and regression may occur because the cells have been incompletely transformed or because of the development of immunity to the tumour. These considerations are speculative but they open possible lines for investigation.

LUNDIN *et al.* (1964) have pointed out that the first pregnancy is important in exposing the squamo-columnar junction to a noxious agent and this is supported by the colposcopic studies of COPPLESON and REID (1967). Moreover, it is just this area that morphological studies indicate as the site of predilection of dysplasia and carcinoma *in situ*. However, it must be remembered that the studies of ASHLEY (1966b) and others (see chapter 3) indicate that all invasive carcinomas may not progress through all these precancerous stages or, if they do, they progress very rapidly; this is particularly true of tumours occurring later in life. Thus, it seems probable that the socioeconomic and other epidemiological factors which relate to the earlier occurring carcinomas do not necessarily relate to those of late onset.

The part played by steroids in the genesis of these abnormalities is difficult to assess. The experimental evidence is inconclusive and contradictory and the evidence in the human subject unclear. CLEMMESEN's (1965) suggestion that the association of cervical carcinoma with the early beginning of sexual activity might be conditioned by a high level of oestrogen needs to be considered.

The evidence discussed in this chapter suggests that cervical neoplasia has a multifactorial aetiology. The effect of any factor is dependent on the age of the individual at the time of exposure, and the time relationship between the exposure to one factor and exposure to others is of great importance. It is probable that some aetiological factors, or agents, are important in initiating the malign process and others in promoting the neoplastic change. BARRON and RICHART (1971) suggest that the progression of cervical neoplasia involves a sequence of discrete events and the transition from one stage to another may involve different factors.

It seems probable that the decline in mortality from cervical carcinoma which started before mass cytological screening was introduced is largely due to control of one of these aetiological factors by some general trend in public hygiene or social custom.

References

ABEL, M. R., GOSLING, J. R. G.: Intraepithelial and infiltrative carcinoma of the vulva: Bowen's Type. Cancer (Philad.) **14**, 319—330 (1961).

ACHENBACH, R. R., JOHNSTONE, E., HERTIG, A. T.: The validity of vaginal smear diagnosis in carcinoma in situ of the cervix. A report of 60 cases. Amer. J. Obstet. Gynec. **61**, 385—392 (1951).

ALAUDDIN, S., ZAMAN, H.: The fate of 20-methylcholanthrene induced dysplasia of the mouse uterine cervix. Acta cytol. (Philad.) **11**, 211—216 (1967).

ALEXANDER, E. R.: Maternal and neonatal infection with Cytomegalovirus in Taiwan. Pediatrics **1**, 210 (1967).

ALFERT, M.: Variations in cytochemical properties of cell nuclei. Exp. Cell Res. Suppl. **6**, 227—235 (1958).

ALLEN, E., GARDNER, W. U.: Cancer of the cervix of the uterus in hybrid mice following long-continued administration of estrogen. Cancer Res. **1**, 359—366 (1941).

AMARAL FERREIRA, C.: In: Symposium on Sex Chromatin. Acta cytol. (Philad.) **6**, 93—94 (1962).

AN, S. H.: Herpes simplex virus infection detected on routine gynecology cell specimens. Acta cytol. (Philad.) **13**, 354—358 (1969).

ANDERSON, S. G., LINTON, E. B.: The diagnostic accuracy of cervical biopsy and cervical conization. Amer. J. Obstet. Gynec. **99**, 113—116 (1967).

ANDERSON, W. A., GUNN, S. A.: A comparative study of patient-obtained vaginal irrigation and physician-obtained aspiration and cervical scrape smears in cancer of the cervix. C A (N. Y.) **15**, 158—160 (1965).

ANTOINE, T., GRÜNBERGER, V.: Die Auflichtmikroskopie in der Gynäkologie. Klin. Med. (Wien) **4**, 15, 575—579 (1949).

ANTOINE, T., GRÜNBERGER, V.: Atlas der Kolpomikroskopie. Stuttgart: Georg Thieme 1956.

ARMITAGE, P.: Statistical Methods in Medical Research. Oxford: Blackwell 1971.

ASBOE-HANSEN, G.: The mast cell. Int. Rev. Cytol. **3**, 399—436 (1954).

ASCHOFF, L.: Zur Frage der atypischen Epithelwucherung und der Entstehung pathologischer Drüsenbildungen. Nachr. v. d. k. Gesellsch. d. Wissensch. zu Göttingen. Mathem.-phys. Kl. 250—260 (1894).

ASCHOFF, L.: Zur Cervixfrage: Nachtrag zu der Arbeit des Herrn Hofmeier. Mschr. Geburtsh. Gynäk. **22**, 611—615 (1905).

ASCHOFF, L.: Über die Berechtigung und Notwendigkeit des Begriffes Isthmus uteri. Verh. dtsch. path. Ges. (Jena) **12**, 314—322 (1908).

ASHLEY, D. J. B.: The biological status of carcinoma *in situ* of the uterine cervix. J. Obstet. Gynaec. Brit. Cwlth. **73**, 373—381 (1966a).

ASHLEY, D. J. B.: Evidence for the existence of two forms of cervical carcinoma. J. Obstet. Gynaec. Brit. Cwlth. **73**, 382—389 (1966b).

ASHRAF, M., ZAMAN, H.: The effect of bilateral adrenalectomy and ovariectomy on the induction of carcinoma of the mouse uterine cervix. Acta cytol. (Philad.) **13**, 347—351 (1969).

ASHWORTH, C. T., LUIBEL, F. J., SANDERS, E.: Epithelium of normal cervix uteri studied with electron microscopy and histochemistry. Amer. J. Obstet. Gynec. **79**, 1149—1160 (1960).

ASHWORTH, C. T., STEMBRIDGE, V. A., LUIBEL, F. J.: A study of basement membranes of normal epithelium, carcinoma *in situ* and invasive carcinoma of the uterine cervix utilizing electron microscopy and histochemical methods. Acta cytol. (Philad.) **5**, 369—382 (1961).

ATKIN, N. B.: Symposium on Nuclear Sex, New York: Interscience Publishers, Inc. pp. 168—176 1958.

ATKIN, N. B.: Nuclear size in premalignant conditions of the cervix uteri. Nature (Lond.) **202**, 201 (1964a).

ATKIN, N. B.: Nuclear size in carcinoma of the cervix: its relation to DNA content and to prognosis. Cancer (Philad.) **17**, 1391—1399 (1964b).

ATKIN, N. B.: The influence of nuclear size and chromosome complement on prognosis of carcinoma of the cervix. Proc. roy. Soc. Med. **59**, 979—982 (1966a).

ATKIN, N. B.: Sex chromatin abnormalities in carcinoma of the cervix uteri. Acta cytol. (Philad.) **10**, 392 (1966b).

ATKIN, N. B.: A high incidence of cells with a condensed (telophase) chromatin pattern in human tumors and carcinoma *in situ*. Acta cytol. (Philad.) **11**, 81—85 (1967a).

ATKIN, N. B.: Sex chromatin in cervical smears. Acta cytol. (Philad.) **11**, 435—436 (1967b).

ATKIN, N. B.: Triple sex chromatin and other sex chromatin anomalies in tumours of females. Brit. J. Cancer **21**, 40—47 (1967c).

ATKIN, N. B., BAKER, M. C.: A nuclear protrusion in a human tumor associated with an abnormal chromosome. Acta cytol. (Philad.) **8**, 431—433 (1964).

ATKIN, N. B., BAKER, M. C.: Chromosomes in carcinoma of the cervix. Brit. med. J. **1**, 522—523 (1965).

ATKIN, N. B., BAKER, M. C.: Chromosome abnormalities as primary events in human malignant disease: evidence from marker chromosomes. J. nat. Cancer Inst. **36**, 539—557 (1966).

ATKIN, N. B., BAKER, M. C., WILSON, S.: Stem-line karyotypes of 4 carcinomas of the cervix uteri. Amer. J. Obstet. Gynec. **99**, 506—514 (1967).

ATKIN, N. B., MATTISON, G., BAKER, M. C.: A comparison of the DNA content and chromosome number of fifty human tumours. Brit. J. Cancer **20**, 87—101 (1966).

ATKIN, N. B., RICHARDS, B. M., ROSS, A. J.: The desoxyribonucleic acid content of carcinoma of the uterus: an assessment of its possible significance in relation to histopathology and clinical course, based on data from 165 cases. Brit. J. Cancer **13**, 773—787 (1959).

AUERBACH, S. H., PUND, E. R.: Squamous metaplasia of the cervix uteri. Amer. J. Obstet. Gynec. **49**, 207—213 (1945).

AUERSPERG, N., COREY, M. J., WORTH, A.: Chromosomes in pre-invasive lesions of the human uterine cervix. Cancer Res. **27**, 1394—1401 (1967).

AUERSPERG, N., WORTH, A.: Growth patterns *in vitro* of invasive squamous carcinomas of the cervix. A correlation of cultural, histologic, cytogenetic and clinical features. Int. J. Cancer **1**, 219—238 (1966).

AVERETTE, H. E., WEINSTEIN, G. D., FROST, P.: Autoradiographic analysis of cell proliferation kinetics in human genital tissues. Amer. J. Obstet. Gynec. **108**, 8—17 (1970).

AYRE, J. E.: The vaginal smear. "Precancer" cell using a modified technique. Amer. J. Obstet. Gynec. **58**, 1205—1219 (1949).

AYRE, J. E., REYNER, F. C., FAGUNDES, W. B., LEGUERRIER, S. M.: Oral progestins and regression of carcinoma *in situ* and cervical dysplasia. Obstet. and Gynec. **34**, 545—560 (1969).

BADER, G. M., SIMON, T. R., KOSS, L. G., DAY, E.: A study of the detection tampon method as a screening device for uterine cancer. Cancer (Philad.) **10**, 332—337 (1957).

BAJARDI, F.: Histomorphology of carcinoma *in situ*. Acta cytol. (Philad.) **5**, 271—273 (1961a).

BAJARDI, F.: Symposium on Malignant Cervical Lesions (Nomenclature of the atypical epithelium). Acta cytol. (Philad.) **5**, 344—348 (1961b).

BAJARDI, F.: In: Symposium on Malignant Cervical Lesions (The atypical noninvasive zones around invasive cervical carcinoma). Acta cytol. (Philad.) **5**, 355—358 (1961c).

BAMFORD, S., MITCHELL, G. W., DAVID, J., SPERBER, A., CASSIN, C.: Size variation of the late-replicating X-chromosome in leucocytes of individuals with hyperplastic and malignant lesions of the uterine epithelium. Acta cytol. (Philad.) **13**, 238—245 (1969).

BANGLE, R., BERGER, M., LEVIN, M.: Variations in morphogenesis of squamous cell carcinoma of the cervix. Cancer (Philad.) **16**, 1151—1159 (1963).

BARILE, M. F., BLUMBERG, J. M., KRAUL, C. W., YAGUCHI, R.: Penile lesions among U.S. Armed Forces personnel in Japan. The prevalence of herpes simplex and the role of pleuropneumonia-like organisms. Arch. Derm. **86**, 273—281 (1962).

BARR, M. L., BERTRAM, E. G.: A morphological distinction between neurones of the male and female, and the behaviour of the nucleolar satellite during accelerated protein synthesis. Nature (Lond.) **163**, 679—680 (1949).

BARR, M. L., CARR, D. H.: Correlations between sex chromatin and sex chromosomes. Acta cytol. (Philad.) 6, 34—45 (1962).

BARRON, B. A., RICHART, R. M.: An epidemiologic study of neoplastic disease, based on a self-selected sample of 7,000 women in Barbados, West Indies. Cancer (Philad.) 27, 978—986 (1971).

BASERGA, R., HENEGAR, G. C., KISIELESKI, W. E., LISCO, H.: Uptake of tritiated thymidine in human tumors *in vivo*. Lab. Invest. 11, 360—364 (1962).

BEATO, M., CASTAÑO-ALMENDRAL, A., BARCELLOS, J. M.: Die Frühstadien des Plattenepithelcarcinomas des Collum uteri. Arch. Gynäk. 205, 1410—1427 (1968).

BECHTOLD, E., REICHER, N. B.: The relationship of Trichomonas infestation to false diagnosis of squamous carcinoma of the cervix. Cancer (Philad.) 5, 442—457 (1952).

BELL, E. B., WOOD, A.: Heterogeneity of isoantisera against spermatozoa in hyperimmunized mice. Nature (Lond.) 220, 508—509 (1968).

BELL, J. L., EGERTON, M. E.: 6-phosphogluconate dehydrogenase estimation in vaginal fluid in the diagnosis of cervical cancer. J. Obstet. Gynaec. Brit. Cwlth. 92, 603—609 (1965).

BELLER, F. K., KHATAMEE, M.: Evaluation of punch biopsy of the cervix under direct colposcopic observation (target punch biopsy). Obstet. and Gynec. 28, 622—625 (1966).

BENNETT, H. S.: Morphological aspects of extracellular polysaccharides. J. Histo. Cytochem. 11, 14—23 (1963).

BERENBLUM, I.: In: General Pathology; ed. H. W. FLOREY, Chapters 21 and 24. London: Lloyd-Luke 1970.

BERGER, J. VON: Die Feinstruktur des electronmikroskopisch darstellbaren Basalmembran des normalen mehrschichtigen Plattenepithels der Portio vaginalis uteri und deren angrenzenden Gebiete. Gynaecologia (Basel) 152, 208—223 (1961a).

BERGER, J. VON: Histochemistry of reserve cell hyperplasia, basal cell hyperplasia and dysplasia. Acta cytol. (Philad.) 5, 253—256 (1961b).

BERGER, J., NEIDITSCH, L. A., MUMPRECHT, E.: Electronenmikroskopische Untersuchungen von Plattenepithelveränderungen der Portio vaginalis uteri. Geburtsh. u. Frauenheilk. 18, 510—516 (1958).

BERNSTINE, J. B., RAKOFF, A. E.: Vaginal infections, infestations and discharges. New York: Blakiston 1953.

BERTALANFFY, F. D.: Aspects of cell formation and exfoliation related to cytodiagnosis. Acta cytol. (Philad.) 7, 362—371 (1963).

BERTALANFFY, F. D.: Aspects of cell formation and exfoliation. Acta cytol. (Philad.) 8, 373—374 (1964).

BERTALANFFY, L., BERTALANFFY, F. D.: Fluorescence microscopy of cervical cells and macrophages. Acta cytol. (Philad.) 4, 298 (1960).

BERTALANFFY, L., BERTALANFFY, F. D., GOODWIN, A. M.: Fluorescence microscopy of hyperplasia in gynecological cytodiagnosis. Acta cytol. (Philad.) 5, 256—257 (1961).

BERTINI, B., HORSTEIN, M.: The epidemiology of trichomoniasis and the role of infection in the development of carcinoma of the cervix. Acta cytol. (Philad.) 14, 325—332 (1970).

BIBBO, M., KEEBLER, C. M., WIED, G. L.: Prevalence and incidence rates of cervical atypia. J. Reproductive Med. 6, 184—188 (1971).

BIVENS, M. D., FLEETWOOD, H. O.: A 10-year survey of cervical carcinoma in Indians of the Southwest. Obstet. and Gynec. 32, 10—16 (1968).

BLANK, H., BUERK, M. S., WEIDMAN, F.: The nature of the inclusion body of verruca vulgaris: a histochemical study of the nucleotids. J. invest. Derm. 16, 19—30 (1951).

BLEICH, A. R.: Prophylaxis of penile carcinoma. J. Amer. med. Ass. 143, 1054—1057 (1950).

BLOCH, D. P., GODMAN, G. C.: A microphotometric study of the synthesis of desoxyribonucleic acid and nuclear histone. J. biophys. biochem. Cytol. 1, 17—28 (1955).

BLONK, D. I.: Cytochemical examination of lactic dehydrogenase and glucose-6-phosphate dehydrogenase in smears from the uterine cervix. Acta cytol. (Philad.) 13, 266—269 (1969).

BODDINGTON, M. M., SPRIGGS, A. I., WOLFENDALE, M. R.: Cytogenetic abnormalities in carcinoma in situ and dysplasias of the uterine cervix. Brit. med. J. 1, 154—158 (1965).

BOLTEN, K. A.: Introduction to Colposcopy. New York-London: Grune and Stratton 1960.

BOLTEN, K. A.: Practical colposcopy in early cervical and vaginal cancer. Clin. Obstet. Gynec. 10, 808—837 (1967).

BONHAM, D. G.: A new test for the diagnosis of gynaecological cancer, 6-phosphogluconate dehydrogenase activity in the vaginal fluid. Triangle (En.) 6, 157—162 (1964).

BONHAM, D. G., GIBBS, D. F.: A new test for gynaecological cancer, 6-phosphogluconate dehydrogenase activity in vaginal fluid. Brit. med. J. 2, 823—824 (1962).

BOTTELLA, J., NOGALES, F., MONTALVO, L.: The polysaccharide content of the human vagina as a
criterion of the action of sex hormones. Acta cytol. (Philad.) 2, 363—366 (1958).

BOUDA, J., DOHNAL, V.: Zur Frage der Krebsprophylaxe durch Elektrokoagulation bei Ektopie
und Umwandlungszone. Geburtsh. u. Frauenheilk. 25, 1186—1194 (1965).

BOYD, J. T., DOLL, R.: A study of the aetiology of carcinoma of the cervix uteri. Brit. J. Cancer
18, 419—434 (1964).

BOYES, D. A., FIDLER, H. K., LOCK, D. R.: Significance of in situ carcinoma of the uterine cervix.
Brit. med. J. 1, 203—205 (1962).

BOYES, D. A., WORTH, A. J., FIDLER, H. K.: The results of treatment of 4386 cases of pre-clinical
cervical squamous cell carcinoma. J. Obstet. Gynaec. Brit. Cwlth. 77, 769—780 (1970).

BRADFIELD, J. R. G.: Glycogen of the vertebrate epidermis. Nature (Lond.) 167, 40—41 (1951).

BRAUN-FALCO, O.: Histochemische und morphologische Studien an normalen und pathologisch
veränderten Haut. Arch. Dermat. Syph. (Berl.) 198, 111—198 (1954).

BRAUN-FALCO, O.: The histochemistry of psoriasis. Ann. N.Y. Acad. Sci. 73, 936—976 (1958).

BREATNACH, A. S.: The cell of Langerhans. Int. Rev. Cytol. 18, 1—28 (1965).

BREDAHL, E., KOCK, F., STAKEMANN, G.: Cancer detection by cervical scrapings, vaginal pool
smears and irrigation smears. A comparative study. Acta cytol. (Philad.) 9, 189—193 (1965).

BREDAHL, E., LEFEVRE, H.: Value of routine vaginal cytology in gynecologic pathology in order
to detect tumor cells. Acta obstet. gynec. scand. 44, 348—356 (1965).

BREMER, J. L.: Congenital anomalies of the viscera. Cambridge: Harvard University Press 1957.

BRESCIANI, F.: Cell proliferation in cancer. Europ. J. Cancer 4, 343—366 (1968).

BRET, J., COUPEZ, F.: Colposcopie. Paris: Masson et Cie. 1960.

BRIAND, P.: Thesis (1967) quoted by S. N. Pederson (1968).

BRODERS, A. C.: Carcinoma: Grading and practical application. Arch. Path. Lab. Med. 2, 376—381
(1926)

BRODERS, A. C.: Carcinoma in situ contrasted with benign penetrating epithelium. J. Amer.
med. Ass. 99, 1670—1674 (1932).

BRODY, I.: Different staining methods for electronmicroscopic elucidation of the tonofibrillar differentiation in normal epidermis. In: W. MONTAGNA and W. C. LOBITZ, The Epidermis, pp. 251—
274. New York and London: Academic Press 1964a.

BRODY, I.: Cytoplasmic components in the psoriatic horny layers with special reference to electronmicroscopic findings. In: W. MONTAGNA and W. C. LOBITZ, The Epidermis, pp. 551—572.
New York and London: Academic Press 1964b.

BRUNSCHWIG, A.: A method for mass screening for cytological detection of carcinoma of the cervix
uteri. Cancer (Philad.) 7, 1182—1184 (1954).

BRYAN, W. R.: Some biological considerations of tumor viruses. In: P. EMMELOT and O. MÜHLBOCK,
Cellular Control Mechanisms and Cancer, pp. 330—355. Amsterdam: Elsevier 1964.

BRYANS, T. E., BOYES, D. A., FIDLER, H. K.: The influence of a cytological screening program upon
the incidence of invasive squamous cell carcinoma of the cervix in British Columbia. Amer. J.
Obstet. Gynec. 88, 898—903 (1964).

BUCKINGHAM, J. C., BUETHE, R. A., DANFORTH, D. N.: Collagen-muscle ratio in clinically normal
and clinically incompetent cervices. Amer. J. Obstet. Gynec. 91, 232—237 (1965).

BUCKINGHAM, J. C., SELDEN, R., DANFORTH, D. N.: Connective tissue changes in the cervix during
pregnancy and labor. Ann. N.Y. Acad. Sci. 97, 733—742 (1962).

BULLOUGH, W. S., LAURENCE, E. B., IVERSEN, O. H., ELGJO, K.: The vertebrate epidermal chalone.
Nature (Lond.) 214, 578—580 (1967).

BULMER, D.: The development of the human vagina. Journ. Anat. 91, 490—509 (1957).

BUNTING, H., STRAUSS, M. J., BANFIELD, W. G.: The cytology of skin papillomas that yield virus-like
particles. Amer. J. Path. 28, 985—993 (1952).

BURGHARDT, E.: Latest aspects of precancerous lesions in squamous and columnar epithelium of the
cervix. Int. J. Gynec. Obstet. 8, 573—580 (1970).

BUTLER, E. B.: Carcinoma of the cervix in pregnancy. Proceedings of XIII Congreso Chileno de
Obstetricia y Ginecologia. Symposium Cancer de Cuello Uterino y Embarago. November 1969.

BUTLER, E. B.: Problems in diagnostic cytology. Chapter 13. In: H. Fox and F. A. LANGLEY, Postgraduate Obstetrical and Gynaecological Pathology. Oxford: Pergamon 1973.

BUTLER, E. B., LANGLEY, F. A.: (1969) unpublished observations.

CALABRESI, D., STOVALL, W. D.: Cytological screening for uterine cancer through physicians' offices. J. Amer. med. Ass. 168, 243—247 (1958).

CAMPO-AASEN, I., PEARSE, A. G. E.: Enzymologia de la célula Langerhans. Med. Cutánea (Barcelona) 1, 35—44 (1966).

CARMICHAEL, R., JEAFFRESON, B. L.: Basal cells in the epithelium of the human cervical canal. J. Path. Bact. 49, 63—68 (1939).

CARMICHAEL, R., JEAFFRESON, B. L.: Squamous metaplasia of the columnar epithelium of the human cervix. J. Path. Bact. 52, 173—186 (1941).

CARROW, L., HILKER, R. R. J. ELESH, R. H., EGGUM, P. R.: Evaluation of the vaginal irrigation smear technique. Amer. J. Obstet. Gynec. 97, 821—826 (1967).

CARSTEN, P.-M., MERKER, H.-J., MOSLENER, C.: Electronenmikroskopische Untersuchungen am menschlichen Portioepithel. Arch. Gynäk. 197, 72—92 (1962).

CASPERSSON, O.: Quantitative cytochemical studies on normal, malignant, premalignant and atypical cell populations from the human uterine cervix. Acta cytol. (Philad.) 8, 45—60 (1964).

CASTAÑO-ALMENDRAL, A., BEATO, M.: Die Frühstadien des Plattenepithelcarcinoms des collum Uteri. II. Histometrische Untersuchungen. Arch. Gynäk. 205, 428—451 (1968).

CHAPMAN, G. B., MANN, E. C., WEGRYN, R., HULL, C.: The ultrastructure of human cervical epithelial cells during pregnancy. Amer. J. Obstet. Gynec. 88, 3—16 (1964).

CHARLES, A.: Electronmicroscope observations on the human wart. Dermatologia (Basel) 121, 193—203 (1960).

CHIANG, W. T., ALEXANDER, E. R., WEI, P. Y., FRESH, J. W.: Genital infection with TRIC agents in Taiwan. Amer. J. Obstet. Gynec. 100, 422—431 (1968).

CHRISTOPHERSON, W. M.: The control of cervix cancer. Acta cytol. (Philad.) 10, 6—10 (1966).

CHRISTOPHERSON, W. M., BROGHAMER, W.: Progression of experimental cervical dysplasia in the mouse. Cancer (Philad.) 14, 201—204 (1961).

CHRISTOPHERSON, W. M., MENDEZ, W. M., AHUJA, E. M., LUNDIN, F. E., PARKER, J. E.: Cervix cancer control in Louisville, Kentucky. Cancer (Philad.) 26, 29—38 (1970).

CHRISTOPHERSON, W. M., PARKER, J. E.: A study of the relative frequency of carcinomas of the cervix in the Negro. Cancer (Philad.) 13, 711—713 (1960).

CHRISTOPHERSON, W. M., PARKER, J. E.: Chapter 13 in: Dysplasia, Carcinoma in situ and Microinvasive Carcinoma of the Cervix Uteri, ed. L. A. GRAY. Springfield: Thomas 1964.

CHRISTOPHERSON, W. M., PARKER, J. E.: Relation of cervical cancer to early marriage and childbearing. New Engl. J. Med. 273, 235—239 (1965).

CHRISTOPHERSON, W. M., PARKER, J. E., DRYE, J. C.: Control of cervical cancer: Preliminary report on community program. J. Amer. med. Ass. 182, 179—182 (1962).

CLARK, E. R., CLARK, E. L.: Microscopic observations on the growth of blood capillaries in the living animal. Amer. J. Anat. 64, 251—301 (1939).

CLEAVER, J. E.: Thymidine Metabolism and Cell Kinetics. Amsterdam: North-Holland Publishing Co. 1967.

CLEMMESEN, J.: Statistical Studies in the Aetiology of Malignant Neoplasms. København: Munksgaard 1965.

CLEMMESEN, J., NIELSEN, A.: The social distribution of cancer in Copenhagen, 1943 to 1947. Brit. J. Cancer 5, 159—171 (1951).

COCKER, J., FOX, H., LANGLEY, F. A.: Consistency in the histological diagnosis of epithelial abnormalities of the cervix uteri. J. clin. Path. 21, 67—70 (1968).

COHART, E. M.: Socieconomic distribution of cancer of the female sex organs in New Haven. Cancer (Philad.) 8, 34—41 (1955).

COHEN, S., WAY, S.: Histochemical demonstration of pentose shunt activity in smears from the uterine cervix. Brit. med. J. 1, 88—89 (1966).

COMAN, D. R.: Decreased mutual adhesiveness, a property of cells from squamous cell carcinomas. Cancer Res. 4, 625—627 (1944).

COMAN, D. R.: Mechanisms responsible for origin and distribution of blood-borne tumor metastases: review. Cancer Res. 13, 397—404 (1953).

COPPLESON, M.: Carcinoma of the cervix: Epidemiology and aetiology. Brit. J. Hosp. Med. **2**, 961—980 (1969).

COPPLESON, M., PIXLEY, E., REID, B.: Colposcopy. Springfield, Illinois: Charles C. Thomas 1971.

COPPLESON, M., REID, B.: A colposcopic study of the cervix during pregnancy and the puerperium. J. Obstet. Gynaec. Brit. Cwlth. **73**, 575—585 (1966).

COPPLESON, M., REID, B.: Preclinical carcinoma of the cervix uteri. Oxford: Pergamon 1967.

COTTE, G., MILEFF, A., MEYER, C.: Sur l'action de la folliculine sur la muqueuse vaginale de la femme. Rev. franç. Gynéc. **32**, 683—702 (1937).

CRAMER, H.: Die Kolposkopie in der Praxis. Stuttgart: Thieme 1956.

CROMPTON, A. C.: Doctoral thesis. Manchester University 1971.

CROSS, H. E., KENNEL, E. E., LILIENFELD, A. M.: Cancer of the cervix in an Amish population. Cancer (Philad.) **21**, 102—108 (1968).

CULLEN, T. S.: Cancer of the Uterus. New York: Appleton 1900.

CUYLER, W. K., KAUFMANN, L. A., CARTER, B. A., ROSS, R. A., THOMAS, W. L., PALUMBO, L.: Genital cytology in obstetric and gynecologic patients. A four year study. Amer. J. Obstet. Gynec. **62**, 262—278 (1951).

DALIAN, G., SIMATOS, A., NUOVO, V. M.: Exfoliative cytology of dysplasia during pregnancy. Acta cytol. (Philad.) **3**, 80—82 (1959).

DANFORTH, D. N.: The fibrous nature of the human cervix and its relation to the isthmic segment in gravid and non-gravid uteri. Amer. J. Obstet. Gynec. **53**, 541—557 (1947).

DANFORTH, D. N.: The distribution and functional activity of the cervical musculature. Amer. J. Obstet. Gynec. **68**, 1261—1270 (1954).

DANFORTH, D. N., BUCKINGHAM, J. C.: Connective tissue mechanisms and their relation to pregnancy. Obstet. gynec. Surv. **19**, 715—732 (1964).

DANFORTH, D. N., BUCKINGHAM, J. C., RODDICK, J. W.: Connective tissue changes incident to cervical effacement. Amer. J. Obstet. Gynec. **80**, 939—945 (1960).

DANFORTH, D. N., CHAPMAN, J. C. F.: The incorporation of the isthmus uteri. Amer. J. Obstet. Gynec. **59**, 979—988 (1950).

DARDIN, V. J.: Metaplasia. Georgetown Med. Bull. **9**, 13 (1955).

DAVIDSOHN, I., KOVARIK, S.: Isoantigens A, B and H in benign and malignant lesions of the cervix. Arch. Path. **87**, 306—314 (1969).

DAVIES, J., KUSAMA, H.: Developmental aspects of the human cervix. Ann. N.Y. Acad. Sci. **97**, 534—550 (1962).

DAVIS, H.: A comment on Ashley's paper. Obstet. gynec. Surv. **22**, 176—177 (1967).

DAVIS, H. J.: The irrigation smear: accuracy in detection of cervical cancer. Acta cytol. (Philad.) **6**, 459—467 (1962a).

DAVIS, H. J.: The irrigation smear. A cytologic method for mass population screening by mail. Amer. J. Obstet. Gynec. **84**, 1017—1023 (1962b).

DAVIS, H., JONES, H. W.: Cervical control with irrigation smears. Obstet. gynec. Surv. **24**, 927—935 (1969).

DAWSON, I. M., FILIPE, M. I.: The value of enzyme histochemical studies in the histological and cytological diagnosis of uterine cervical lesions. J. Obstet. Gynaec. Brit. Cwlth. **74**, 432—441 (1967).

DE BRUX, J. A.: Do administered estrogens stimulate growth and maturity of the epithelium directly or indirectly through stimulation of the nervous system and enzyme system? Acta cytol. (Philad.) **2**, 343—346 (1958).

DE BRUX, J. A., DUPRÉ-FROMENT, J.: Differentiation of endocervical glandular and metaplastic cells. Acta cytol. (Philad.) **4**, 299—303 (1960).

DE BRUX, J. A., DUPRÉ-FROMENT, J.: In: Symposium on premalignant cervical lesions. Acta cytol. (Philad.) **5**, 136—142 (1961a).

DE BRUX, J. A., DUPRÉ-FROMENT, J.: Interrelationship: Reserve cell hyperplasia, basal cell hyperplasia, dysplasia and cervical carcinoma. Acta cytol. (Philad.) **5**, 265—269 (1961b).

DE BRUX, J. A., DUPRÉ-FROMENT, J.: Cytomorphology of carcinoma *in situ*. Acta cytol. (Philad.) **5**, 422—424 (1961c).

DE BRUX, J. A., DUPRÉ-FROMENT, J.: Junctional areas in squamous cell carcinoma of the cervix. Amer. J. Obstet. Gynec. **93**, 181—192 (1965).

DE BRUX, J. A., WENNER-MANGEN, H.: In: Symposium on malignant cervical lesions. Acta cytol. (Philad.) 5, 349—351 (1961).

DEFENDI, V., STOKER, M.: Growth regulating substances for animal cells in culture. Wistar Institute Symposium Monograph. No. 7, Philadelphia: Wistar Institute Press 1967.

DE GIROLAMI, E.: Perinuclear halo versus koilocytotic atypia. Obstet. and Gynec. 29, 479—487 (1967).

DEMETRAKOPOULOS, N. S., GREENE, R. R.: Lymph follicles in the cervix uteri. Surg. Gynec. Obstet. 106, 729—733 (1958).

DERKSEN, J. C., HERINGA, G. C., WEIDINGER, A.: Acta neerl. Morph. 1, 31 (1937) quoted by Odland (1964).

DE ROBERTIS, E. D. P., NOWINSKI, W. W., SAEZ, F. A.: Cell Biology, 4th Edition. Philadelphia and London: Saunders 1966.

DE WITT, S. H.: Chromocenters resembling sex chromatin. Acta cytol. (Philad.) 6, 95—97 (1962).

DIERKS, K.: Der normale menstruale Zyklus der Vaginalschleimhaut. Arch. Gynäk. 130, 46—69 (1927).

DIOSI, P., BABUSCEAC, L., NEVINGLOSCHI, O., KUNSTOICI, G.: Cytomegalic virus infection associated with pregnancy. Lancet 1967 II, 1063—1066.

DITO, W. R., BATSAKIS, J. G.: Norethynodrel-treated endometriosis: a morphological and histochemical study. Amer. J. Obstet. Gynec. 81, 1—12 (1961).

DOLL, R., PAYNE, P., WATERHOUSE, J.: Cancer incidence in five continents. (U.I.C.C.) Berlin: Springer 1966.

DORN, H. F., CUTLER, S. J.: Morbidity from Cancer in United States. Public Health Monograph. 56. Washington: U.S. Gov't Printing Office 1959.

DOUGHERTY, C. M.: The cytomorphology of the endocervix. Acta Cytol. (Philad.) 4, 293—296 (1960).

DOUGHERTY, C. M., Low, E. M.: The fine structure of the basement membrane of the uterine cervical epithelium. Amer. J. Obstet. Gynec. 76, 839—850 (1958).

DOUGHERTY, C. M., MOORE, W. R., COTTEN, N.: Histologic diagnosis and clinical significance of benign lesions of the non-pregnant cervix. Ann. N.Y. Acad. Sci. 97, 683—702 (1962).

DUNN, J. E.: The relationship between carcinoma in situ and invasive cervical carcinoma. Cancer (Philad.) 6, 873—886 (1953).

DUNN, J. E.: Preliminary findings of the Memphis-Shelby County uterine cancer study and their interpretation. Amer. J. publ. Hlth. 48, 861—872 (1958).

DUNN, J. E.: The presymtomatic diagnosis of cancer with special reference to cervical cancer. Proc. roy. Soc. Med. 59, 1198—1204 (1966).

DUNN, J. E., MARTIN, P. L.: Morphogenesis of cervical cancer. Findings from San Diego County cytology registry. Cancer (Philad.) 20, 1898—1906 (1967).

DUNN, J. E., ROWAN, J. C., ERIKSON, C., SIEGLER, E.: Uterine cancer morbidity data. Memphis-Shelby County, Tennessee. Publ. Hlth. Rep. (Wash.) 69, 269—274 (1954).

DUNN, J. E., SLATE, T. A., MERRITT, N. W., MARTIN, P. L.: Findings for uterine cancer from one or more cytologic examinations of 33,750 women. J. nat. Cancer Inst. 23, 507—529 (1959).

DUPERROY, G.: Morphological study of the endocervical mucosa in relation to the menstrual cycle and leucorrhea. Gynaecologia (Basel) 131, 73—86 (1951).

EBNER, H. J., DIENSBACH, F., SANDRITTER, W.: The effects of nor-progesterone on experimental cancer of the cervix. Germ. med. Mthl. 13, 41 (1968).

EDWARDS, J. I.: A study of adult human cervical epithelia and human foetal skin maintained in organ culture. M. Sc. Thesis. University of Manchester (1971).

EDWARDS, J. I., LANGLEY, F. A.: Unpublished observations (1971).

EICHHOLZ, P.: Quoted by Fluhmann, 1964, Inaug. Diss. Königsberg (1902).

EPPERSON, J. W. W., HELLMAN, L. M., GALBIN, G. A., BUSBY, T.: The morphological changes in the cervix during pregnancy, including intraepithelial carcinoma. Amer. J. Obstet. Gynec. 61, 50—61 (1951).

EPSTEIN, W. L., CONANT, M. A., KRASNOBROD, H.: Molluscum contagiosum: Normal and virus-infected epidermal cell kinetics. J. invest. Derm. 46, 91—103 (1966).

ETON, B., VINCE, S. W.: Colpomicroscopy, a new method of study of the cervix in the living. J. Obstet. Gynaec. Brit. Cwlth. 68, 357—360 (1961).

EVANS, D. M. D.: In: Cytology Automation, proceedings of Second Tenovus Symposium, pp. 5—13. Edinburgh: Livingstone 1970.

FARQUHAR, M. G., PALADE, G. E.: Cell junctions in amphibian skin. J. cell Biol. **26**, 263—291 (1965).

FAWCETT, D. W.: Surface specializations of absorbing cells. J. Histochem. Cytochem. **13**, 75—91 (1965).

FEIT, J., STANIČEK, J.: Histoautoradiographical investigation of DNA synthesis in precancerous states and carcinomas of the uterine cervix in bioptical material. Neoplasma (Bratisl.) **14**, 499—505 (1967).

FELL, H. B.: The experimental study of keratinization in organ culture. pp. 61—82. The Epidermis (ed. W. MONTAGNA and W. C. LOBITZ). New York: Academic Press. (1964).

FENNELL, R. H.: Carcinoma *in situ* with early invasive changes. Cancer (Philad.) **8**, 302—309 (1955).

FENNELL, R. H. J.: Carcinoma *in situ* of the uterine cervix; report of 118 cases. Cancer (Philad.) **9**, 374—384 (1956).

FETTIG, O.: Zur morphologischen und klinischen Problematik des Mikrocarcinoms (Collumcarcinom Stadium Ia). Arch. Gynäk. **199**, 571—608 (1964).

FETTIG, O., OEHLERT, W.: Autoradiographische Untersuchungen der DNS- und Eiweiß-Neubildung im gynäkologischen Untersuchungsmaterial. Arch. Gynäk. **199**, 649—662 (1964).

FETTIG, O., SIEVERS, R.: 3 H-Index und mittlere Generationszeit des menschlichen Portiokarzinoms und seiner Vorstufen (autoradiographische Untersuchungen mit 3 H-Thymidin). Beitr. path. Anat. **133**, 83—100 (1966).

FIDLER, H. K., BOYD, J. R.: Occult invasive squamous carcinoma of the cervix. Cancer (Philad.) **13**, 764—771 (1960).

FIDLER, H. K., BOYES, D. A.: Patterns of early invasion of carcinoma *in situ*. Cancer (Philad.) **12**, 673—680 (1959).

FIDLER, H. K., BOYES, D. A., WORTH, A. J.: Cervical cancer detection in British Columbia. J. Obstet. Gynaec. Brit. Cwlth. **75**, 392—404 (1968a).

FIDLER, H. K., BOYES, D. A., WORTH, A. J.: Screening for malignant disease by means of exfoliative cytology. In: Presymptomatic Detection and Earlier Diagnosis (ed. C. L. E. H. SHARP and H. KEEN). pp. 295—332. London: Pitman 1968 (b).

FIDLER, H. K., BOYES, D. A., WORTH, A. J.: quoted by FIDLER *et al.* (1968b), Lying-in **1**, 128 (1968c).

FIELD, E. O.: Editorial. Cell Tissue Kinetics **1**, 1 (1968).

FIENBERG, R., COHEN, R. B.: Enzymes of glycogen metabolism in the squamous epithelium of the cervix. A histochemical study. Obstet. and Gynec. **31**, 608—617 (1968).

FIGGE, D. C., DE ALVAREZ, R. R., BROWN, D., FULLINGTON, W. R.: Long-range studies of the biologic behavior of the human uterine cervix. Amer. J. Obstet. Gynec. **84**, 638—647 (1962).

FILIPE, M. I., DAWSON, I. M.: Qualitative and quantitative enzyme histochemistry of the human endometrium and cervix in normal and pathological conditions. J. Path. Bact. **95**, 243—258 (1968).

FISHMAN, W. H.: β-Glucuronidase and the action of steroid hormones. Ann. N.Y. Acad. Sci. **54**, 548—557 (1951).

FISHMAN, W. H., GREEN, S., HOMBURGER, F., KASDON, S. C., NIEBURGS, H. E., McINNIS, G., PUND, E. R.: β-Glucuronidase studies in women; VII, premenopausal vaginal fluid-β-glucuronidase values in relation to *in-situ* cancer of the cervix. Cancer (Philad.) **7**, 729—743 (1954).

FISHMAN, W. H., MITCHELL, G. W.: Studies in vaginal enzymology. Ann. N.Y. Acad. Sci. **83**, 105—121 (1959).

FISHMAN, W. H., MITCHELL, G. W., BORGES, P. R. T., LADVE, K. T., HAYASHI, M.: Enzymorphology of cancer of the cervix. Cancer (Philad.) **16**, 118—125 (1963).

FISHMAN, M., SHEAR, M. J., FRIEDMAN, H. F., STEWART, H. L.: Studies in carcinogenesis. XVII. Local effect of repeated application of 3,4-benzpyrene and of human smegma to the vagina and the cervix of mice. J. nat. Cancer. Inst. **2**, 361—365 (1942).

FITZGERALD, P. J., YERMAKOV, V., SOBIN, L., LEVINE, L.: The mass of cancer *in situ* cells of the human cervix uteri as compared to normal cervical cells. Acta Un. int. Cancr. **15**, 296—302 (1959).

FLEISCHMAJER, R., BILLINGHAM, R. E.: Epithelial-mesenchymal interactions. 18th Hahnemann Symposium. Baltimore: Williams and Wilkins 1968.

FLEISSNER, E.: In: Gynaecological Oncology (ed. H. R. K. BARBER and E. A. GRABER), Amsterdam: Excerpta Medica Foundation 1970.

FLESCH, P., ESODA, E. C. J.: Chemical anomalies in pathological horny layers. In: The Epidermis, pp. 539—550, (ed. W. MONTAGNA and W. C. LOBITZ). New York and London: Academic Press 1964.

FLETCHER, C. M., OLDHAM, P. D.: Problem of consistent radiological diagnosis in coal miners' pneumoconiosis; experimental study. Brit. J. industr. Med. **6**, 168—183 (1949).

FLETCHER, C. M., OLDHAM, P. D.: Use of standard films in radiological diagnosis of coal-workers' pneumoconiosis. Brit. J. industr. Med. **8**, 138—149 (1951).

FLUHMANN, C. F.: Comparative studies of squamous metaplasia of the cervix uteri and endometrium. Amer. J. Obstet. Gynec. **68**, 1447—1462 (1954).

FLUHMANN, C. F.: The glandular structures of the cervix uteri during pregnancy. Amer. J. Obstet. Gynec. **78**, 990—1003 (1959).

FLUHMANN, C. F.: The cervix uteri and its diseases. Philadelphia: Saunders 1961.

FLUHMANN, C. F.: The cervix uteri. In: Dysplasia, carcinoma in situ and microinvasive carcinoma of the cervix uteri. (Ed. L. GRAY). Chapter 2. Springfield: Thomas 1964.

FOIX, A., BURR, G. E.: Desarollo y studio histoquimico del canal cervico-vaginal. Obstet. Ginec. lat-amer. **13**, 55—69 (1955).

FOOTE, F. W., Jr., STEWART, F. W. :The anatomical distribution of the intraepithelial epidermoid carcinomas of the cervix. Cancer (Philad.) **1**, 431—440 (1948).

FORAKER, A. G.: Histochemistry of the uterine cervix, normal exocervical, metaplastic, dysplastic, intraepithelial and invasive squamous cell carcinomatous epithelium. Ann. N.Y. Acad. Sci. **97**, 632—637 (1962).

FORAKER, A. G., DENHAM, S. W., AGUILAR CELI, P.: Localization of sites of dehydrogenase activity in the cervix uteri. Cancer (Philad.) **7**, 311—317 (1954).

FORAKER, A. G., MARINO, G.: Glycogen in invasive squamous cell carcinoma of the cervix. Amer. J. Obstet. Gynec. **72**, 400—403 (1956).

FORAKER, A. G., MARINO, G.: Glycogen synthesizing enzymes in the uterine cervix. Obstet. and Gynec. **17**, 311—315 (1961).

FORAKER, A. G., WINGO, W. J.: Protein-bound sulfhydryl and disulfide groups in squamous cell carcinoma of the uterine cervix. Amer. J. Obstet. Gynec. **71**, 1182—1188 (1956).

FORD, D. K., FIDLER, H. K., LOCK, D. R.: Dysplastic lesions of the bronchial tree. Cancer (Philad.) **14**, 1226—1234 (1961).

FORNI, A., MILES, C. P.: Sex chromatin abnormalities in carcinoma of the cervix uteri. Acta cytol. (Philad.) **10**, 200—204 (1966).

FRANK, R. T.: Gynecological and obstetrical pathology. New York: Appleton 1931.

FRAENKEL-CONRAT, H.: The chemistry and biology of viruses. New York: Academic Press 1969.

FRANKLIN, R. R., DUKES, C. D.: Antispermatozoal antibody and unexplained infertility. Amer. J. Obstet. Gynec. **89**, 6—9 (1964).

FREEDMAN, A., AL-HUSSAINI, M. K., DUNLOP, E. M. C., et al.: Infection by TRIC agent and other members of the Bedsonia group. Trans. ophthal. Soc. U.K. **86**, 313—320 (1966).

FREINKEL, R. K.: Carbohydrate metabolism in the skin. In: The Epidermis, Chapter 24. (Ed. W. MONTAGNA and W. C. LOBITZ). New York: Academic Press 1964.

FRIEDRICH, E. R., COLE, W., MIDDLEKAMP, J. N.: Herpes simplex. Clinical aspects and electron-microscopic findings. Amer. J. Obstet. Gynec. **104**, 758—779 (1969).

FROST, J. K.: Trichomonas vaginalis and cervical epithelial changes. Ann. N.Y. Acad. Sci. **97**, 792—795 (1962).

FROST, J. K.: Diagnostic accuracy of "cervical smears". Obstet. gynec. Surv. **24**, 893—908 (1969).

FUNCK-BRENTANO, P., MORICARD, R., ROBERT, H.: Des modifications de l'endocol après implantation oestrogène chez la femme ménopausée; problème du diagnostic differentiel des métaplasies des glandes endocervicales (glycogène et mucine). Bull. Fed. Soc. Gynéc. Obstét. franç. **3**, 381—387 (1951).

GAGNON, F.: Contribution to study of etiology and prevention of cancer of the cervix of the uterus. Amer. J. Obstet. Gynec. **60**, 516—522 (1950).

GANSE, R.: Das normale und pathologische Gefäßbild der Portio vaginalis uteri. Berlin: Akademie-Verlag 1958.

GANSE, R.: Einführung in die Kolposkopie. Jena: Fischer 1963.

GARDNER, H. L., KAUFMAN, R. H.: Condyloma acuminatum. Clin. Obstet. Gynec. **8**, 938—945 (1965).

GELLER, F. C.: Über atypische Epithelwucherung an Gebärmutterhalse. Zbl. Gynäk. **47**, 406—411 (1923).

GENET, P., HENRY, R., VANDEL, S., DESFOSSES, B., JAYLE, M.-F.: Comparaison de l'activité biologique de l'oestrone, de la 16α-hydroxyoestrone et de l'oestriol. Ann. Endocr. (Paris) **23**, 693—704 (1962).

GERE, J. B., ABEL, A. R., SHIELDS, D.: Observations on the bronchial epithelium of infants and children. Cancer (Philad.) 15, 118—121 (1962).

GESCHICKTER, C. F., FERNANDEZ, F.: Epidermidization of the cervix. Ann. N.Y. Acad. Sci. 97, 638—652 (1962).

GIROUD, A., BULLIARD, H.: Bull. Soc. Chim. biol. (Paris) 14, 278 (1932) quoted by Odland (1964).

GLATTHAAR, E.: Studien über die Morphogenese des Plattenepithelcarcinomas der Portio vaginalis uteri. Basel: Karger 1950.

GLATTHAAR, E.: In: SEITZ-AMREICH, Biologie und Pathologie des Weibes, Vol. 3, p. 911. Berlin: Urban und Schwarzenberg 1955.

GLATTHAAR, E., VOGEL, A.: Electronenmikroskopische Studien am Portioepithel und Portio-karzinom. Geburtsh. u. Frauenheilk. 18, 502—509 (1958).

GLÜCKSMANN, A.: In: Recent Advances in Clinical Pathology, Chapter 33 (ed. S. C. DYKE). London: Churchill 1947.

GLÜCKSMANN, A.: Aspects of cell formation and exfoliation. Acta Cytol. (Philad.) 8, 164 (1964a).

GLÜCKSMANN, A.: Aspects of cell formation and exfoliation. Acta Cytol. (Philad.) 8, 376 (1964b).

GLÜCKSMANN, A.: Microinvasive carcinoma of the uterine cervix. T. norske Laegeforen. 12b, 1267—1270 (1968).

GLÜCKSMANN, A., CHERRY, C. P.: Micro-invasive carcinoma of the cervix; histo-pathological aspects. In: Dysplasia, carcinoma in situ and micro-invasive carcinoma of the cervix uteri. Chapter 15 (ed. L. A. GRAY). Springfield: Thomas 1964.

GOLDBERG, D. M., HART, D. M., WATTS, C.: Distribution of enzymes in human vaginal fluid. Cancer (Philad.) 21, 964—974 (1968).

GOLDMANN, E.: The growth of malignant disease in man and the lower animals with special reference to the vascular system. Proc. roy. Soc. Med. 1, 3, 1—13 (1907—1908).

GOMPEL, C.: Anatomie pathologique gynécologique et obstétricale. Bruxelles: Arscia 1963.

GORE, H., HERTIG, A. T.: In: Dysplasia, carcinoma in situ and micro-invasive carcinoma of the cervix uteri. Chapter 5 (ed. L. A. GRAY). Springfield: Thomas 1964.

GOVAN, A. D. T., BLACK, W. P., SHARP, J. L.: Aberrant glandular polypi of the uterine cervix associated with contraceptive pills: pathology and pathogenesis. J. clin. Path. 22, 84—89 (1969).

GOVAN, A. D. T., HAINES, R. M., LANGLEY, F. A., TAYLOR, C. W., WOODCOCK, A. S.: Changes in the epithelium of the cervix uteri. J. Obstet. Gynaec. Brit. Cwlth. 73, 883—896 (1966).

GOVAN, A. D. T., HAINES, R. M., LANGLEY, F. A., TAYLOR, C. W., WOODCOCK, A. S.: The histology and cytology of changes in the epithelium of the cervix uteri. J. clin. Path. 22, 383—395 (1969).

GRAGERT, O.: Über das Glykogen in der fetalen Vagina. Arch. Gynäk. 128, 43—47 (1926).

GRAHAM, J. B., SOTTO, L. S. J., PALOUCEK, F. P.: Carcinoma of the cervix. Philadelphia: Sanders 1962.

GRAHAM, S., LEVIN, M., LILIENFIELD, A.: The socioeconomic distribution of cancer of various sites in Buffalo, N.Y., 1948—1952. Cancer (Philad.) 13, 180—191 (1960).

GRANBERG, I.: Chromosomes in preinvasive, microinvasive and invasive cervical carcinoma. Hereditas (Lund) 68, 165—218 (1971).

GRAUMANN, W., HEINKE, W., SIEGEL, P.: Die Variationsbreite des histochemischen Verhaltens der Schleimstoffe in der menschlichen Cervix uteri. Acta histochem. (Jena) 23, 288—294 (1966).

GRAY, L. A.: Dysplasia, carcinoma in situ and micro-invasive carcinoma of the cervix uteri. Springfield: Thomas 1964.

GREEN, G. H.: The significance of cervical carcinoma in situ. Aust. N. Z. J. Obstet. Gynaec. 6, 42—44 (1966).

GREEN, G. H., DONOVAN, J. W.: The natural history of carcinoma in situ. J. Obstet. Gynaec. Brit. Cwlth. 77, 1—9 (1970).

GREEN, H. N.: Immunological concept of cancer: preliminary report. Brit. med. J. 2, 1374—1380 (1954).

GREEN, H. N., ANTHONY, H. M., BALDWIN, R. W., WESTROP, J. W.: An immunological approach to cancer. London: Butterworth 1967.

GREIDER, M. H., SCARPELLI, D. G.: The application of electron microscopy to the study of exfoliated cells. Acta Cytol. (Philad.) 8, 39—44 (1964).

GRICOUROFF, G.: Le problème du cancer du col de l'utérus au stade zéro. Presse méd. 60, 743—744 (1952).

GRICOUROFF, G.: La thyroidose métastatique bénigne et ses tumeurs. Bull. Ass. franç. Cancer 49, 300—311 (1962).

GRISWOLD, M. H., WILDER, C. S., CUTLER, S. J., POLLACK, E. S.: Cancer in Connecticut, 1935—1951, p. 23. Hartford, Connecticut: State Department of Health 1955.

GRUBB, C., HACKEMANN, M., HILL, K. R.: Small granules and plasma membrane thickening in human cervical squamous epithelium. J. Ultrastruct. Res. 22, 458—468 (1968).

GRUBB, C., JANOTA, I.: Squamous differentiation in carcinoma in situ of the cervix uteri. J. clin. Path. 20, 7—14 (1967).

GRUENAGEL, H. H.: Die Plattenepithel-Zylinderepithelgrenze an der Portio vaginalis uteri bei unreifen und reifen Neugeborenen, Säuglingen und Kindern bis zu neun Jahren. Frankfurt. Z. Path. 68, 465—496 (1957).

GRUENWALD, P.: Growth and development of the uterus: the relationship of epithelium to mesenchyme. Ann. N.Y. Acad. Sci. 75, 436—440 (1959).

GRUMBACH, M., MORISHIMA, A.: Sex chromatin and the sex chromosomes: on the origin of sex chromatin from a single X chromosome. Acta cytol. (Philad.) 6, 46—60 (1962).

GUHR, L.: quoted by MAQUEO et al. (1966). Selecta 6, 1460 (1964).

GUIN, G. H.: The incidence and anatomical distribution of basal cell hyperactivity and its relationship to carcinoma of the cervix uteri. Amer. J. Obstet. Gynec. 65, 1081—1087 (1953).

GÜRELI, N., DENHAM, S. W., ROOT, S. W.: Cytologic dysplasia related to busulphan (myleran) therapy. Obstet. and Gynec. 21, 466—470 (1963).

GUSBERG, S. B.: Coning biopsy in the detection of early cancer of the cervix: a survey of 500 normal women. Amer. J. Obstet. Gynec. 61, 270—288 (1951).

GUSBERG, S. B., MOORE, D. B.: The clinical pattern of intraepithelial carcinoma of the cervix; and its pathologic background. Obstet and Gynec.. 2, 1—14 (1953).

HABEL, K.: Resistance of polyoma virus-immune animals to transplanted polyoma tumours. Proc. Soc. exp. Biol. (N.Y.) 106, 722—725 (1961).

HABEL, K.: Antigenic properties of cells transformed by polyoma virus. Cold Spring Harbor Symp. 27, 433—439 (1962).

HABEL, K.: Specific complement fixing antigens in polyoma tumour and transformed cells. Virology 25, 55—61 (1965).

HACKEMANN, M., GRUBB, C., HILL, K. R.: The ultrastructure of normal squamous epithelium of the human cervix uteri. J. Ultrastruct. Res. 22, 443—457 (1968).

HAEFELI, K.: Die Früherfassung des Portiokarzinoms an der Universitäts-Frauenklinik Zürich, 1945—1948. Dissertation Zürich (1950).

HAENSZEL, W., HILLHOUSE, M.: Uterine cancer morbidity in New York City and its relation to pattern of regional variation within United States. J. nat. Cancer Inst. 22, 1157—1181 (1959).

HAMBRICK, G. W., LAMBERG, S. I., BLOOMBERG, R.: Observations on keratinization of human skin in vitro. J. invest. Derm. 47, 541—550 (1966).

HAMPERL, H.: Definition and classification of so-called carcinoma in situ. In: Cancer of the Cervix, Ciba Foundation. London: Churchill 1959.

HAMPERL, H.: Über das infiltrierende (invasive) Tumorwachstum (Untersuchungen am Carcinom und am sog. Carcinom in situ). Virchows Arch. path. Anat. 340, 183—205 (1966).

HAMPERL, H., KAUFMANN, C.: The cervix uteri at different ages. Obstet. and Gynec. 14, 621—631 (1959).

HANDLEY, W. S.: The prevention of cancer. Lancet 1936 I, 987—991.

HANSCHKE, H. J.: Chromosomal sex determination in carcinoma of the cervix uteri and in bronchial carcinoma in man. Z. Krebsforsch. 63, 232—235 (1960).

HANSCHKE, H. J., SCHULZ, H.: Electronmikroskopische Befunde an Zellen von Vaginal- und Portioabstrichen. Arch. Gynäk. 192, 393—411 (1960).

HARTMAN, C.: Cyclic changes in the endocervix of the monkey and the origin of cervical mucus. Ann. N. Y. Acad. Sci. 97, 564—570 (1962).

HARVALD, B., HAUGE, M.: Heredity of cancer elucidated by a study of unselected twins. J. Amer. med Ass. 186, 749—753 (1963).

HASHIMOTO, M., YORISATO, M.: Electronenmicroscopic studies on the fine structure of the human uterine cervix. J. Jap. obstet. gynaec. Soc. 6, 99—107 (1959).

HAY, E. D., REVEL, J. P.: Autoradiographic studies of the origin of the basement lamella in Ambystoma. Develop. Biol. 7, 152—168 (1963).

HEDBERG, G. T.: The alkaline phosphatase activity in the cervical mucosa. Gynaecologia (Basel)
129, 239—246 (1950).

HEINS, H. C., DENNIS, E. J., PRATT-Thomas, H. R., CHARLTON, S. C.: Possible role of smegma in
carcinoma of cervix. Amer. J. Obstet. Gynec. 76, 726—735 (1958).

HELD, E.: Intracervicale Lokalisation des nicht invasiven, atypischen Plattenepithels (Oberflächen-
karzinom, Carcinoma in situ) und des beginnenden Pflasterzellkarzinoms. Arch. Gynäk. 188, 376
— 390 (1957).

HELLMAN, L. M., ROSENTHAL, A. H., KISTNER, R. W., GORDON, R.: Some factors influencing the
proliferation of reserve cells in the human cervix. Amer. J. Obstet. Gynec. 67, 899—911 (1954).

HEROVICI, C.: In Symposium: Effects of endogenous estrogens on the vaginal epithelium. Acta
cytol. (Philad.) 4, 51—58 (1960a).

HEROVICI, C.: Cytochemistry of normal and abnormal endocervix. Acta Cytol. (Philad.) 4, 297
1960b).

HERTIG, A. T., GORE, H.: Tumors of the female sex organs. Part 2. Tumors of the vulva, vagina
and uterus. Washington: Armed Forces Institute of Pathology (1960).

HILL, G. B., ADELSTEIN, A. M.: Cohort mortality from carcinoma of the cervix. Lancet 1967 II,
605—606.

HILLEMANNS, H. G.: Serological and immunological studies on the pathogenesis of cervical cancer.
Z. Naturforsch. 17b, 240—261 (1962).

HILLEMANNS, H. G., FRÖHLICH, D., PRESTEL, E.: Zellzahl und Mitosefrequenz bei Entstehung des
Cervixcarcinoms (zum Carcinoma in situ und Mikrocarcinom der Cervix). Arch. Gynäk. 206,
292—319 (1968a).

HILLEMANNS, H. G., PRESTEL, E.: Karyometrie mit den Teilchengrößenanalysator (TGZ) am Bei-
spiel des Cervixcarcinoms und seiner Vorstufen. Z. Krebsforsch. 71, 316—319 (1968).

HILLEMANNS, H. G., SIXTUS-KLUG, B., PRESTEL, E.: Cytoplasma-Kernrelationen der Malignitäts-
stufen des Cervixepithels, gemessen mit dem Integrationsocular I zum Carcinoma in situ und
Mikrocarcinom der Cervix. Arch. Gynäk. 206, 82—97 (1968b).

HINSELMANN, H.: Verbesserung der Inspektionsmöglichkeiten von Vulva, Vagina und Portio.
Münch. med. Wschr. 72, 1733 (1925).

HINSELMANN, H.: Der Nachweis der aktiven Ausgestaltung der Gefäße beim jungen Portikarzinom
als neues differentialdiagnostische Hilfsmittel. Zbl. Gynäk. 64, 1810—1814 (1940).

HISAW, F. L., LENDRUM, F. C.: Squamous metaplasia in the cervical glands of monkeys following
oestrin administration. Endocrinology 20, 228—229 (1936).

HOFFMAN, R. L., MERRITT, J. W.: 6-phosphogluconate dehydrogenase in uterine cancer detection.
Amer. J. Obstet. Gynec. 92, 650—657 (1965).

HOPMAN, B. C.: Histochemical methods applied to benign and malignant squamous epithelium of
the cervix uteri. Amer. J. Obstet. Gynec. 79, 346—369 (1960).

HORSTMANN, E., STEGNER, H. E.: Handbuch der microskopischen Anatomie des Menschen VII/1.
Berlin: Springer 1966.

HOWARD, L., ERICKSON, C. C., STODDARD, L.: A study of the histogenesis of endocervical metaplasia
and intra-epithelial carcinoma. Amer. J. Path. 25, 794—795 (1949).

HOWARD, L., ERICKSON, C. C., STODDARD, L. D.: A study of the incidence and histogenesis of
endocervical metaplasia and intraepithelial carcinoma; observations on 400 uteri removed for
noncervical disease. Cancer (Philad.) 4, 1210—1233 (1951).

HOWATSON, A. F.: Viruses connected with tumours and warts. Brit. med. Bull. 18, 193—198 (1962).

HUGHESDON, P. E.: The fibromuscular structure of the cervix and its changes during pregnancy
and labour. J. Obstet. Gynaec. Brit. Emp. 59, 763—776 (1952).

ILIYA, F. A., AZAR, H. A.: Radioautographic studies in neoplasia of the uterine cervix. Amer. J.
Obstet. Gynec. 99, 515—521 (1967).

INTERNATIONAL COMMITTEE ON HISTOLOGICAL DEFINITIONS (1961): Editorial in Acta cytol. (Philad.)
6, 235—236 (1962).

ISHIHARA, M., HASEGAWA, G., MORI, M.: Histochemical observations of oxidative enzymes in
malignant tumors of female genital organs. Amer. J. Obstet. Gynec. 90, 183—194 (1964).

ISHIHARA, M., YAMADA, H., CHAYA, I., NOBATA, G.: Histochemical study of aminopeptidase in
malignant neoplasms of the female genitals. Amer. J. Obstet. Gynec. 102, 525—530 (1968).

IVERSEN, O. H.: Mast cells in the myometrium of the human cervix uteri and changes caused by
androgenic and estrogenic hormones. Acta path. microbiol. scand. 49, 337—343 (1960).

IVERSEN, O. H.: Effect of epidermal chalone on human epidermal mitotic activity *in vitro*. Nature 219, 75 (1968).

IVERSEN, O. H., BJERKNES, R., DEVIK, F.: Kinetics of cell renewal, cell migration and cell loss in hairless mouse dorsal epidermis. Cell Tissue Kinet 1, 351—367 (1968).

JARRETT, A., RILEY, P. A.: Esterase activity in dendritic cells. Brit. J. Derm. 75, 79—81 (1963).

JARRETT, A., SPEARMAN, R. I. C., RILEY, P. A.: Dermatology: A functional introduction. London: English Universities Press 1966.

JIMERSON, G. K., MERRILL, J. A.: Multicentric squamous malignancy involving both cervix and vulva. Cancer (Philad.) 26, 150—153 (1969).

JOHNSON, H. A., BOND, V. P.: A method of labeling tissues with tritiated thymidine in vitro and its use in comparing rates of cell proliferation in duct epithelium, fibroadenoma and carcinoma of the human breast. Cancer (Philad.) 14, 639—643 (1961).

JOHNSON, H. A., HAYMAKER, W. E., RUBINI, J. R., FLIEDNER, I. M., BOND, V. P., CRONITE, E. P., HUGHES, W. L.: A radioautographic study of human brain and glioblastoma multiforme after the uptake of tritiated thymidine. Cancer (Philad.) 13, 636—642 (1960a).

JOHNSON, H. A., RUBINI, J. R., CRONKITE, E. P., BOND, V. P.: Labeling of human tumor cells in vivo with tritiated thymidine. Lab. Invest. 9, 460—465 (1960b).

JONEK, J., SKALBA, H., KLIMLIEWICZ, Z., DZIECIUCHOWICZ, L.: Histoenzymatic studies on the behavior of succinic acid dehydrogenase, NADH2 tetrazolium reductase, ATP-ase and alkaline phosphatase in cancer of the uterine cervix in women. Pol. med. J. 5, 614—621 (1966a).

JONEK, J., SKALBA, H., KLIMKIEWICZ, Z., DZIECIUCHOWICZ, L.: Histoenzymatic studies on the localization of some enzymes in uterine cervix cancer in women. Pol. med. J. 5, 622—629 (1966b).

JONES, B. R., Al-HUSSAINI, M. K., DUNLOP, E. M.: Genital infection in association with TRIC virus infection of the eye. I Isolation of virus from urethra, cervix and eye. Brit. J. vener. Dis. 40, 19—24 (1964).

JONES, H. W., Jr., DAVIS, H. J., FROST, J. K., PARK, I. J., SALIMI, R., TSENG, P. Y., WOODRUFF, J. D.: The value of the assay of chromosomes in the diagnosis of cervical neoplasia. Amer. J. Obstet. Gynec. 102, 624—641 (1968).

JONES, H. W., KATAYAMA, K. P., STAFL, A., DAVIS, H. J.: Chromosomes of cervical atypia, carcinoma in situ, and epidermoid carcinoma of the cervix. Obstet. and Gynec. 30, 790—805 (1967).

JORDAN, M. J., BADER, G. M., DAY, E.: Carcinoma in situ of the cervix and related lesions. An 11-year prospective study. Amer. J. Obstet. Gynec. 89, 160—182 (1964).

JORDAN, S. W., MUNSICK, R. A., STONE, R. S.: Carcinoma of the cervix in American Indian women. Cancer (Philad.) 23, 1227—1232 (1969).

JOSEY, W. E., NAHMIAS, A. J., NAIB, Z. M.: Genital infection with type 2 herpesvirus. Amer. J. Obstet. Gynec. 101, 718—729 (1968).

JÜTTING, G., KUSS, E., MARTIUS, G.: Ist eine Diagnose von Genitalcarcinomen durch Bestimmung der 6-Phosphogluconat-Dehydrogenase-Aktivität des Vaginalsekretes möglich? Klin. Wschr. 43, 1037—1060 (1965).

KAISER, R. F., ERICKSON, C. C., EVERETT, B. E., GILLIAM, A. G., WALTON, M., SPRUNT, D. H.: Initial effect of community-wide cytologic screening on clinical stage of cervical cancer detected in an entire community; results of Memphis-Shelby County, Tennessee, Study. J. nat. Cancer Inst. 25, 863—881 (1960).

KAHN, R. H.: Vaginal keratinization in vitro. Ann. N.Y. Acad. Sci. 83, 347—355 (1959).

KAMINETZKY, H. A.: Methylcholanthrene-induced cervical dysplasia and sex steroids. Obstet. and Gynec. 27, 489—493 (1966).

KAMINETZKY, H. A., JAGIELLO, G. M.: Differential chromosomal effects of carcinogenic and noncarcinogenic substances. Amer. J. Obstet. Gynec. 98, 349—353 (1967).

KAMINETZKY, H. A., McGREW, E. A.: The effect of podophyllin on the human endocervix. Obstet. and Gynec. 18, 255—258 (1961).

KAMINETZKY, H. A., SWERDLOW, M.: Experimental cervical dysplasia in the rhesus monkey. Amer. J. Obstet. Gynec. 102, 404—413 (1968).

KAPLAN, A. S.: Herpes simplex and pseudorabies viruses. Virology Monograph. 6, New York: Springer 1969.

KARRER, H.: Cell intercommunications in normal human cervical epithelium. J. biophys. biochem. Cytol. 7, 181—184 (1960).

KASHGARIAN, M.: The concepts of prevalence and incidence as applied to the study of development and duration of disease. Method. Inform. Med. **7**, 111—117 (1968).

KASHGARIAN, M., DUNN, J. E.: The duration of intraepithelial and pre-clinical squamous cell carcinoma of the uterine cervix. J. Epidemiology **92**, 211—222 (1970).

KASPER, T. A., SMITH, E. S. O., COOPER, P., CLAYTON, J., TODD, D.: An analysis of the prevalence and incidence of gynecologic cancer cytologically detected in a population of 175,767 women. Acta cytol. (Philad.) **14**, 261—269 (1970).

KAUFMANN, W., ADHAM, M., TARDIF, L.: An evaluation of colpomicroscopy in the diagnosis of carcinoma in situ of the cervix. Surg. Gynec. Obstet. **114**, 261—266 (1962).

KAUFMANN, C., OBER, K. G.: The morphological changes in the cervix uteri with age and their significance in the early diagnosis of carcinoma. In: Cancer of the Cervix, Diagnosis and early Forms (ed. G. E. W. WOLSTENHOLME and M. O'CONNOR), pp. 61—65. London: Churchill 1959.

KAY, S., FRABLE, W. J., HUME, D. H.: Cervical dysplasia and cancer developing in women on immunosuppression therapy for renal homotransplantation. Cancer (Philad.) **26**, 1048—1052 (1970).

KEMP, R. B.: Effect of the removal of cell surface sialic acids on cell aggregation in vitro. Nature (Lond.) **218**, 1255—1256 (1968).

KERN, G., ZANDER, J.: Gefäßveränderungen im Verlauf der Carcinogenese. Z. Krebsforsch. **63**, 168—183 (1959).

KERR, L. M. H., CAMPBELL, J. L., LEVVY, G. A.: β-Glucuronidase and tissue damage. Nature. (Lond.) **160**, 572 (1947).

KIRKLAND, J. A.: Atypical epithelial changes in the uterine cervix. J. clin. Path. **16**, 151—154 (1963)

KIRKLAND, J. A., STANLEY, M. A., CELLIER, K. M.: Comparative study of histologic and chromosomal abnormalities in cervical neoplasia. Cancer (Philad.) **20**, 1934—1952 (1967).

KIRSCHNER, R. H., ESTERLY, J. R.: Pulmonary lesions associated with busulphan therapy of chronic myelogenous leukemia. Cancer (Philad.) **27**, 1074—1080 (1971).

KLAVINS, J. V.: Intra-epithelial carcinoma with differentiated surface cells and dysplasia. Definition and separation of these lesions. Acta cytol. (Philad.) **7**, 350—356 (1963).

KLEGER, M. S., PRIER, J. E., ROSATO, D., McGINNIS, A. E.: Herpes simplex infection of the female genital tract. I. Incidence of infection. Amer. J. Obstet. Gynec. **102**, 745—748 (1968).

KLIGMAN, A. M.: The biology of the stratum corneum. In: The Epidermis (ed. W. H. MONTAGNA and W. C. LOBITZ), pp. 387—437. New York: Academic Press 1964.

KLIONSKY, B., COHEN, M.: Quality control in cytology — a proposed method for selection of slides for review. Acta cytol (Philad.) **15**, 54—56 (1971).

KNOX, E. G.: In: Problems and Progress in Medical Care, chapter 10 (ed. M. McLACHLAN). London: Oxford University Press 1966.

KNOX, E. G.: In: Screening in Medical Care. Nuffield Provincial Hospital Trust, chapter 4. London: Oxford University Press 1968.

KOFF, A.: Development of the vagina in the human foetus. Contr. Embryol. Carneg. Instn. **24**, 59—91 (1933).

KOLLER, O.: The Vascular Patterns of the Uterine Cervix. Oslo: University Press 1963.

KOLLER, O., KOLSTAD, P.: A colpophotographic study of carcinoma in situ and of early invasive carcinoma of the cervix. Acta Un. int. Cancr. **19**, 1390—1393 (1962).

KOLSTAD, P.: Vascularization, oxygen tension and radiocurability in cancer of the cervix. Oslo: University Press 1964.

KOS, J.: Gefäßanordnung in der Portio vaginalis cervix uteri unter normalem gesundem Plattenepithel. Zbl. Gynäk. **82**, 1849—1855 (1960).

KOS, J.: Blood Capillaries in Normal and Pathological Conditions. Čs. Morfol. **9**, 17—33 (1961).

KOS, J.: Darstellung der Gefäßkapillaren an Exzisionen aus der Cervix uteri auf histochemischem Wege. Zbl. Gynäk. **84**, 538—541 (1962).

KOS, J., LANÉ, V.: Die Architektonik der terminalen Blutgefäße an der Cervix uteri. Kolposkopische und zytologische Studien in zwangloser Folge, Heft 9 (ed. Prof. Dr. R. GANSE). Leipzig: VEB Georg Thieme 1963.

KOSS, L. G.: Diagnostic cytology and its histopathologic bases. 1st ed. Philadelphia: Lippincott 1961.

KOSS, L. G.: In: Dysplasia, carcinoma in situ and micro-invasive carcinoma, chapter 9 (ed. L. A. GRAY). Springfield: Thomas 1964.

Koss, L. G.: Diagnostic cytology and its histopathologic bases. 2nd edition. Philadelphia: Lippincott 1968.

Koss, L. G., Melamed, M. R., Mayer, K.: The effect of busulfan on human epithelia. Amer. J. clin. Path. **44**, 385—397 (1965).

Koss, L. G., Stewart, F. W., Foote, F. W., Jordan, M. J., Bader, G. M., Day, E.: Some histological aspects of behavior of epidermoid carcinoma *in situ* and related lesions of the uterine cervix. Cancer (Philad.) **9**, 1160—1211 (1963).

Kotcher, E., Gray, L. A., James, Q. C., Frick, C. A., Bottorff, D. W.: Cervical cell inclusion bodies and viral infections of the cervix. Ann. N.Y. Acad. Sci. **97**, 571—580 (1962).

Kotin, P., Falk, H. L., McCammon, C. J.: Experimental induction of pulmonary tumors and changes in respiratory epithelium in C 57 BL mice following their exposure to an atmosphere of ozonized gasoline. Cancer (Philad.) **11**, 473—481 (1958).

Kottmeier, H. L.: Carcinoma of the female genitalia. The Abraham Flexner Lecture Series. Number **11**. Baltimore: Williams and Wilkins 1953.

Kottmeier, H. L., Karlsstedt, K., Santesson, L., Moberger, G.: In: Cancer of the Cervix. Ciba Foundation. London: Churchill 1959.

Kraatz, H.: Farbfiltervorschaltung zur leichteren Erlernung der Kolposkopie. Zbl. Gynäk. **42**, 2307—2309 (1939).

Kramer, W. M., Kay, S.: Anaplasia clinic. Cancer (Philad.) **20**, 202—207 (1967).

Krantz, K. E., Phillips, W. P.: Anatomy of the human uterine cervix, gross and microscopic. Ann. N.Y. Acad. Sci. **97**, 551—563 (1962).

Kreyberg, L.: Über präcanceröse Gefäßveränderungen. Virchows Arch. path. Anat. **273**, 367—440 (1929).

Kury, G., Rev-Kury, L. H., Friedell, G. H.: Metabolism of human cervical tissues. A radioautographic study. Amer. J. Obstet. Gynec. **98**, 767—772 (1967).

Ladinsky, J. L., Peckham, B. M.: The kinetics of the generative compartment of the estrogen dependent vaginal epithelium. Exp. Cell Res. **40**, 447—455 (1965).

Laguens, R. P., Lagrutta, J., Koch, O. R., Francisco, Q.: Fine structure of human endocervical epithelium. Amer. J. Obstet. Gynec. **98**, 773—780 (1967).

Lamb, E. J., Fucilla, I., Greene, R. R.: Basement membranes in the female genital tract. Amer. J. Obstet. Gynec. **79**, 79—85 (1960).

Lang, W. R.: Benign cervical erosion in non-pregnant women of childbearing age. A colposcopic study. Amer. J. Obstet. Gynec. **74**, 993—999 (1957).

Langerhans, P.: Über die Nerven der menschlichen Haut. Virchows Arch. path. Anat. **44**, 325—337 (1868).

Langley, F. A.: Unpublished observations (1959).

Langvad, E., Pedersen, S. N.: LDH-isoenzyme patterns in the non-malignant and malignant uterine cervix. Cancer (Philad.) **23**, 1171—1175 (1969).

Lapan, B., Friedman, M. M.: Glycogen and reducing substances in cervical mucus. Gestational and cyclical variations. Amer. J. Obstet. Gynec. **59**, 921—923 (1950).

Lapid, L. S., Goldberger, M. A.: Exfoliative dyskaryotic cells associated with atypical cervical lesions. Amer. J. Obstet. Gynec. **61**, 1324—1328 (1951).

Latner, A. L., Turner, D. M., Way, S. A.: Enzyme and isoenzyme studies in pre-invasive carcinoma of the cervix. Lancet **1966 II**, 814—816.

Lawson, J. G.: Cancer of the Cervix. Ciba Foundation Symposium. London: Churchill 1959 (a).

Lawson, J. G.: Vaginal fluid β-glucuronidase — with special reference to cancer of the cervix. J. Obstet. Gynaec. Brit. Emp. **66**, 946—953 (1959 b).

Lawson, J. G.: Biochemical factors and cervical epithelial abnormalities. In: Dysplasia, carcinoma in situ and microinvasive carcinoma of the cervix uteri, pp. 110—123 (ed. L. A. Gray). Springfield: Thomas 1964.

Lawson, J. G., Watkins, D. K.: Vaginal fluid enzymes in relation to cervical cancer. J. Obstet. Gynaec. Brit. Cwlth. **72**, 1—8 (1965).

Leuchtenberger, C., Leuchtenberger, R., Doolin, P. F.: Correlated histological, cytological and cytochemical study of the tracheobronchial tree and lungs of mice exposed to cigarette smoke. Cancer (Philad.) **11**, 490—560 (1958).

Linhartová, A., Štafl, A.: Zur Morphologie des Ectropiums an der Portio vaginalis uteri. Arch. Gynäk. **200**, 131—141 (1964).

LINHARTOVÁ, A., ŠTAFL, A.: Morphologische Befunde an der Umwandlungszone der Portio vaginalis uteri. Arch. Gynäk. **200**, 590—600 (1965a).

LINHARTOVÁ, A., ŠTAFL, A.: Weiterer Beitrag zur Pathogenese der Felderung an der Portio vaginalis uteri. Arch. Gynäk. **200**, 678—688 (1965b).

LIPPMAN, M.: Glycosaminoglycans and cell division. In: Epithelial-mesenchymal Interactions, pp. 208—229 (eds. R. FLEISHMAJER and R. E. BILLINGHAM). Baltimore: Williams and Wilkins 1968.

LISKA, M.: Häufigkeit des Geschlechtschromatin-Vorkommens bei Karzinomen und bei Präkanzerosen portionis cervices uteri. Neoplasma (Bratisl.) **8**, 411—420 (1961).

LIU, W.: Positive smears in previously screened patients (Certain cytologic findings of public health importance). Acta cytol (Philad.) **11**, 193—198 (1967).

LOGAN, W. P. D.: Social class variation in mortality. Brit. J. prev. soc. Med. **8**, 128—137 (1954).

LOHE, K.: Vergleichende Untersuchungen zu Sitz und Ausdehnung von Dysplasien und Carcinomata in situ der Cervix. Arch. Gynäk. **207**, 470—479 (1969).

LONGNECKER, D. S., WHITE, C. A.: Trial of a simplified vaginal fluid 6-phosphogluconic dehydrogenase assay method in screening for cancer. Acta cytol. (Philad.) **11**, 202—204 (1967).

LOUIS, C. J.: A histochemical study by fluorescence technique of the epithelial tumors of the cervix and uterus. Amer. J. Obstet. Gynec. **79**, 336—345 (1960).

LUNDIN, F. E., ERICKSON, C. C., SPRUNT, D. H.: Socio-economic distribution of cervical cancer in relation to early marriage and pregnancy. Public Health Monograph 73, Dept. Health, Education and Welfare. Public Health Service. Washington 1964.

LUSTED, L. B.: Introduction to Medical Decision Making. Springfield: Thomas 1968.

MACGREGOR, J. E.: A study of clinically and cytologically detected cervical cancers in the city of Aberdeen. Acta cytol. (Philad.) **10**, 246—247 (1966).

MACGREGOR, J. E., BAIRD, D.: Detection of cervical carcinoma in the general population. Brit. med. J. **1**, 1631—1636 (1963).

MACPHERSON, I.: Reversion in hamster cells transformed by Rous sarcoma virus. Science **148**, 1731—1733 (1965).

McKAY, D. G., TERJANIAN, B., PASCHYACHIODA, D., YOUNGE, P. A., HERTIG, A. T.: Clinical and pathologic significance of anaplasia (atypical hyperplasia) of the cervix uteri. Obstet. and Gynec. **14**, 2—21 (1959).

McLAREN, H. C.: The normal menopause. J. Obstet. Gynaec. Brit. Emp. **48**, 1—40 (1941).

MAJEWSKI, A.: Die Noradrenalinprobe als neues Hilfsmittel der Kolposkopie. Geburtsh. u. Frauenheilk. **20**, 983 (1960).

MALIPHANT, R. G.: Incidence of cancer of uterine cervix. Brit. med. J. **1**, 978—982 (1949).

MANNAN, A. H. M. A., ZAMAN, H.: Effect of ovariectomy on the fate of 20-methylcholanthrene induced dysplasia of the mouse uterine cervix. Acta cytol. (Philad.) **12**, 243—250 (1968).

MAQUEO, M., AZUELA, J. C., CALDERON, J. J., GOLDZIEHER, J. W.: Morphology of the cervix in women treated with synthetic progestins. Amer. J. Obstet. Gynec. **96**, 994—998 (1966).

MARTIN, C. E.: Marital and coital factors in cervical cancer. Amer. J. publ. Hlth. **57**, 803—814 (1967).

MARTZLOFF, K. H.: Leucoplakia of the cervix uteri: a manifestation of early malignant change. Amer. J. Obstet. Gynec. **24**, 57—67 (1932).

MARTZLOFF, K. H.: Discussion to SCHEFFEY, LANG and TATARIAN. Amer. J. Obstet. Gynec. **70**, 886 (1955).

MASSON, P.: Tumeurs humaines. Paris: Librairie Malone (1956).

MATĚJKA, M.: Studien über die Histogenese der Plattenepithel-Zylinderepithelgrenze an der Portio vaginalis uteri des Menschen, unter Berücksichtigung der Bedeutung der phylogenetischen Faktoren für die Ontogenese. Anat. Anz. **112**, 426—446 (1963).

MATHER, K.: Statistical analysis in biology. London: Methuen 1943.

MATTER, R.: Histochemische Untersuchungen an der menschlichen Vaginalschleimhaut. Z. Geburtsh. Gynäk. **151**, 225—246 (1958).

MEISELS, A.: Dysplasia and carcinoma of the uterine cervix. IV. A correlated cytologic and histologic study with special emphasis on vaginal microbiology. Acta cytol. (Philad.) **13**, 224—231 (1969).

MELAMED, M. R., KOSS, L. G., FLEHINGER, B. J., KELISKY, R. P., DUBROW, H.: Prevalence rates of uterine cervical carcinoma in situ for women using the diaphragm or contraceptive oral steroids. Brit. med. J. **3**, 195—200 (1969).

MELCZER, N., HAMAR, M.: The repeated isolation of an altered adenovirus type 3 from uterine fibromyomas. Oncologia (Basel) 19, 401—416 (1965).

MESSELT, D. T.: Diagnosis of cancer in the female genital organs by smears. Acta obstet. gynec. scand. 34, 345—365 (1955).

MESTWERDT, G.: Atlas der Kolposkopie. 2nd Edition. Jena: Fischer 1953.

MESTWERDT, G., WESPI, H. J.: Atlas der Kolposkopie. 3. Aufl. Stuttgart: Fischer 1961.

MEYER, J., MEDAK, H.: Keratinization of the oral mucosa. In: Fundamentals of Keratinization. No. 70, p. 81, (ed. E O. BUTCHER and R. F. SOGMAS). Washington: Amer. Ass. Advanc. Sci. 1961.

MEYER, J. S., DONALDSON, R. C.: Growth kinetics of squamous cell carcinoma in man. Arch. Path. 87, 479—490 (1969).

MEYER, R.: Die Epithelentwicklung der Cervix und Portio vaginalis uteri und die Pseudoerosio Congenita. Arch. Gynäk. 91, 579—598 (1910a).

MEYER, R.: Der Erosion und Pseudoerosion der Erwachsenen. Arch. Gynäk. 91, 658—691 (1910b).

MEYER, R. K., ALLEN, W. H.: Production of mucification of vaginal epithelium in rodents by oestrogenic hormone. Science 75, 111—112 (1932).

MILLER, E. M., VON HAAM, E.: Comparison of vaginal aspiration and cervical scraping technics in the screening process for uterine cancer. Acta cytol. (Philad.) 5, 214—216 (1961).

MISHIMA, Y., PINKUS, H.: Electron microscopy of keratin layer stripped human epidermis. J. invest. Derm. 50, 89—107 (1968).

MORGAN, H., BALDUZZI, P. C.: Isolation of cytomegalovirus from tissues of condyloma acuminatum. Amer. J. clin. Path. 47, 734—737 (1967).

MORI, M., MIYAJI, T., MURATA, I., MURAKAMI, M.: Histochemical observations of alpha-glycero-phosphate dehydrogenase activity in human tumors. Cancer Res. 23, 1685—1688 (1963).

MORICARD, R., CARTIER, R.: Topographie orificielle des dystrophies et de l'épithélioma intra-épithélial du col utérin. Bull. Féd. Soc. Gynéc. Obstet. franç. 8, 314—339 (1956).

MORICARD, R., CARTIER, R.: Chromosomal and cytoplasmic cytopathology of intra-epithelial squamous-cell epithelioma of the cervix uteri (optical and electron microscopy). In: Cancer of the Cervix. Ciba Foundation, p. 28. London: Churchill 1959.

MORICARD, R., CARTIER, R.: Chromosomal and fine structures, cytopathology. In: Dysplasia, carcinoma in situ and micro-invasive carcinoma of the cervix uteri, pp. 124—175 (ed. L. A. GRAY). Springfield: Thomas 1964.

MORICARD, R., HINGLAIS-GUILLAUD, N., CARTIER, R.: Cytologie comparée en microscopie optique et électronique de l'épithélium pavimenteux cervical normal et pathologique. Gynéc. et Obstét. 57, 453—489 (1958).

MORICARD, R., PAPATHEODOROU, B.: Les anomalies de nombre et de position des chromosomes comme nouvelle méthode de diagnostic des épithéliomas intra-épithéliaux pavimenteux du col utérine en dehors de la gestation. Gynéc. et Obstét. 55, 251—257 (1953).

MOUKHTAR, M., HIGGINS, G.: The early diagnosis of carcinoma of the female genital tract. Part I. 6-phosphogluconate dehydrogenase activity and carcinoma of the female genital tract. J. Obstet. Gynaec. Brit. Cwlth. 72, 677—690 (1965).

MUEENUDDIN, G., ZAMAN, H.: Effect of ovariectomy on the induction by 20-methylcholanthrene of carcinoma of the mouse uterine cervix. Acta cytol. (Philad.) 11, 205—210 (1967).

MUIR, G. G., CANTI, G., WILLIAMS, D.: Use of 6-phosphogluconate dehydrogenase as a screen test for cervical carcinoma in normal women. Brit. med. J. 2, 1563—1565 (1964).

MUIR, G. G., VALTERIS, G.: Vaginal fluid enzyme patterns in benign and malignant lesions of the female genital tract. J. clin. Path. 22, 593—597 (1969).

MURPHY, E. D.: Studies on carcinogen-induced carcinoma of the cervix in mice. Amer. J. Path. (Abstract) 29, 608 (1953).

MUSSEY, E., SOULE, E. H., WELCH, J. S.: Microinvasive carcinoma of the cervix. Amer. J. Obstet. Gynec. 104, 738—744 (1969).

NAHMIAS, A. J., DOWDLE, W. R.: Antigenic and biologic differences in herpesvirus hominis. Progr. med. Virol. 10, 110—159 (1968).

NAHMIAS, A. J., JOSEY, W. E., NAIB, Z. M., LUCE, C. F., DUFFREY, A.: Antibodies to *Herpesvirus hominis* types 1 and 2 in humans. II. Women with cervical cancer. Amer. J. Epidem. 91, 539—546 (1970).

NAIB, Z. M.: Exfoliative cytology of viral cervico-vaginitis. Acta cytol (Philad.) 10, 126—129 (1966).

NAIB, Z. H., NAHMIAS, A. J., JOSEY, W. E.: Cytology and histopathology of herpes simplex infection. Cancer (Philad.) 19, 1026—1031 (1966).

NAUJOKS, H.: Sex chromatin in exfoliated cells of cervical carcinoma in situ. Acta cytol. (Philad.) 13, 634—636 (1969).

NAVRATIL, E.: Colposcopy. In: Dysplasia, Carcinoma in Situ and Micro-invasive Carcinoma of the Cervix, pp. 228—283, (ed. L. A. GRAY). Springfield: Thomas 1964.

NAVRATIL, E., BURGHARDT, E., BAJARDI, F., NASH, W.: Simultaneous colposcopy and cytology used in screening for carcinoma of the cervix. Amer. J. Obstet. Gynec. 75, 1292—1297 (1958).

NERDRUM, H. J.: The activity of 6-phosphogluconic acid dehydrogenase in vaginal secretions. A comparative study of the activity in women with and without gynaecological cancer. Scand. J. clin. Lab. Invest. 16, 563—569 (1964).

NESBITT, R. E. L., Jr., HELLMAN, L. M.: The histopathology and cytology of the cervix in pregnancy. Surg. Gynec. Obstet. 94, 10—20 (1952).

NICHOLS, T. M., BOYES, D. A., FIDLER, H. K.: Advantages of routine step serial sectioning of cervical cone biopsies. Amer. J. clin. Path. 49, 342—346 (1968).

NICHOLSON, G. W., Sebaceous glands in the cervix uteri. J. Path. Bact. 22, 252—254 (1919).

NIEBURGS, H.: Detection of cancer in the cervix uteri. Use of new method of cell collection. Obstet. and Gynec. 7, 10 (1956).

NIEBURGS, H. E., STERGUS, I., STEPHENSON, E. M., HARBIN, B. L.: Mass screening of the total female population of a county for cervical carcinoma. J. Amer. med. Ass. 164, 1546—1551 (1957).

NIELSEN, A., CLEMMESEN, J.: Twin studies in the Danish cancer registry. Brit. J. Cancer 11, 327—336 (1957).

NG, A. B. P., REAGAN J. E. Micro-invasive carcinoma of the uterine cervix. Amer. J. clin. Path. 52, 511—529 (1969).

NG, A. B., REAGAN, J. W., LINDNER, E.: The cellular manifestations of primary and recurrent herpes genitalis. Acta cytol. 14, (Philad.) 124—129 (1970).

NORTH WEST OF ENGLAND: Collaborative Study. Cytomegalovirus infection in the North West of England. Arch. Dis. Childh. 45, 513—522 (1970).

NOZAKA, K., SIMPSON, W. L.: Mast cells in the human pylorus and cervix. Anat. Rec. 142, 263 (1962).

OBER, K. G., BONTKE, E.: Sitz und Ausdehnung des Carcinoma in situ. Arch. Gynäk. 192, 55—68 (1959).

ODLAND, G. F.: The fine structure of the interrelationship of cells in the human epidermis. J. biophys. biochem. Cytol. 4, 527—539 (1958).

ODLAND, G. F.: Tonofilaments and keratohyalin. In: The Epidermis, pp. 237—250, (ed. W. MONTAGNA and W. C. LOBITZ). New York and London: Academic Press 1964.

OETTLÉ, A. G.: Malignant neoplasms of the uterus in the white, "coloured", Indian and Bantu races of the Union of South Africa. Acta Un. int. Cancr. 17, 915—933 (1961).

OLD, J. W., WIELENGA, G., VON HAAM, E.: Squamous carcinoma in situ of the uterine cervix. I. Classification and histogenesis. Cancer (Philad.) 18, 1598—1612 (1965).

OLSON, A. W., NICHOLS, E. E.: Colposcopic examination in a combined approach for early diagnosis and prevention of carcinoma of the cervix. Obstet. and Gynec. 15, 372—381 (1960).

OLSON, A. W., NICHOLS, E. E.: Leukoplakia of the cervix, the mosaic and papillary pattern. Amer. J. Obstet. Gynec. 82, 895—902 (1961).

ORTIZ, R., NEWTON, M., LANGLOIS, P. L.: Colposcopic biopsy in the diagnosis of carcinoma of the cervix. Obstet. and Gynec. 34, 303—306 (1969).

OSTERGARD, D. R., GONDOS, B.: The incidence of false negative cervical cytology as determined by colposcopically directed biopsies. Acta cytol. (Philad.) 15, 292—293 (1971).

OVERHOLZER, M. D., ALLEN, E.: Atypical growth induced in cervical epithelium of monkey by prolonged injection of ovarian hormone combined with chronic trauma. Surg. Gynec. Obstet. 60, 129—136 (1935).

PAPANICOLAOU, G. N.: The sexual cycle in the human female as revealed by vaginal smears. Amer. J. Anat. 52 (Supp), 519—637 (1933).

PAPANICOLAOU, G. N., TRAUT, H. E., MARCHETTI, A. A.: The epithelium of woman's reproductive organs. New York: Commonwealth Fund 1948.

PARK, I. J., JONES, H. W.: Glucose-6-phosphate dehydrogenase and the histogenesis of epidermoid carcinoma of the cervix. Amer. J. Obstet. Gynec. 102, 106—109 (1968).

PARK, H. Y., KOPROWSKA, I.: A comparative *in vitro* and *in vivo* study of induced cervical lesions in mice. Cancer Res. **28**, 1478—1489 (1968).

PARKER, J. D., BANATVALA, J. E.: Herpes genitalis; clinical and virological studies. Brit. J. vener. Dis. **43**, 212—216 (1967).

PARMENTIER, R., DUSTIN, P.: On the mechanism of mitotic abnormalities induced by hydroquinone in animal tissues. Rev. belge Path. **23**, 20—30 (1954).

PATTEN, S. F.: Dysplasia of the uterine cervix. In: New Concepts in Gynecologic Oncology, pp. 33—44, (ed. G. C. LEWIS, W. B. WENTZ and R. M. JAFFE). Philadelphia: Davis 1966.

PATTEN, S. F.: Diagnostic cytology of the uterine cervix. Basel: Karger 1969.

PATTEN, S. F., HUGHES, C. P., REAGAN, J. W.: An experimental study of the relationship between *Trichomonas vaginalis* and dysplasia of the uterine cervix. Acta cytol. (Philad.) **7**, 187—190 (1963).

PAYLING WRIGHT, G.: Introduction to Pathology. London: Longman, Green & Co. 1950.

PAYNE, E. A.: Free Churchmen, unrepentant and repentant. pp. 30—45. London: Carey Kingsgate Press 1965.

PEARSE, A. G. E.: Histochemistry. 3rd Edition. London: Churchill 1968.

PEDERSEN, S. N.: Respiration and glycolysis in malignant and non-malignant tissue of the human cervix uteri. Acta obstet. gynec. scand. **47**, 469—481 (1968).

PEMBERTON, F. A., SMITH, G. V. S.: The early diagnosis and prevention of carcinoma of the cervix. A clinical pathologic study of borderline cases treated at the Free Hospital for Women. Amer. J. Obstet. Gynec. **17**, 168—176 (1929).

PETERS, H.: Cytologic smears from the mouth. Cellular changes in diseases and after irradiation. Amer. J. clin. Path. **29**, 219—225 (1958).

PETERSON, O.: Precancerous changes of the cervical epithelium, in relation to manifest cervical carcinoma. Acta radiol. (Stockh.) **127**, 1—168 (1955).

PETRY, G., OVERBECK, L., VOGEL, W.: Vergleichende elektronen- und lichtmikroskopische Untersuchungen am Vaginalepithel in Schwangerschaft. Z. Zellforsch. **54**, 382—401 (1961).

PIERCE, G. B.: The development of basement membranes in the mouse embryo. Develop. Biol. **13**, 231—249 (1966).

PIERCE, G. B., BEALS, T. F., RAM, J. S., MIDGELY, A. R.: Basement membranes. IV. Epithelial origin and immunologic cross reactions. Amer. J. Path. **45**, 929—961 (1964).

PICK, J.: Über ein Mikroskop zur Lebenduntersuchung der ungefärbten und vitalgefärbten Schleimhaut menschlicher Körperhöhlen. Wien. klin. Wschr. **50**, 1449—1451 (1937).

PINCUS, G.: Some effects of progesterone and related compounds upon reproduction and early development in mammals. Acta Endocr. **28**, Suppl. 28, 18—36 (1956).

PINCUS, G.: In discussion in: R. W. WISSLER, T. L. DAO and S. WOOD, Endogenous factors influencing host-tumor balance. pp. 137—146. Chicago: Chicago University Press 1967.

PIXLEY, E.: See M. COPPLESON (1969) and M. COPPLESON and B. L. REID. Preclinical carcinoma of the cervix uteri. London: Pergamon 1967.

PLAUT, A., KOHN-SPEYER, A. C.: The carcinogenic action of smegma. Science **105**, 391—392 (1947.

POLAK, M.: Transformación de la "barrera epithelial argentófilia" de la mucosa exocervical en capa melanoblástica (Nota previa). Soc. argent. Anat. norm. pat. Buenos Aires (1949).

PRATT THOMAS, H. R., HEINS, H. C., LATHAM, E., DENNIS, E. J., McIVER, F. A.: The carcinogenic effect of human smegma: An experimental study. Cancer (Philad.) **9**, 671—680 (1956).

PRZYBORA, L. A.: Varieties of carcinogenesis. Oncologia (Basel) **20**, 39—53 (1966).

PRZYBORA, L. A., PLUTOWA, A.: Histological topography of carcinoma *in situ* of the cervix uteri. Cancer (Philad.) **12**, 263—277 (1959).

PUNDEL, J. P.: Les frottis vaginaux endocriniens. Paris: Masson 1952.

PUNDEL, J. P.: The so-called diastase-resistant PAS-positive material in the human vaginal epithelium. A cyto- and histochemical study. Acta cytol. (Philad.) **10**, 428—439 (1966).

PUNDEL, J. P., MOITZHEIM, P., BECKIUS, C.: La membrane basale de l'épithélium pavimenteux du vagin et du col utérin. Étude comparative histologique et histochimique. Gynéc. Obstét. (Paris) **66**, 125—143 (1967).

RAURAMO, L.: The significance of β-glucuronidase content in the vaginal fluid of patients with cancer of the uterus. J. clin. Invest. **11**, 285—289 (1959).

RAWLS, W. E., TOMPKINS, W. A. F., FIGUEROA, M. E., MELNICK, J. L.: Herpesvirus Type 2. Association with carcinoma of the cervix. Science **161**, 1255—1256 (1968).

RAWLS, W. E., TOMPKINS, W. A. F., MELNICK, J. L.: The association of herpesvirus Type 2 and carcinoma of the uterine cervix. Amer. J. Epidem. 89, 547—554 (1969).

REAGAN, J. W.: In: Dysplasia, Carcinoma in-situ and micro-invasive Carcinoma, Chapter 12 (ed. L. A. GRAY). Springfield: Thomas 1964.

REAGAN, J. W., BELL, B. A., NEUMAN, J. L., SCOTT, R. B., PATTEN, S. F.: Dysplasia in the uterine cervix during pregnancy: An analytical study of the cells. Acta cytol. (Philad.) 5, 17—29 (1961).

REAGAN, J. W., HARMONIC, M. J.: The cellular pathology of carcinoma *in situ*. A cytohistopathological correlation. Cancer (Philad.) 9, 385 (1956a).

REAGAN, J. W., HARMONIC, M. J.: Dysplasia of the uterine cervix. Ann. N.Y. Acad. Sci. 63, 1236—1244 (1956b).

REAGAN, J. W., HICKS, D. J.: A study of *in situ* and squamous cell cancer of the uterine cervix. Cancer (Philad.) 6, 1200—1214 (1953).

REAGAN, J. W., HICKS, J. D., SCOTT, R. B.: Atypical hyperplasia of the uterine cervix. Cancer (Philad.) 8, 42—52 (1955).

REAGAN, J. W., PATTEN, S. F.: Dysplasia: a basic reaction to injury in the uterine cervix. Ann. N.Y. Acad. Sci. 97, 662—682 (1962).

REAGAN, J. W., SEIDEMANN, I. B., PATTEN, S. F.: Developmental stages of *in situ* carcinoma of the uterine cervix: An analytical study of the cells. Acta cytol. (Philad.) 6, 538—546 (1962).

REAGAN, J. W., SEIDEMAN, I. L., SARACUSA, Y.: The cellular morphology of carcinoma *in situ* and dysplasia or atypical hyperplasia of the uterine cervix. Cancer (Philad.) 6, 224—235 (1953).

REAGAN, J. W., WENTZ, W. B.: Changes in the mouse cervix antedating induced cancer. Cancer (Philad.) 12, 389—395 (1959).

REDDY, D. G., BARUAH, I. K.: Carcinogenic action of human smegma. Arch. Path. 75, 414—420 (1963).

REID, B. L.: H³ thymidine incorporation studies in human uterine cervix epithelium. Med. Res. 1, 49 (1962).

REID, B. L.: Autoradiographic analysis of uptake of tritiated thymidine and S³⁵ cystine by cultured human cervical explants undergoing metaplasia. J. nat. Cancer Inst. 32, 1059—1073 (1964a).

REID, B. L.: The behaviour of human sperm toward cultured fragments of human cervix uteri. Lancet 1964 Ib, 21—23.

REID, B. L.: Interaction between homologous sperm and somatic cells of the uterus and peritoneum in the mouse. Exp. Cell Res. 40, 679—683 (1965a).

REID, B. L.: Cancer of the cervix uteri: review of causal factors with an hypothesis as to its origin. Med. J. Aust. 1, 375—383 (1965b).

REID, B. L.: The fate of nucleic acid of sperm phaged by regenerating cells. Aust. N.Z. J. Obstet. Gynaec. 6, 30—34 (1966).

REID, B. L., COPPLESON, M.: Autoradiographische Untersuchungen an normalem und atypischem Plattenepithel der menschlichen Cervix und Vagina. Arch. Gynäk. 200, 172—179 (1964).

REID, B. L., SINGER, A., COPPLESON, M.: The process of cervical regeneration after electrocauterization. II. Histochemical, autoradiographic and pH study. Aust. N. Z. J. Obstet. Gynaec. 7, 125—143 (1967).

RIBBERT, H.: Über das Gefäßsystem und die Heilbarkeit der Geschwültse. Dtsch. med. Wschr. 30, 801—803 (1904).

RICHART, R. M.: A radioautographic analysis of cellular proliferation in dysplasia and carcinoma in situ of the uterine cervix. Amer. J. Obstet. Gynec. 86, 925—930 (1963).

RICHART, R. M.: Evaluation of the true false negative rate in cytology. Amer. J. Obstet. Gynec. 89, 723—726 (1964).

RICHART, R. M.: Colpomicroscopic studies of the distribution of dysplasia and carcinoma in situ on the exposed portion of the human uterine cervix. Cancer (Philad.) 18, 950—954 (1965).

RICHART, R. M.: Colpomicroscopic studies of cervical intraepithelial neoplasia. Cancer (Philad.) 19, 395—405 (1966).

RICHART, R. M.: The natural history of cervical intraepithelial neoplasia. Clin. Obstet. Gynec. 10, 748—784 (1967).

RICHART, R. M.: A theory of cervical carcinogenesis. Obstet. Gynec. Surv. 24, 874—879 (1969).

RICHART, R. M., BARRON, B. A.: The intrauterine device and cervical neoplasia. A prospective study of patients with cervical dysplasia. J. Amer. med. Ass. 199, 817—819 (1967).

RICHART, R. M., BARRON, B. A.: A follow-up study of patients with cervical dysplasia. Amer. J. Obstet. Gynec. **105**, 386—393 (1969).

RICHART, R. M., CORFMAN, P. A.: Chromosome number and morphology of a human pre-invasive neoplasm. Science **144**, 65—67 (1964).

RICHART, R. M., SCIARRA, J. J.: Treatment of cervical dysplasia by out-patient electrocauterization. Obstet. and Gynec. **101**, 200—205 (1968).

RICHART, R. M., VAILLANT, H. W.: The irrigation smear: false negative rates in a population with cervical neoplasia. J. Amer. med. Ass. **192**, 199—202 (1965).

RICHART, R. M., WILBANKS, G. D.: The chromosomes of human intraepithelial neoplasia. Cancer Res. **26**, 60—74 (1966).

RIES, E.: Erosion, leukoplakia and the colposcope in relation to carcinoma of the cervix. Amer. J. Obstet. Gynec. **23**, 393—399 (1932).

RITCHIE, A. C., SAFFOITTI, V.: Orally administered 2-acetylaminofluorene as initiator and as promoter in epidermal carcinogenesis in mouse. Cancer Res. **15**, 84—88 (1955).

ROBERTS, G. P., GUPTA, S. K.: Use of galactose oxidase in the histochemical examination of mucus-secreting cells. Nature (Lond.) **207**, 425—426 (1965).

ROCKEY, E. E., KUSCHNER, M., KOSAK, A. L., MAYER, E.: Effect of tobacco tar on the bronchial mucosa of dogs. Cancer (Philad.) **11**, 466—472 (1958).

RØJEL, J.: Interrelation between uterine cancer and syphilis. Acta path. microbiol. scand. Suppl. **97**, (1953).

ROSA, C. G., VELARDO, J. T.: Histochemical localization of vaginal oxidative enzymes and mucins in rats treated with estradiol and progesterone. Ann. N.Y. Acad. Sci. **83**, 122—144 (1959).

ROSENTHAL, A. H., HELLMAN, L. M.: Epithelial changes in the fetal cervix, including the role of "reserve cells". Amer. J. Obstet. Gynec. **64**, 260—270 (1952).

ROSS, M. H., GRANT, L.: On the structural integrity of basement membranes. Exp. Cell Res. **50**, 277—285 (1968).

ROTKIN, I. D.: Relation of adolescent coitus to cervical cancer risk. J. Amer. med. Ass. **179**, 486—491 (1962).

ROTKIN, I. D.: Sexual characteristics of a cervical cancer population. Amer. J. publ. Hlth. **57**, 815—829 (1967).

ROY, S., WOLMAN, L.: Electron microscopic observations on the virus particles in herpes simplex encephalitis. J. clin. Path. **22**, 51—59 (1969).

ROYSTON, I., AURELIAN, L.: The association of genital herpesvirus with cervical atypia and carcinoma in situ. Amer. J. Epidem. **91**, 531—538 (1970).

RUBIN, I. C.: Pathological diagnosis of incipient carcinoma of uterus. Amer. J. Obstet. Gynec. **62**, 668—676 (1910).

RYAN, G. M., CRAIG, J., REID, D. E.: Histology of the uterus and ovaries after long-term cyclic norethynodrel therapy. Amer. J. Obstet. Gynec. **90**, 715—725 (1964).

SAGIROGLU, N.: Progression and regression studies of precancer (anaplastic or dysplastic) cells, and the halo test. Amer. J. Obstet. Gynec. **85**, 454—469 (1963).

SALERNO, E. V.: La "barrera epitelial argentofilia" de Polak en la vagina de la mujer durante et ciclo genital normal. Obstet. Ginec. lat.-amer. **2**, 913—926 (1944).

SANDRITTER, W.: Ultraviolettmikrospectrophotometrische Untersuchungen an Plattenepithel. Frankfurt. Z. Path. **64**, 520—530 (1953).

SANDRITTER, W.: Cytophotometrische Untersuchungen am Portiocarcinom und seinen Vorstufen. Verh. dtsch. Ges. Path. **48**, 34—43 (1964).

SANDRITTER, W., CARL, M., RITTER, W.: Cytophotometric measurements of the DNA content of human malignant tumor cells by means of the Feulgen reaction. Acta cytol. (Philad.) **10**, 26—30 (1966).

SANI, G.: Studio istochimico dei mucopolisaccharidi nella vagina in condizionzi normali e sperimentali. Rev. Ital. Gineologia **34**, 473—504 (1953).

SAPHIR, O., LEVENTHAL, M. L., KLINE, T. S.: Podophyllin-induced dysplasia of the cervix uteri. Amer. J. clin. Path. **32**, 446—456 (1959).

SCHADE, R. O. K., SWINNEY, J.: Pre-cancerous changes in the bladder epithelium. Lancet **1968 II**, 943—946.

SCHAUENSTEIN, W.: Histologische Untersuchungen über atypisches Plattenepithel an der Portio und an der Innenfläche der Cervix uteri. Arch. Gynäk. **85**, 576—616 (1908).

Scheffey, L. C., Lang, W. R., Tatarian, G.: An experimental program with colposcopy. Amer. J. Obstet. Gynec. **70**, 876—886 (1955).

Schellhas, H. F.: Cell renewal in the human cervix uteri. Amer. J. Obstet. Gynec. **104**, 617—632 (1969).

Schmidt, W. J.: Die Bausteine des Tierkörpers. Bonn: Cohen 1924. Quoted by G. F. Odland (1964).

Schottlaender, J., Kermauner, F.: Zur Kenntnis des Uteruskarzinoms; monographische Studie über Morphologie, Entwicklung, Wachstum, nebst Beiträgen zur Klinik der Erkrankung. Berlin: Karger 1912.

Schröder, R.: Ergebnisse scheidenbiologischer Forschungen. Arch. Gynäk. **125**, 403—406 (1925).

Schröder, R.: Die weiblichen Genitalorgane. In: Handbuch der mikroscopischen Anatomie des Menschen, Vol. 7, Part 1. (Ed. W. U. Möllendorff). Berlin: Springer 1930.

Scott, R. B.: Problems in the diagnosis of cervical lesions. In: New Concepts in Gynecologic Oncology, pp. 91—101 (ed. G. C. Lewis, W. B. Wentz and R. M. Jaffe). Philadelphia: Davis 1966.

Scott, R. B., Ballard, L. A.: Problems of cervical biopsy. Ann. N.Y. Acad. Sci. **97**, 767—781 (1962).

Scott, R. B., Brown, A. M., Reagan, J. W.: Comparative results of the routine Papanicolaou and Draghi tampon cytologic studies in atypical hyperplasia of the cervix and uterine cancer. Amer. J. Obstet. Gynec. **73**, 349—353 (1957).

Selye, H.: The mast cell. Washington: Butterworths 1965.

She, M. P., Cheng, F. L., Liu, T. H., T'Sai, H. Y., Liu, C. M., Wu, E. R.: Cancer Research, Shanghai: Shanghai Scientific and Technical Publishers 1962. Quoted by Boyd and Doll (1964).

Shingleton, H. M., Richart, R. M., Wiener, J., Spiro, D.: Human cervical intraepithelial neoplasia: fine structure of dysplasia and carcinoma in-situ. Cancer Res. **28**, 695—706 (1968).

Siegel, P.: Histochemische Untersuchungen an den Schleimstoffen der Cervix uteri. Z. Geburtsh. Gynäk. **167**, 1967.

Siegler, E. E.: Microdiagnosis of carcinoma *in situ* of the uterine cervix. A comparative study of pathologists' diagnoses. Cancer (Philad.) **9**, 463—469 (1956).

Simeckova, A., Lonser, E., Nichols, E. E., Rubinstein, I. N.: Chronic trichomoniasis and cervical cancer. Obstet. and Gynec. **20**, 410—412 (1962).

Simon, T. R., Sheehan, J. F.: Reversible atypia of cervical epithelium. Proc. 1st Int. Congr. Exfol. Cytol., pp. 116—120. Philadelphia: Lippincott 1961.

Sjorgren, H. O., Hellstron, I., Klein, G.: Transplantation of polyoma induced tumours in mice. Cancer Res. **21**, 329—337 (1961).

Sjövall, A.: Untersuchungen über die Schleimhaut der Cervix Uteri. Acta obstet. gynec. scand. **18**, Suppl. 4 (1938).

Skinner, G. R. B., Thouless, M. E., Jordan, J. A.: Antibodies to Type 1 and Type 2 herpes virus in women with abnormal cervical cytology. J. Obstet. Gynaec. Brit. Cwlth. **78**, 1031—1038 (1971).

Slate, T. A.: Symposium on cancer cytology during pregnancy. Acta cytol. (Philad.) **3**, 29—31 (1959).

Slate, T. A., Martin, P. L., Merritt, J. W.: Pathological detection of uterine cancer in private obstetrical and gynecological practice. Amer. J. Obstet. Gynec. **66**, 878—890 (1953).

Slate, T. A., Merritt, J. W.: The behavior of cervical atypia and carcinoma *in situ* in pregnancy. A study of 120 patients. Proc. 1st Int. Congr. Exfol. Cytol., pp. 128—132. Philadelphia: Lippincott 1961.

Slavin, H. B., Gavett, E.: Primary herpetic vulvovaginitis. Proc. Soc. exp. Biol. (N.Y.) **63**, 343—345 (1946).

Smith, J. W., Townsend, D. E., Sparkes, R. S.: Genetic variants of glucose-6-phosphate dehydrogenase in the study of carcinoma of the cervix. Cancer (Philad.) **28**, 529—532 (1971).

Song, J.: The human uterus: morphogenesis and embryological basis for cancer. Springfield: Thomas 1964.

Song, Y. S., Fanger, H., Murphy, T. H.: Significance of performing dual smear examinations in a mass screening survey for uterine cancer. Amer. J. Obstet. Gynec. **78**, 1309—1311 (1959).

Spriggs, A. I., Boddington, M. M., Clarke, C. M.: Carcinoma *in situ* of the cervix uteri. Some cytogenetic observations. Lancet **1962 I**, 1383—1384.

Štafl, A., Dohnal, V., Linhartová, A.: Über kolposkopische, histologische und Gefäßbefunde an der krankhaft veränderten Portio. Geburtsh. Frauenheilk. **23**, 438—445 (1963).

Štafl, A., Linhartová, A., Dohnal, V.: Das kolposkopische Bild der Felderung und seine Pathogenese. Arch. Gynäk. **199**, 223—242 (1963).

Stanton, M. F., Stewart, S. E., Eddy, B. E., Blackwell, R. H.: Oncogenic effect of tissue-culture preparations of polyoma virus on fetal mice. J. nat. Cancer. Inst. **23**, 1441—1475 (1959).

Stemshorn, W.: Zur Frage des menstruellen Zyklus der menschlichen Vaginalschleimhaut. Zbl. Gynäk. **52**, 2387—2392 (1928).

Stern, E.: Epidemiology of dysplasia. Obstet. gynec. Surv. **24**, 711—723 (1969).

Stern, E., Dixon, W. J.: Cancer of the cervix — a biometric approach to etiology. Cancer (Philad.) **14**, 153—160 (1961).

Stern, E., Lachenbruch, P. A., Dixon, W. J.: Cancer of the uterine cervix. II. A biometric approach to etiology. Cancer (Philad.) **20**, 190—201 (1967).

Stern, E., Longo, L. D.: Identification of herpes simplex virus in a case showing cytological features of viral vaginitis. Acta cytol. (Philad.) **7**, 295—299 (1963).

Stern, E., Neely, P. M.: Carcinoma and dysplasia of the cervix: a comparison of rates for new and returning populations. Acta cytol. (Philad.) **7**, 357—361 (1963).

Stewart, F. W.: Factors influencing curability of cancer. In: Proceedings of the Third National Cancer Conference, pp. 62—73. Philadelphia: Lippincott 1957.

Stoker, M.: New growth and viruses. Brit. med. J. **3**, 541—545 (1970).

Strauss, M. J., Bunting, H., Melnick, J. L.: Eosinophilic inclusion bodies and cytoplasmic masses in verrucae. J. invest. Derm. **17**, 209—211 (1951).

Sugihara, S.: The morphological study of blood vessels in cervical carcinoma. Acta Med. Okayama **12**, 261—280 (1958).

Sutcliffe, R. G., Emery, A. E.: Lactate dehydrogenase isoenzymes in carcinoma of the cervix. Manchester Med. Gaz. **47**, 22 —23 (1968).

Tavares, A. S.: Sex chromatin in tumor cells. Acta cytol. (Philad.) **6**, 90—94 (1962).

Taylor, C. W.: In: Symposium on malignant cervical lesions. Acta cytol. (Philad.) **5**, 358 (1961).

Taylor, H. B., Irey, N. S., Norris, H. J.: Atypical endocervical hyperplasia in women taking oral contraceptives. J. Amer. med. Ass. **202**, 637—639 (1967).

Teplitz, R. L., Valco, Z., Rundall, T.: Comparative sequential cytologic changes following in vitro infection with herpesvirus Type I and II. Acta cytol. (Philad.) **15**, 455—459 (1971).

Terris, M.: Epidemiology of cervical cancer. Ann. N.Y. Acad. Sci. **97**, 808—813 (1962).

Terris, M., Wilson, F., Smith, H., Sprung, E., Nelson, J. H.: The relationship of coitus to carcinoma of the cervix. Amer. J. publ. Hlth. **57**, 840—846 (1967).

Thiele, J.: Zellkernmorphologische Geschlechtserkennung am Portiokarzinom und an der Adenomyomatose der Prostata. Zbl. Path. **110**, 363—366 (1967).

Thiersch, C.: Der Epithelialkrebs namentlich der Haut. Leipzig: Engelmann 1865.

Thiery, M., Willighagen, R. G.: Enzyme histochemistry of induced and transplanted squamous cell carcinoma of the uterine cervix. Brit. J. Cancer **13**, 582—591 (1964).

Thiery, M., Willighagen, R. G.: Enzyme histochemistry of squamous carcinoma of the uterine cervix. Amer. J. Obstet. Gynec. **95**, 1059—1067 (1966).

Thorarinsson, A., Jensson, O., Bjarnason, O.: Screening for uterine cancer in Iceland. Acta cytol. (Philad.) **13**, 304—308 (1969).

Timonen, S.: Prophase index in the diagnosis of gynaecological cancer. Ann. Chir. Gynaec. Fenn. **4**, 222—233 (1955).

Tjio, J. H., Puck, T. T.: The somatic chromosomes of man. Proc. nat. Acad. Sci. (Wash.) **44**, 1229—1237 (1958).

Topkins, P.: The histological appearance of the endocervix during the menstrual cycle. Amer. J. Obstet. Gynec. **58**, 654—665 (1949).

Towne, J. E.: Carcinoma of the cervix in nulliparous and celibate women. Amer. J. Obstet. Gynec. **69**, 606—613 (1955).

Townsend, D. E., Ostergard, D. R.: Cryocauterization for preinvasive cervical neoplasia. J. Reproductive Medicine **6**, 4 (1971).

Townsend, D. E., Ostergard, D. R., Mishell, D. R., Hirose, F. M.: Abnormal Papanicolaou smears evaluated by colposcopy, biopsies and endocervical curettage. Amer. J. Obstet. Gynec. **108**, 429 —434 (1970).

TRAUT, H. F., BLOCH, P. W., KUDER, A.: Cyclical changes in the human vaginal mucosa. Surg.
    Gynec. Obstet. 63, 7—15 (1936).
TREBBIN, H.: Die Häufigkeit der Barrschen Zellkernkörper bei Karzinomen der weiblichen Genitale.
    Geburtsh. u. Frauenheilk. 28, 193—197 (1968).
TURNER, D. M.: Proc. Ass. clin. Biochem. 111, 14 (1964). Quoted by LATNER et al. (1966).
TWEEDALE, D. N., RODDICK, J. W.: Histologic types of squamous cell carcinoma in situ of the cervix.
    Obstet. and Gynec. 33, 35—40 (1969).
ULLERY, J. C., VON HAAM, E., MILLER, E.: Early diagnosis and treatment in a cancer survey program.
    Obstet. and Gynec. 10, 371—377 (1957).
UYEDA, C. K., DAVIS, H. J., JONES, H. W., Jr.: Nuclear protrusions and giant chromosome anomalies
    in cervical neoplasia. Acta cytol. (Philad.) 10, 331—334 (1966).
VALERI, V., CRUZ, A. R., BRANDÃO, H. J., LISON, L.: Relationship between cell nuclear volume and
    deoxyribonucleic acid of cells of normal epithelium of carcinoma in situ and of invasive carcinoma
    of the uterine cervix. Acta cytol. (Philad.) 11, 488—496 (1967).
VAN NIEKERK, W. A.: Cervical cytological abnormalities caused by folic acid deficiency. Acta cytol.
    (Philad.) 10, 67—73 (1966).
VANTSA, N., BEVERIDGE, G. C., FORAKER, A. G.: The uterine cervix at term: Glycogen, mast
    cells and connective tissue elements: Obstet. and Gynec. 22, 108—114 (1963).
VELLIOS, F., GRIFFIN, J.: The pathogenesis of dimethylbenanthracene induced carcinoma of the
    cervix of rats. Cancer Res. 17, 364—366 (1957).
VENDRELY, C., VENDRELY, R.: Localisation de l'acide ribonucléique dans les différents tissus et
    organes de vertébrés. In: Handbuch der Histochemie, Vol. III, Nucleoproteids. Stuttgart:
    Gustav Fischer 1959
VILLASANTA, U.: Malignant potential of cervical dysplasia. Sth. med. J. (Bgham, Ala.) 61, 1018—1022
    (1968).
VON HAAM, E.: Animal experiments. In: Symposium on premalignant cervical lesions. Acta cytol.
    (Philad.) 5, 258 (1961).
VON HAAM, E., OLD, J. W.: Reserve cell hyperplasia, squamous metaplasia and epidermidization.
    In: Dysplasia, Carcinoma in situ and microinvasive Carcinoma of the Cervix Uteri, pp. 41—52.
    (Ed. L. A. GRAY). Springfield: Thomas 1964.
VON HAAM, E., SCARPELLI, D. G.: Experimental carcinoma of the cervix: A comparative cytologic
    and histology study. Cancer Res. 15, 449—453 (1955).
VONWILLER, P.: Die Auflichtmikroskopie, ihre Entwicklung, Anwendung, Ergebnisse und Zukunfts-
    aussichten in der Biologie und Medizin. Wien. klin. Wschr. 59, 693—696 (1947).
WAHI, P. N., MALI, S., LUTHRA, U. K.: Factors influencing cancer of the cervix in North India.
    Cancer (Philad.) 25, 1221—1226 (1969).
WAKEFIELD, J.: The family doctor and cervical cytology. Health Trends (Dept. of Health and
    Social Security and the Welsh Office) 3, 25—29 (1971).
WAKONIG-VAARTAJA, R.: Chromosomes in gynaecological malignant tumours. Aust. N. Z. J.
    Obstet. Gynaec. 3, 170—177 (1963).
WAKONIG-VAARTAJA, R., HUGHES, D. T.: Chromosomal anomalies in dysplasia, carcinoma in situ
    and carcinoma of cervix uteri. Lancet 1965 II, 756—759.
WALZ, W.: Erfahrungsbericht über die Früherfassung des Portiokarzinoms unter besonderer Be-
    rücksichtigung der Kolmomikroskopie. Z. Geburtsh. Gynäk. 144, 2, 117—154 (1955).
WALZ, W.: Über die Genese der sogenannten indirekten Metaplasie im Bereich des Müllerschen
    Gang-Systems. Z. Geburtsh. Gynäk. 151, 1—21 (1958).
WALZ, W.: Colpomicroscopy of ectopy, ectropion and epidermidization. Acta cytol. (Philad.) 5,
    91—94 (1961).
WARONSKI, W.: Histochemische Untersuchungen über die Aktivität der sauren Desoxyribonuklease
    bei Carcinoma colli uteri. Zbl. Gynäk. 86, 862—868 (1964).
WARREN, J. W., DOCKERTY, M. B., WILSON, R. B., WELCH, J. S.: Basement membrane in the uterine
    cervix. Amer. J. Obstet. Gynec. 95, 23—20 (1966).
WATSON, P. G., GAIRDNER, D.: TRIC agent as a cause of neonatal eye sepsis. Brit. med. J. 3, 527—528
    (1968).
WATTS, C., GOLDBERG, D. M.: New observations on β-glucuronidase in human cervical cancer.
    Europ. J. Cancer 5, 465—473 (1969).

WEAVER, J. M., DE LA PUENTE, J.: Sequential analysis and quality control — an aid to the cyto-pathologist. Acta cytol. (Philad.) **8**, 270—273 (1964).

WEBER, G.: Some aspects of the carbohydrate metabolism enzymes in the human epidermis under normal and pathological conditions. In: The Epidermis, pp. 453—470, (ed. W. MONTAGNA and W. C. LOBITZ). New York and London: Academic Press 1964.

WEINSTEIN, G. D., FROST, P., HSIA, S. L.: In vitro interconversion of estrone and 17 β-estradiol in human skin and vaginal mucosa. J. invest. Derm. **51**, 4—10 (1968).

WEISS, M. C., EPHRUSSI, B., SCALETTA, L. J.: Loss of T-antigen from somatic hybrids between mouse cells and SV 40-transformed human cells. Proc. nat. Acad. Sci. (Wash.) **59**, 1132—1135 (1968).

WENTZ, W. D.: Significance of mucosal lesions antedating mouse cervical cancer. Amer. J. Obstet. Gynec. **84**, 1506—1511 (1962).

WENTZ, W. B., REAGAN, J. W.: Survival in cervical cancer with respect to cell type. Cancer (Philad.) **12**, 384—388 (1959).

WIDY, K., KIERSKI, J.: Succinic, lactic and glucose-6-phosphate dehydrogenases in precancerous and cancerous stages in the uterine cervix. Acta cytol. (Philad.) **11** 231—235 (1967).

WIED, G. L.: Quality control mechanism for cytology programs. Acta cytol. (Philad.) **9**, 407—412 (1965).

WIED, G. L., MESSINA, A. M., ROSENTHAL, E.: Comparative quantitative DNA-measurements on Feulgen-stained cervical epithelial cells. Acta cytol. (Philad.) **10**, 31—37 (1966).

WILBANKS, G. D., RICHART, R. M.: The in vitro interaction of epithelial neoplasia, normal epithelium and fibroblasts from the adult human uterine cervix. Cancer Res. **26**, 1641—1647 (1966).

WILBANKS, G. D., RICHART, R. M., TERNER, J. Y.: DNA content of cervical intraepithelial neoplasia studied by two-wavelength Feulgen cytophotometry. Amer. J. Obstet. Gynec. **98**, 792—799 (1967).

WILBANKS, G. D., SHINGLETON, H. M.: Normal human cervical squamous epithelium in vitro fine structural differences from in vivo cells. Acta cytol. (Philad.) **14**, 182—186 (1970).

WILLIAMS, J.: Cancer of the uterus. Harveian Lectures for 1886. London: Lewis 1888.

WILLIS, R. A.: The Borderland of Embryology and Pathology. London: Butterworth 1958.

WILLIS, R. A.: Pathology of Tumours. 3rd ed. London: Butterworth 1960.

WISLOCKI, G. B.: The staining of the intercellular bridges of the stratified squamous epithelium of the oral and vaginal mucosa by Sudan black B and Baker's haematein method. Anat. Rec. **109**, 128—129 (1951).

WISLOCKI, G. B., BUNTING, H., DEMPSEY, E. W.: The chemical histology of the human uterine cervix with supplementary notes on the endometrium. In: Menstruation and its Disorders, (ed. E. T. ENGLE). Springfield: Thomas 1950.

WOLINSKA, W. H., MELAMED, M. R.: Herpes genitalis in women attending planned parenthood of New York City. Acta cytol. (Philad.) **14**, 239—242 (1970).

WOLLNER, A.: The histological correlations of endometrial and cervical biopsies with comment on the etiology of endometriosis. Amer. J. Obstet. Gynec. **36**, 10—21 (1938).

WOLLNER, A.: The early diagnosis of cervical carcinoma. Surg. Gynec. Obstet. **68**, 147—154 (1939).

WOMACK, N. A., GRAHAM, E. A.: Epithelial metaplasia in congenital cystic disease of lung; its possible relation to carcinoma of bronchus. Amer. J. Path. **17**, 645—654 (1941).

WYNDER, E. L., CORNFIELD, J., SCHROFF, P. D., DORAISWAMI, K. K.: Study of environmental factors in carcinoma of the cervix. Amer. J. Obstet. Gynec. **68**, 1016—1052 (1954).

YEN, S. S. C., REAGAN, J. W., ROSENTHAL, M. S.: Herpes simplex infection in female genital tract. Obstet. and Gynec. **25**, 479—492 (1965).

YOUNES, M. S., ROBERTSON, E. M., BENCOSME, S. A.: Electron microscope observations on Langerhans cells in the cervix. Amer. J. Obstet. Gynec. **102**, 397—403 (1968).

YOUNES, M. S., STEELE, H. D., ROBERTSON, E. M., BENCOSME, S. A.: Correlative light and electron microscope study of the basement membrane of the human ectocervix. Amer. J. Obstet. Gynec. **92**, 163—171 (1965).

YULE, R.: Personal communication (1971).

ZELICKSON, A. S., HARTMAN, S.: An electronmicroscopic study of normal human non-keratinizing oral mucosa. J. invest. Derm. **38**, 99—107 (1962).

ZINSER, H. K., ROSENBAUER, K. A.: Untersuchungen über die Angioarchitektonik der normalen und pathologisch veränderten Cervix uteri. Arch. Gynäk. **194**, 73—112 (1960).

ZWILLENBERG, L. O.: The dendritic cell system and mast cells in non-epidermal stratified squamous epithelium. Nature (Lond.) **181**, 1343 (1958).

ZWILLENBERG, L. O.: Beiträge zur Kenntnis des geschichten Pflasterepithels. Acta anat. (Basel), Suppl. **35, 36, 37**, 1—127 (1959).

ZWILLENBERG, L. O., BERGER, J.: Einige morphologische Beobachtungen am normalen und pathologischen Pflasterepithel der Portio vaginalis uteri. Oncologia (Basel) **10**, 1—10 (1957).

Subject Index

Recent Results
in Cancer Research

Sponsored by the Swiss League against Cancer
Editor in chief: P. Rentchnick, Genève

---

* Distribution rights for U. K., Commonwealth and the Traditional British Market (excluding Canada): W. Heinemann, Medical Books Ltd., London.